Praise for *Nou*

"*Nourish* is simply *the* book for any family wanting
when companies marketing junk foods are spending ____ ___ children hooked
for life, and confusion reigns about the pros and cons of various diets, you have cause for
gratitude. This wonderful book will fortify you and your whole family against the predatory
practices of industrial food companies, and it is also jam-packed with useful and practical
guidance that is 100 percent supported by science. Get it, read it, and heed it... and it will
guide you and your family on a delicious, convenient, and exquisitely health-promoting food
journey. If you want your children to thank you for the rest of their lives, get this book."

—**John Robbins**, bestselling author and president
of 650,000+ member Food Revolution Network

"*Nourish* takes the mystery out of eating for optimal wellness—not only for yourself but
for those you love and nurture. Plan on keeping this book nearby as a trusted resource and
constant companion. No one makes healthful, compassionate eating as clear and concise
as Brenda and Reshma."

—**Colleen Patrick-Goudreau**, author of
The 30-Day Vegan Challenge and *The Joyful Vegan*

"Just when you think a comprehensive guide to adopting plant-based eating could not
be made fun and family friendly, along comes *Nourish* by seasoned pediatrician Dr. Reshma
Shah and renowned registered dietitian Brenda Davis. This book tenderly introduces us to
arguably the most important concepts in health, ecology, and ethics today with a tone that
is clear, enlightening, and empowering. The authors—who are both parents and working
professionals—courageously explore the aspects of making plant-based diets work in the
real world, from shopping on tight food budgets and unforgiving time crunches, to feeding
picky eaters and growing toddlers. *Nourish* provides a sane, reassuring, and practical path
to evolving your food choices to those that will deliciously transform your life, the lives of
those you love, and all of our futures. It will be the go-to book that I suggest for my patients
who need to make the plant-based transition. Savor the life-affirming journey that *Nourish*
offers—you are in good hands."

—**Michael Klaper, MD**, program director of Moving Medicine Forward Initiative

"*Nourish* is the definitive resource we've been waiting for. Brenda and Reshma couple
research and experience with a practical, welcoming approach so that nutritious plant-based
meals can be on every family's table. From nutritional specifics to practical concerns, *Nourish*
delivers with expert support and guidance."

—**Dreena Burton**, author of *Plant-Powered Families*

"Reassuring and packed with essential information, this is the book all parents need to
ease their family's transition to a plant-based diet. Writing with warmth and enthusiasm,
Reshma and Brenda provide the tools and the knowledge that will allow anyone to confi-
dently choose a more compassionate and healthy way of eating."

—**Virginia Messina, MPH, RD**, author of *Vegan for Life*

"*Nourish,* by Reshmah Shah, MD, MPH, and Brenda Davis, RD, is an outstanding guide for families adopting plant-based diets and for health professionals who want accurate, up-to-date, and reader-friendly nutrition information. This book is exceptionally well written and provides carefully researched scientific material plus a wealth of practical tips. *Nourish* guides readers expertly through the potential challenges of pregnancy, lactation, childhood, and adolescence. It includes helpful information on meal planning along with recipes that the whole family will enjoy.

—**Vesanto Melina, MS, RD**, lead author of the current position paper
on vegetarian diets of the Academy of Nutrition and Dietetics

"What we eat in our childhood has far-reaching and powerful effects on our health throughout our entire life. *Nourish* is a well-researched and authoritative work that gives parents the most accurate information to assure their child's well-being. But more than that, this book can help anyone at any age understand and apply the foundational principles of nutritional excellence to prevent health problems, support our emotional well-being, and even protect our planet.

—**Joel Fuhrman, MD**, *New York Times* bestselling author
and president of Nutritional Research Foundation

"Evidence continuously supports the myriad advantages that a plant palate proffers. Dr. Reshma Shah and Brenda Davis have gifted the world with this comprehensive, conscientious, and caring guide to help families navigate a plant-based diet safely, healthfully, and effectively. *Nourish* is an informationally dense tome that belongs in every family's library.

—**Julieanna Hever, MS, RD, CPT**, author of *The Healthspan Solution*
and *Plant-Based Nutrition (Idiots Guides)*

"In *Nourish,* parents will finally find what they have been looking for—the complete guide to a plant-based lifestyle for the whole family from experts they can trust. Beautifully written and relatable, this book is the perfect nutrition guide for kids. Parents, this is the book you've been waiting for."

—**Dr. Gemma Newman**

"*Nourish* will give you and your family the info, answers, recipes, and *umph* to maximize your plant-based lifestyle with 100 percent confidence. With Brenda and Reshma at the helm, you can rest assured that no stone will be left unturned as you and your loved ones set sail to the plant-strong promised land!"

—**Rip Esselstyn**, founder of Plant-Strong by Engine 2

"This year, if you had only one book to help you and your family reach optimal health, it would be *Nourish*. Based on science and written to be easily applied to your life, we assure you this book will be a life-changing gift."

—**Ayesha Sherzai, MD, and Dean Sherzai, MD**, co-directors of the
Alzheimer's Prevention Program at Loma Linda University
Medical Center and authors of *The Alzheimer's Solution*

nourish

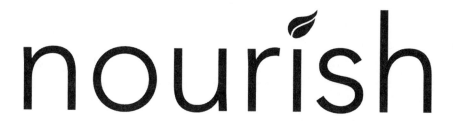

nourish

The Definitive Plant-Based Nutrition Guide for Families

Reshma Shah, MD, MPH, and
Brenda Davis, RD

Health Communications, Inc.
Boca Raton, Florida

www.hcibooks.com

Library of Congress Cataloging-in-Publication Data
is available through the Library of Congress

© 2020 Reshma Shah, MD, MPH, and Brenda Davis, RD

ISBN-13: 978-07573-2362-1 (Paperback)
ISBN-10: 07573-2362-6 (Paperback)
ISBN-13: 978-07573-2363-8 (ePub)
ISBN-10: 07573-2363-4 (ePub)

Publisher: Health Communications, Inc.
          1700 NW 2nd Avenue
          Boca Raton, FL 33432-1653

Cover design and illustrations by Larissa Hise Henoch
Interior design and formatting by Lawna Patterson Oldfield
Cover photo by Rakhee Yadav

"The openness of our hearts and minds can be measured by how wide we draw the circle of what we call family."

—*Mother Teresa*

To our families

Daniel, Maya, and Owen (Reshma)

Paul, Leena, and Cory (Brenda)

Contents

Foreword   xi

Acknowledgments   xv

Introduction   1

Part I: CONSIDERATION

CHAPTER 1   Health   7

CHAPTER 2   Home   33

CHAPTER 3   Heart   43

Part II: CARE

CHAPTER 4   Managing Macronutrients and Fiber   55

CHAPTER 5   Micronutrients   93

CHAPTER 6   What Makes a Healthy Diet?   145

CHAPTER 7   Pregnancy and Lactation   169

CHAPTER 8   Childhood and Adolescence   191

Part III: CONFIDENCE

CHAPTER 9   Principles of Feeding: Setting the Table   237

CHAPTER 10 Family Meals   253

CHAPTER 11 Weighty Matters   265

CHAPTER 12 Raising a Veg Leaning Family   285

Part IV: CONNECTION

CHAPTER 13 Shopping, Planning, and Prepping   305

CHAPTER 14 Sample Menus   317

CHAPTER 15 Recipes   323

Resources   393

References   397

Index   425

Foreword

FOOD FOR LOVE: *WHAT, WHY, AND HOW*

We all know the expression "food for thought." The case could be made—and, indeed, I have made it more than once—that, if anything, we "think" a bit too much about food. We parse and we argue, debate and probe—and all the while, the fundamental truths that matter most hide in plain sight. The essential elements of eating vastly better were famously distilled into just seven words by Michael Pollan: "eat food, not too much, mostly plants."

Pollan's insight stuck with us, like hearty food to the ribs, not because it was pithy, but because it was correct. An overwhelming body of evidence of stunning diversity and staggering consistency tells us that plant-predominant diets of wholesome foods in sensible assemblies foster longevity and vitality alike. They favor equity, social justice, kindness across the spectrum of biodiversity, and sustainability as well. And while important, the "not too much" tends to take care of itself when such dietary patterns are achieved. Calories count, but counting them is a tedious enterprise. Get the quality of their sourcing right, and the quantity of calories consumed tends to itself. Achieve "not too much" as a byproduct of putting the right stuff on your table.

I have devoted a nearly thirty-year career and more total pages in writing than I have tallied to assessing that "right stuff." With that view from altitude, I see it as an entirely settled matter. Sure, there are many details left to learn and even some rarefied questions we may never lay fully to rest. But just as we know the profound benefits of routine physical activity without necessarily knowing whether biking or hiking is "better," so, too, and with comparable conviction, we know the basic theme of feeding Homo sapiens well.

That we are all Homo sapiens is important, by the way. Much is made these days of "precision" or "personalized" nutrition, as if that is somehow an alternative to eating fundamentally well. It is not.

Rather, personalization is an overlay of inclination, preference, and intentions on a common foundation of dietary choices good for our kind of animal. Consider how cavalierly we accept that all horses can eat like horses, all dolphins can eat fish, all koalas can eat eucalyptus leaves. Don't we need the genomic profile of a given koala first? Of course not; there is a set of dietary adaptations that pertains to that kind of animal. So, too, for the kind of animal we are.

As noted, we think too much and mostly in all the wrong ways about food. We think far too little about food for love.

Food, after all, is the construction material for the growing bodies of our children. It is the source material for the daily refurbishments our bodies make every day throughout life. Food is sustenance, sharing, generosity, and celebration. There is no place in any of that for junk; but there is a compelling case for love.

Food, often, is an expression of love. So, it is time to think of food for love, and I know of no more expert guidance for that critical transition than this book: *Nourish*.

Nourish establishes and validates the "what" of optimal eating—a plant-predominant dietary pattern of wholesome, high quality foods in balanced, sensible assemblies. There is no dogma or ideology here, a refreshing distinction! There is just a calm, convincing, engaging, evidence-based case. From my point of view, it is ironclad.

The value proposition of getting the basic theme of diet right is all but inestimable: more years in our lives, more life in our years; the chance to pay such blessings forward to those we love; an opportunity to help save the oceans and aquifers, glaciers and rainforests; means to protect the awesome treasure of Earth's biodiversity; a kinder, gentler, more equitable dietary footprint; making sure a wholesome diet is still an option for the generations that follow.

The "what" and the "why" of optimal eating reside there, and populate the early pages of *Nourish*. But Reshma and Brenda do not leave us there; they take us into all of the particulars of "how." From macronutrients and micronutrients to picky eaters; from family dinners to shopping lists; from neophobia (fear of the new) to breast feeding—our hands are held here by expert guides. You will know "what" with confidence; you will know the overwhelming "why;" and you will be empowered with the many practical expressions of "how." That is a full menu.

The emphasis here is on families, and that is just right. The emphasis is on engaging children in the lifelong benefits of eating well, and that is just right. The emphasis is on the rightful place of diet in the health of people and planet alike, on the confluence of nourishment and sustainability and kindness, on solidarity and celebration. That is just right.

In the end, what sets *Nourish* apart is not that it is expert; it is. Not that it is insightful; it is. Not that it is wise, comprehensive, or evidence-based; it is all that.

What sets *Nourish* apart is that it is all about food for love. Embrace this book, and it all but literally embraces you back. Is it a book or a hug? Maybe both.

Lean in, and let this beautiful book nourish your understanding, your motivation, your will-power and skill-power alike. Lean in—and taste the love.

What could be more nourishing than that?

—*David L. Katz, MD, MPH*

Acknowledgments

Sincere gratitude to those who made this book possible: Our literary agent, Marilyn Allen, for her wisdom and support; our publisher, HCI, for embracing our proposal and being so accommodating every step of the way; HCI editorial director, Christine Belleris, for her expertise and enthusiasm, HCI typesetter, Lawna Patterson Oldfield, for her beautiful interior book design, and HCI director of pre-press services, Larissa Henoch, for her remarkable artistic talent and flexibility.

Deep appreciation to our PR team: HCI public relations director, Allison Janse, for her guidance and grace, PR by the Book publicist, Leslie Barrett, for her leadership and expertise, and our publicity strategist, Marika Flatt, for her skill and vision.

Special thanks to our foreword author: Distinguished colleague, David Katz, for his brilliant and eloquent words and his decades of leadership and sheer genius in health and nutrition.

Heartfelt gratitude to our recipe testers: Daneen Agecoutay, Kelle Auld, Rohini Bajekal, Barbara Bangert, Anne Bridges, Sonya Buys, Lori Calman, Tina Caskey, Margie Colclough, Janet Duffy, Rosemary Erickson, Lorraine Esman, Anne-Renee Feldman, Sydney Feldman, Lani Hnatiuk, Jennifer Hughes, Carol Hunter, Valerie Ingram, Lynn Isted, Palissa Kelley, Mary Jean Kersey, Monika Mendels, Heidi Moore, Karoline Mueller, Sarah Mulligan, Amy Otterspoor, Dave Roitner, Jeanne Rosner, Caitlin Selle, Michael Serrano, Dana Smith, Nicole Stammer, Tara Tanaka, Sarah, Tranter, Liliana Cruz Vallejo, Sarah Valor, Sandra Vermeulen, Shelly Vossen, Jennifer Whitmire, and Paula Wilson, for their dedication, time, resources, and boundless energy. Your care and attention to detail made the recipes in this book appealing, tasty, and easy to follow. Special thanks to Leena Markatchev for creating the awesome baby treats.

Reshma Shah

A big thank you to cherished friends that are more like family for offering your love and endless encouragement—Lindsay Flack, Michelle McMacken, and Tonya Passarelli I am so fortunate to know you. Teru Clavel, Kari Greenfield, and Kaarina Roberto thank you for your wisdom and friendship. Heartfelt gratitude to Ann Ming Yeh and the Stanford Pediatric Integrative Medicine Program for inviting me to be a part of such a creative, inspiring community.

To my parents, Mahendra and Aruna Shah, for teaching me about the value of family, that it's never too late to do what you love, and of course everything I know about cooking. To Anish, Dhwani, Ashna, and Navya Shah for your enthusiasm, love, and support.

Dan, Maya, and Owen words cannot express the depth of my love and care for you. Time around our dinner table is always the most cherished part of my day.

And finally, to Brenda Davis. It's rare that you meet a person that is so gifted and bright and also has such a kind and loving spirit. I have long admired and respected you and now, am so grateful to call you my friend. Working with you has been a true joy and great honor.

Brenda Davis

Eternal gratitude to Vesanto Melina and Margie Colclough, for their advice, consideration, and endless encouragement. Sincere appreciation to Joel Fuhrman, Michael Greger, Julieanna Hever, Michael Klaper, Reed Mangels, Ginny Messina, and Jack Norris for their insights and inspiration.

Love and gratitude to my cherished family: my husband, Paul, my children Leena and Cory, their spouses, Nayden and Josie, my grandchildren, Mila and Violet, my mom, Doreen Charbonneau, my mother-in-law, Linda Davis, my brother, Andy Charbonneau, and my sisters-in-law, Jaclyn Labchuk and Peggy Davis. Your ongoing love, support, encouragement, and understanding set the foundation of my resolve.

To my remarkable co-author, Reshma Shah. It is both an honor and a privilege to work with you. You never cease to amaze me with your talents. You are kind, courageous, and incredibly gifted. This book is just the beginning of a long working relationship, and a forever friendship.

Introduction

No one precise way of eating guarantees a life free of disease, and many dietary approaches can allow for vibrant health. Indeed, nutrition is just one aspect of health. Sleep, stress management, movement, relationships, a sense of purpose, and community all contribute to an overall sense of well-being. Why then, another book about food? Is there anything new and noteworthy to add to the conversation? We would offer that with the growing rates of chronic diseases (expanding even into many countries in the developing world), dire concerns around climate change, and increasing rates of childhood and adolescent health issues (from type 2 diabetes to anxiety), food sits at the center of so many of the conversations that matter most to parents. Not only does diet play an essential role in our health, but it also has the power to connect and serve as an expression of our culture and values. We propose a way of eating and feeding that is centered around plants and at the dinner table. This approach is health-promoting, sustainable, and compassionate, not to mention abundant and delicious.

The evidence overwhelmingly supports a plant-centered diet as the foundation for promoting health. With clarity and care, we will outline the specifics of a plant-based diet to optimize health, beginning by establishing its safety for children. We offer an evidence-based approach to understand the vast benefits of a plant-based diet for disease prevention and longevity while addressing common concerns as they relate to minimizing or eliminating animal foods in the diet. The broad strokes of disease prevention and overall health will be reinforced with more detailed information regarding nutrients, supplements, and age-specific nutritional recommendations. The real actionable steps for parents will be to focus

The real actionable steps for parents will be to focus on maximizing the consumption of whole, plant foods as far as is possible and practical within a given family.

on maximizing the consumption of whole, plant foods as far as is possible and practical within a given family.

Additionally, while the primary focus will be on the health-promoting aspects of a plant-based diet, we will also discuss the many benefits beyond our individual plates. Sustainability, compassion, and allocation of resources may seem outside the typical realm of a book by two health care professionals, but we contend that because of our roles in caring for families, this is precisely the place where such a conversation should be had. We will discuss the toll that animal agriculture takes on our environment and the steps we can collectively take to help protect our planet. It's alarming to know that nearly 70 percent of the world's farmable land is used for animal agriculture with an additional 10 percent used to grow grains to feed livestock. Beef production alone uses about three-fifths of the Earth's farmland but yields less than 5 percent of the world's protein.[1] Animal agriculture is the leading cause of species extinction, ocean dead zones, water pollution, and habitat destruction.

The health benefits and environmental advantages could alone support the recommendation to adopt a plant-based diet for all, but perhaps one of the most compelling reasons to favor plants is the call to mitigate animal suffering. Given two equally convenient, delicious, satisfying, and healthful choices, we no doubt would choose the more compassionate alternative. If we concede that a variety of diets can promote health, it seems nonsensical to ignore the horrific acts of violence bestowed upon countless innocent animals every day.

Following a detailed examination of a plant-based diet and its myriad benefits, we will delve deeply into the specific guidance that many parents seek. We will provide age-specific recommendations to optimize growth and development, review nutrient requirements and the role of supplements, as well as address many of the common nutrition questions about which parents often worry. Again, the information will be evidence-based, while at the same time accessible and practical.

Information is critical, but knowledge can only be put into practice if our values support it, and we have the resources to implement it. After exploring the health and safety issues, we will address many of the concerns families face around their dinner tables. Busy sports schedules and after-school activities may make family dinner nearly impossible most nights; we will provide data to support why, despite these challenges, family dinner is perhaps one of the single best practices parents can adopt. Picky eaters and family tension may make peace the priority at mealtimes. Some families may commit to becoming vegan or vegetarian. Others may value eating locally or supporting fair trade and sustainably grown foods. Preserving culture and tradition will be incredibly valuable to some families. Taste, ease, cost, and availability will be top on the list for other families. From picky eaters to childhood obesity, disordered eating, and more, we hope to show that *how* we feed our families may matter as much as *what* we feed our families. As parents ourselves, we understand all too well the challenges that families face around their dinner tables and hope that a thoughtful conversation around these topics will work to introduce greater joy and connectedness.

The last section of the book is dedicated to resources for families. Whether it's time, money, cooking skills, or availability of food, a family's strengths and limitations will determine how the knowledge that we gain and the values that we embrace show up at our dinner tables. While it would be wonderful to assert that "healthy" eating is always within arm's reach (easy, affordable, satisfying, pleasurable, and appealing to everyone in the family), the reality is that for many families, a scarcity of any of these resources represents genuine impediments to health and joy when it comes to food. It can be difficult or impossible to clear all of these obstacles. We wish it were not the case, but for many families, increasing fruit and vegetable intake is a substantial strain on their budget. Busy work lives often leave little time for shopping and cooking. The best we can do is to work within our constraints and prioritize our resources. A shift in knowledge and values ultimately provides the framework for us to utilize our resources to the best of our abilities. We offer strategies for families to begin making the shift at whatever pace is reasonable. We will provide tips for menu planning and shopping as well as simple, accessible (and delicious!) recipes. Our experience with families has taught us that starting with small changes that are accessible and enjoyable is the easiest and most sustainable way to begin the path forward. The future of food is plants. We provide a path for families to get there.

> The future of food is plants. We provide a path for families to get there.

Whether for health, our environment, or ethics, we aim to start the conversation around why our food choices matter. However, we recognize that each individual and each family will have a unique journey. This means acknowledging that change may be brisk for some and more gradual for others. At whatever pace we choose, perhaps what matters most is that we move forward with both attention and intention. As our awareness and compassion grow, change will surely follow. Little by little, meal by meal, we have an incredible capacity to direct our choices towards health, sustainability, compassion, and, of course, joy. If the choices we make around food have the power to care for our health, our planet, and sentient beings all at once, why not move in the direction of love?

Part I

CONSIDERATION

Nourish has been organized into four key sections: Consideration, Care, Confidence, and Connection. This first section addresses the fundamental question of why families should consider a plant-based approach to feeding their families. Parents will learn the specifics of a plant-based diet as a way to optimize health. First, the safety of plant-based diets for children will be firmly established. We will then offer an evidence-based approach to understand the vast benefits of plant-based diets in terms of disease prevention and longevity while also addressing common concerns about minimizing or eliminating animal foods in the diet. Additionally, while this section primarily focuses on the health-promoting aspects of a plant-based diet, readers will also learn many of the benefits beyond their individual plates, such as caring for our planet and mitigating animal suffering.

Chapter 1

Health

"Nothing will benefit human health and increase the
chances for survival of life on Earth as much
as the evolution to a vegetarian diet."

— Albert Einstein

W hen it comes to feeding children, our topmost priority must always be to optimize their growth, development, and well-being. Not only does this endeavor require sufficient calories, the recommended amounts of macro and micronutrients, but also a sense of connection and love. We affirm that there is, in fact, an approach to eating and feeding that is health-promoting, not just safe and adequate but preferred, and that the conversations around our food choices and their broader implications are not only acceptable but imperative. Perhaps the most extraordinary feature of a plant-based approach to feeding our families is the realization that they are all connected—our health, the health of our planet, and compassion for all living beings. Because no other dietary strategy can claim to address all of these critical points, this approach is, at a minimum, worthy of our

Perhaps the most extraordinary feature of a plant-based approach to feeding our families is the realization that they are all connected — our health, the health of our planet, and compassion for all living beings.

7

consideration. We propose this way of eating knowing that when our hearts and minds align in love, we have the tremendous opportunity to nourish ourselves, our families, and the world at large. But, rest assured, perfection is not a prerequisite. Too often, the demand for exactitude and controversy around the benefits and risks of a specific food or nutrient shifts our attention away from a more thoughtful consideration of our food choices. Arguing over whether high fructose corn syrup is the single most harmful compound we can ingest, instead of merely encouraging more whole, plant foods, is a distraction away from the work ahead of us. Luckily for us, this way of eating is not a mystery, nor is it out of reach. A plant-based approach to feeding ourselves and our families is health, compassion, and sustainability wrapped together into one beautiful package.

WHAT'S IN A NAME?

Before delving into the health benefits and potential safety concerns around plant-based diets, let's review some terminology to bring clarity to the conversation. What, you may ask, exactly is a plant-based diet? Simply stated, a plant-based diet, which can include both vegetarian and vegan diets, is essentially a diet that focuses on maximizing the consumption of whole, plant foods such as vegetables, fruits, legumes, whole grains, nuts, and seeds. It also aims to minimize the intake of animal-based foods (meat, egg, seafood, poultry, and dairy) as well as heavily processed and refined foods (pastries, soda, etc.). While animal products may play a role in some plant-based diets, they tend to appear only occasionally or as flavorings.

In short, if you aim to maximize whole, plant foods and minimize animal-based and heavily processed foods, you are, in fact, a plant-based eater. The degree to which your family may "maximize and minimize" these foods will depend on a variety of factors. It matters the place from which you are beginning. It matters what sorts of resources and supports surround you. Your cultural background, your family's tastes and preferences, likes and dislikes, and comfort with cooking will all influence your approach and pace. Wherever labels can be of use and support your efforts, we encourage you to embrace them. If a label seems too heavy a responsibility or somehow disingenuous, don't feel obligated to carry it. For instance, asking for the "vegan" option at a restaurant or when attending a function can simplify ordering, and give the food preparer a clearer idea of your request. Joining a "vegetarian" or "vegan" group may provide support and a sense of community. If you are still learning, exploring, or even unsure, we encourage you not to allow any specific categorization or label hold you back.

There is no single definition of a plant-based diet. On one end of the spectrum you have flexitarian, also known as semi-vegetarian diets (predominantly plant-based with only occasional consumption of meat, poultry, fish, dairy, eggs, or other animal products), to pescatarian (includes fish), lacto-ovo-vegetarian (includes dairy and eggs) to vegan or plant-exclusive diets, often called complete or pure vegetarian (eliminates all animal sources of food). There are even many variations within these realms, such as raw vegan diets (diets that are at least 75 percent uncooked food by weight).

As you can see, there is a broad spectrum of diets that qualify as "plant-based." Table 1.1 provides a list of some of the most common types of plant-based diets.

Table 1.1: Plant-Based Diet Definitions

TYPE OF PLANT-BASED DIET	DIET DESCRIPTION
Vegan, pure vegetarian, complete vegetarian, plant-exclusive	Free of all animal products, including flesh foods, eggs, dairy products, and sometimes honey.
Raw vegan	Vegan with at least 75% uncooked foods.
Lacto-ovo vegetarian	Free of flesh foods but includes eggs and dairy products.
Lacto-vegetarian	Excludes flesh foods and eggs but includes dairy products.
Ovo-vegetarian	Excludes flesh foods and dairy products but includes eggs.
Pescatarian or pesco-vegetarian	Vegetarian or vegan plus fish.
Semi-vegetarian, plant-predominant, flexitarian	Include small amounts or occasional use of meat, poultry, fish, dairy, eggs, or other animal products, but plant foods predominate.

We provide this information not to create barriers or confusion but rather because when talking about the research, benefits, and potential risks, these distinctions can matter. Many early studies grouped all of the above categories (including ones that ate meat "occasionally") into one broad, vegetarian category. This information can seem even more complicated when we introduce the term whole-food, plant-based (WFPB). Let us explain. A person following a strict vegan diet is someone who aims to eliminate ALL animal-based foods without necessarily considering how processed a food may be. People following a vegan diet may also extend their practices beyond their plates by avoiding animal products in clothing and household items. Their primary aim is to avoid all animal-based products. A person adopting a whole-food, plant-based diet is someone who aims to eat foods that are minimally processed and come from whole, plant sources, often eliminating foods such as refined grains and oils. There can be quite a bit of overlap, and if you are eating a WFPB diet that is entirely devoid of all animal products, you would also be following a vegan diet. It's important to note, however, that not all vegan diets are health-promoting. While a vegan diet may go a long way towards curtailing animal suffering and harm to our environment, a vegan diet that relies on heavily processed foods would not be considered health-promoting. The following research demonstrates this concept more clearly.

A study published in the *Journal of the American College of Cardiology* in 2017 reviewed data from three large prospective studies, the Nurses' Health Study, the Nurses' Health Study 2, and the Health Professionals Follow-Up Study, to examine the incidence of coronary heart disease in more than 200,000 health professionals in the United States.[1] The researchers devised a system to interpret dietary data and created a plant-based dietary index (PDI). They further subdivided this index into a healthful plant-based diet index (hPDI) and unhealthful plant-based diet index (uPDI). They created eighteen food categories, divided into healthy plant foods (fruits, vegetables, whole grains, legumes), less healthy plant foods (sugar-sweetened beverages, refined grains), and animal foods (dairy, meat, eggs). The results are not entirely surprising. The pooled data showed that overall, the PDI was modestly inversely associated with coronary heart disease, meaning more plant foods, less heart disease. But, when they analyzed hPDI and uPDI separately, they found a stronger inverse relationship with the hPDI and a *positive* association (meaning more heart disease) with the uPDI. The overall summary from this large prospective investigation is that PDI is inversely related to heart disease (more plant-based, less heart disease) but that the distinction between the types of plant foods consumed does matter when

A healthful plant-based diet is even more protective, and the unhealthful plant-based diet can be harmful.

it comes to heart health. When separated out, a healthful plant-based diet is even more protective, and the unhealthful plant-based diet can be harmful.

Again, the point of going through this particular study is to clarify that when we speak of a plant-based diet, we mean to emphasize health-promoting foods, such as vegetables, fruits, whole grain, beans, nuts, and seeds. Much of the confusion around the health benefits of vegan diets stems from this distinction. When comparing the standard American diet to its vegan equivalent, the difference in health outcomes will likely be marginal. To avoid confusion and to be as inclusive as possible, we use the term plant-based to emphasize the focus on real, whole, plant foods. We recognize that working towards adopting a plant-based diet is going to look different for different families, and we encourage you not to allow any specific label or perceived "requirements" deter you. Even though there are no vegan police, there can be quite a bit of criticism, judgment, and comparison.

Regardless of where you are, you can begin. The basic principle, then, of a plant-based diet, is to include as many whole plant foods as you can, and at the same time, limit animal-based and heavily processed foods.

The basic principle, then, of a plant-based diet, is to include as many whole plant foods as you can, and at the same time, limit animal-based and heavily processed foods.

One final clarification before we move on to health and safety issues is an explanation of what we mean by "processed" foods. There are two points that we would like to make when it comes to these foods. First, to some degree, most people (our families included!) rely on processed foods daily. Bread, pasta, canned tomatoes or beans, cereals, tortillas, and even whole grains have all been processed to some degree. Not all "processed foods" are created equally. The idea that you should aim for a diet completely devoid of processed foods is neither realistic nor required. In today's modern world, families rely on processed foods. They add convenience to our busy lives and, in some instances, improve the quality of our overall diet. However, whole grain bread with a simple ingredient list is quite different than packaged pastries with an unthinkably long ingredient list and shelf life. Table 1.2 provides a description of various categories of food processing.

Table 1.2: Categories of Processed Foods

DEGREE OF PROCESSING	DESCRIPTION
Unprocessed	Fresh foods as they are picked from the plant. (e.g. whole fresh vegetables, fruits, intact whole grains, legumes, nuts, and seeds)
Minimally Processed	Foods that are only slightly changed from their original form (e.g. canned beans, tofu, tempeh, cut or rolled grains, roasted nuts *or* seeds, nut and seed butters)
Moderately Processed	Foods that have undergone greater processing, but with few added ingredients (e.g. juices, flaked or puffed cereals, whole grain flour products)
Highly/Ultra Processed	Food products that have undergone extensive processing, generally including added fat, sugar, salt, additives and preservatives. (deep fried foods, refined flour products, and soda)

When you think of processed foods, we encourage you to consider the degree to which a food has been processed as well as the frequency with which you serve and consume these foods. Additionally, while we focus on whole, plant foods, such as whole grains, it is necessary to note that using some refined grains and oils may help younger children meet their daily energy and nutrient requirements.[2]

The second point that we would like to make is that being overly and obsessively restrictive when it comes to these foods can create not only confusion but a loss of connection and care in your family. As we consider how we might limit our consumption of highly processed foods, it is critical to exercise caution and move forward with care when it comes to the tone and language we use with our children. The danger in describing foods as "good" or "bad" is that it is not such a far leap to "*I* am good or bad." We will discuss these ideas in greater depth in the chapters on feeding and disordered eating, but addressing this critical point is vital in establishing the tone for the conversation at hand. It's easy to judge and feel judged by the food that shows up in our children's lunchboxes and dinner plates.

Although we will provide ample data and research, such information is only useful at the family level if it can be practical and instructive at the same time. All this to say, that we live, work, and play in the real world. Focusing on what we serve and enjoy most of the time is far more relevant in our minds than expecting or achieving any degree of perfection, especially when it comes to children. When we battle with our children over another bite of broccoli or kale, it's hardly worth the effort if the price we pay is a loss of joy and connection—not to mention the mounds of uneaten broc-

Focusing on what we serve and enjoy most of the time is far more relevant in our minds than expecting or achieving any degree of perfection, especially when it comes to children. When we battle with our children over another bite of broccoli or kale, it's hardly worth the effort if the price we pay is a loss of joy and connection—not to mention the mounds of uneaten broccoli and kale.

coli and kale. We aim to provide a constructive framework and hope to change the architecture of the way in which we feed our families by fostering a sense of competence and well-being. Connection around our dinner tables is undoubtedly a critical pillar. We would add to Michael Pollan's famous dictum to "eat food, mostly (or all!) plants, not too much (and not too little)," *together and with joy*. Our chapter on family meals will highlight the importance of connection around our dinner tables, but even as we consider how to shape our conversations and practices around food in our families and with our children, it is imperative to recognize that how and what we say matters a great deal. More on this to come, but for now, we move on to the health and safety issues as they pertain to a plant-based diet for our families.

ARE PLANT-BASED DIETS SAFE FOR CHILDREN?

Earlier, we emphasized that one of the most critical aspects of feeding children when it comes to nutrition is to ensure their adequate growth and development. So, before we can even begin to tackle the why or how of adopting a plant-based diet, we must address the crucial issue of safety. Is this way of eating safe and appropriate for growing children?

The biggest argument against adopting a plant-based diet for infants and children is that it is simply unsafe. A great deal of attention is paid to the presumed deficiencies of plant-based diets, and strong assertions are often made that it cannot meet the nutritional needs of growing children. Many believe that such a diet cannot provide adequate calories and nutrients such as calcium, iron, essential fatty acids, and of course, protein. We would argue that not only is a plant-based diet safe and appropriate for growing children but, in fact, that we are *more* likely to meet children's nutritional needs by adopting a thoughtfully planned plant-based diet than we are by simply feeding them the standard American diet (SAD).

Let's take a closer look at what we know about children and diets at the top end of the plant-based spectrum—vegetarian and vegan diets. When we look at data regarding the growth of vegetarian/vegan children, there are a few things that we have to keep in mind. First, much of the early research addressing this question studied communities that followed highly restrictive diets that would not be appropriate for growing children (and even most adults). Decades ago, many people following a vegan or vegetarian diet in developed countries were considered to be part of fringe communities. Diets and practices ranged from the refusal of enriched or refined foods, use of homemade infant formulas that were grossly inadequate, refusal of vitamin-mineral supplements, limited (or no) use of healthcare, and raw food only diets, to name a few.[3] As vegetarianism and veganism have become more mainstream, not only are families more aware of precautions that may need to be taken, but health care providers are becoming more comfortable advising and supporting families. Following a vegetarian or vegan diet is no longer considered to be extreme or fringe.

Additionally, there is a greater awareness and availability of nutrient-rich and fortified foods today which makes following a plant-based diet more accessible, while at the same time, less likely to result in nutrient deficiency (this is also true for omnivorous diets when we consider that our food supply is fortified with nutrients such as vitamin D, vitamin A, iodine, and folic acid to name a few). However, the research on vegan and vegetarian diets written decades ago still remains relevant today. What has changed, however, is the notion of the modern vegan. No longer a part of outlying communities espousing fringe beliefs and practices, veg diets are safer and more accessible than ever. Increasing awareness, resources, and availability of foods have made being vegan a part of the cultural norm—if not a member of the majority, certainly a stronger and growing minority voice. This increasing awareness, popularity, and "normalness" of being vegan or vegetarian certainly make it easier to know and practice a healthful way of eating.

GROWTH AND DEVELOPMENT

The Farm Study, published in 1989, is one of the most often cited studies looking at the growth of vegetarian children.[4] This study was unique in that the researchers observed a community in Tennessee that followed a vegan diet and collected annual growth data for the children. Additionally, unlike prior studies that were based on small sample sizes (often fewer than 50 children) and studied populations with a variety of health-related beliefs (not partaking in conventional medical care and refusing vitamin and mineral supplements), the Farm Study followed over 400 children ranging in age from four months to ten years, and the families were generally well-informed regarding issues related to vegetarianism.

Overall, the growth of children in this vegan community was similar to the U.S. reference population and showed no evidence of marked abnormality. More specifically, birth weight and percentage of low birthweight infants were comparable to non-vegan populations in the United States. Children in the Farm Study were shorter between the ages of one and three, but this difference did not persist after age five. One possible explanation for the smaller height between ages one and three is that at the time of the study, growth references were for formula-fed babies, and most Farm infants were breastfed. Healthy breastfed infants typically put on weight more slowly than formula-fed infants in the first year of life.[5] Additionally, the weaning foods of some vegetarian diets can be low in caloric density (such as with fruits and vegetables) which can lead to insufficient caloric intake during the weaning stage. A similar study among British vegan children published in 1988, found that growth among vegan children was typical, and in fact, "children reared as vegans can grow up to be normal children"[6]—which is quite reassuring! As in the Farm study, there was a tendency for vegan children to be smaller at the age of weaning. The key take-home point is that children raised on a vegan diet achieved adequate growth.

> The key take-home point is that children raised on a vegan diet achieved adequate growth.

A study of the Seventh Day Adventist children done in 1990 provides an informative perspective.[7] The California Seventh Day Adventists are a health-conscious community that optimizes health through lifestyle. They tend to lead physically active lives, are socially engaged, don't smoke, and have a large percentage of vegetarians and vegans compared to the general population. Because they share so many "healthy" factors in common but consume varying diets, we can learn about differences in dietary practices in this generally health-conscious community. In other words, (as much as is possible), keeping all things constant, what happens to growth when the only difference is the degree to which a child follows a vegetarian diet? Approximately half of this population consumed some form of a vegetarian diet. One-third of the Adventist children were vegetarian, one third were "low meat-eaters," and the rest were in the "medium/high" meat-consuming category. They also compared these children to children attending state schools in a neighboring community; 92 percent of the state school children were in the medium/high meat-consuming group, 7.6 percent in the low meat group, and only one child was vegetarian. So, what did they find? For all school and diet groups, the average heights were at or above the 50th percentile of the National Center for Health Statistics reference values. For most age categories, the average heights of vegetarian children were similar to or higher than those of children who consumed meat. While the results of this study do not prove that vegetarian children will be taller as adults, at a minimum, it shows that meat (including poultry and fish) is not essential for the healthy growth of children.

Many additional studies have shown that children following a vegetarian/vegan diet grow at least as well as children who ate an omnivorous one.[8, 9] One study examining the dietary intake and nutritional status of vegetarian and omnivorous preschool children in Taiwan found that both groups of children had adequate growth and nutritional status and that "as long as parents can provide an adequate vegetarian diet and care for their preschool children, vegetarian children at each stage can meet their dietary requirements and have normal growth and nutritional status in the same way as omnivorous children do."[10] Another small study in China looking at the growth and nutrition of Chinese, vegetarian children in Hong Kong concluded that an "absence of growth retardation and a low prevalence of nutrient deficiency suggested that a Chinese, vegetarian diet can be suitable for fast-growing children."[11]

A more recent study, the Vegetarian and Vegan Children (VeChi) Study[12] from Germany published in 2019, concluded that vegetarian and vegan diets in early childhood provided sufficient energy and nutrients for adequate growth as these children had similar growth to omnivorous counterparts. However, a small percentage of children in the vegan and vegetarian groups were classified as having stunted growth. In nearly every one of these cases, the children were exclusively breastfed for an extended period of time (ranging from seven to twelve months of age, whereas the introduction of complementary foods should generally begin around six months of age) or had inadequate total energy intakes. These cases highlight the fact that any diet for infants and children needs to be sufficient in calories to optimize growth.

It is important to note that a few studies have reported insufficient growth and nutrient deficiencies in children following "restricted diets" and cite concerns in terms of meeting caloric and nutrient needs in vegetarian children. For instance, the German Nutrition Society (DGE) strongly advocates against vegan and vegetarian diets for infants and children. In its position statement from 2016, the DGE concedes that "it can be assumed that a plant-based diet (with or without low levels of meat) is associated to a reduced risk of nutrition-related diseases in comparison with the currently conventional German diet . . . (and) it is possible to create a vegan diet in which no nutrient deficiency develops."[13] However, despite this acknowledgment, the DGE asserts that a vegan diet is not recommended during pregnancy, lactation, or for children or adolescents of any age. The main objection seems to stem from the idea that plant-based diets need to be well planned and may require supplementation of specific nutrients. On that point, we agree entirely. We will discuss this further at the end of this section, but the bottom line is that when children eating a plant-based diet are provided with sufficient calories, and care is taken to ensure that they obtain necessary nutrients (as is the case for *all* children, regardless of the diet they follow!), they can reasonably meet the appropriate growth milestones. Early studies certainly do support this assertion, and since the 1980s and 1990s, we have had a growing number of resources, information, and research to add to our armamentarium. An expert panel from the Scientific Society for Vegetarian Nutrition in Italy found that " isolated cases of malnutrition in vegan children have been related almost exclusively to the inappropriateness of the diet offered to the infant or to the lack of B12 supplementation."[14] Health care professionals

> The bottom line is that when children eating a plant-based diet are provided with sufficient calories, and care is taken to ensure that they obtain necessary nutrients, they can reasonably meet the appropriate growth milestones.

should take care in advising families that may already be following a largely plant-based diet by providing them with adequate support and information in order to help them succeed.

Plant-based, vegetarian, and vegan diets can be completely safe and adequate for children. As with all diets, consideration must be given to the quality, quantity, and variety of the food that is provided.

Plant-based, vegetarian, and vegan diets can be completely safe and adequate for children. As with all diets, consideration must be given to the quality, quantity, and variety of the food that is provided. Several professional organizations, including the Academy of Nutrition and Dietetics,[15] the American Academy of Pediatrics,[16] the Canadian Paediatric Society,[17] the British Dietetic Association,[18] the Australian Dietary Guidelines,[19] and the Italian Society for Human Nutrition[20] all endorse that appropriately planned vegetarian diets are not only safe for children but may provide certain health advantages. In fact, in its 2016 updated position statement, the Academy of Nutrition and Dietetics announced:

> *"It is the position of the Academy of Nutrition and Dietetics that appropriately planned vegetarian, including vegan, diets are healthful, nutritionally adequate, and may provide health benefits in the prevention and treatment of certain diseases. These diets are appropriate for all stages of the life cycle, including pregnancy, lactation, infancy, childhood, adolescence, older adulthood, and for athletes. Plant-based diets are more environmentally sustainable than diets rich in animal products because they use fewer natural resources and are associated with much less environmental damage."* [21]

Many parents (and health professionals) find themselves stuck on the words "appropriately planned" and fear that such planning is beyond the reach of busy families with limited resources. We contend that *all* diets for children need to be appropriately planned, and while a plant-based diet for children may require some care and consideration, it is no more than any parent would give in feeding their child a balanced and appropriate diet. In Part II, Care, we will discuss many of the nutrients of concern. While it is not

While a plant-based diet for children may require some care and consideration, it is no more than any parent would give in feeding their child a balanced and appropriate diet.

necessary to know the specifics in great detail, we will provide an abundance of information for your ongoing reference. The information will remain relevant regardless of the extent to which you are or plan to be plant-based. However, it is important to remember that nutrient deficiencies exist for many children following a variety of diets, and so our approach to feeding plant-based children is not dramatically different than feeding omnivorous children. In our clinical experience, we have treated children for vitamin D deficiency rickets, iron deficiency anemia, and growth failure due to inadequate caloric intake; the vast majority of these children were following omnivorous diets. The evidence and most preeminent professional organizations support the assertion that appropriately planned plant-based diets are safe for children. The truest thing that we can say is that we are so convinced that we would (and do) feed our own children in this way.

WHAT DO WE EAT?

While it may be reassuring, to know that children eating plant-based diets can and do grow normally, perhaps it is not convincing enough to recommend this way of eating and feeding our families over the more traditional American diet. If we are looking to optimize health and well-being, we must also understand how plant-based diets compare to omnivorous ones and, ultimately, how plant-based diets may, in fact, be more health-promoting. We can begin by examining the current state of what we eat.

The quality of our overall diet is a major contributor to health. In fact, in a 2018 publication in the *Journal of the American Medical Association*, dietary risk was identified as the leading cause of death (ahead of tobacco use and high blood pressure) for Americans.[22] Because dietary habits established in childhood generally persist through adulthood, not only is diet relevant to the current state of children's health, but it also has the potential to mitigate many of the chronic diseases (such as heart disease, diabetes, and cancer) seen in adulthood.

A report published in the *Journal of the Academy of Nutrition and Dietetics* described the diet of US children in relation to the Dietary Guidelines for America (DGA) established by the USDA. They utilized a Healthy Eating Index (HEI), a score ranging from 0–100 based on component food groups (higher scores for fruits and vegetables lower scores for soda and grain-based desserts). While we don't agree entirely with their scoring system (low-fat dairy is not required for health as we will discuss in Chapter 5), this framework can provide an overview of the dietary habits of U.S. children. The report outlines detailed findings by age group; the overall conclusion was that the "total mean HEI-10 scores for all age groups were approximately 50 (80 being the minimum score for disease prevention), indicating diet in childhood is an important target for the prevention of diet-related adult chronic diseases. This study showed that overall diet quality was poor among all age groups and significantly declined for older age groups... there is an urgent need to devise and implement effective dietary quality interventions early on in life, in order to significantly reduce overall risk of chronic diseases like diabetes, cardiovascular disease, and cancer."[23] Specific areas of concern cited by the authors include total vegetables, greens and beans, whole grains, and fatty acids (notice protein and dairy were not identified as major areas of concern).

An earlier report in *The Journal of Nutrition* echoes these findings in the general US population. The report identified "among the food groups, dark green vegetables, orange vegetables, legumes, and whole grains had the poorest showing, with nearly everyone in each sex-age group failing to meet recommendations" and concluded that "nearly the entire U.S. population consumes a diet that is not on par with recommendations."[24] Additionally, looking at specific micronutrient intakes in the US population, we know that fortification (either in foods or via supplements) contributes greatly to our estimated average requirement for many nutrients. A paper published in the *Journal of Nutrition* reported that "most Americans met their recommended nutrient target for the majority of vitamins and minerals evaluated; however, far fewer individuals would have done so without fortification and enrichment. Nevertheless, even after accounting for the contributions of fortification and/or enrichment and dietary supplements, considerable percentages of individuals aged greater than 2 y had intakes that were below the EAR (estimated average requirement) for calcium and vitamin D, and very few consumed the recommended amount of potassium (all nutrients that the 2010 Dietary Guidelines for Americans singled out as being of public health concern). Intakes of magnesium and vitamins A, C, E, and K were also low for a considerable percentage of the population."[25] What these findings suggest is that in addition to a variety of nutrient-dense foods, fortification is often needed to allow us to meet our average nutrient requirements—regardless of the type of diet we follow. The idea that a plant-based diet is nutritionally inadequate because it may require supplementation in the form of fortified foods or specific vitamin and mineral supplements is unfounded because nearly *all* diets in the modern world are fortified in order to meet nutritional requirements and prevent states of deficiency.

We will cover this in greater detail in Part II but suffice it to say that a number of publications support the finding that plant-based diets provide adequate nutritional quality. A study in the journal *Nutrients* concluded that with regards to weight, nutritional intake, nutritional quality, and quantity, "based on different aspects of healthful dietary models, (be it the US Dietary Guidelines for Americans or compliance to a Mediterranean Diet) indicated consistently the vegan diet as the most healthy one."[26]

> The idea that a plant-based diet is nutritionally inadequate because it may require supplementation in the form of fortified foods or specific vitamin and mineral supplements is unfounded because nearly *all* diets in the modern world are fortified in order to meet nutritional requirements and prevent states of deficiency.

People eating a variety of diets, from vegetarian to pescatarian, vegan, and omnivorous, eat an assortment of foods and nutrients. Even within these groups, there exists a variety of intakes. At the population level, focusing on dietary factors such as saturated fat, vitamin D, and folic acid, as well as foods such as fruits, vegetables, and whole grains, can help to improve overall population health. At the individual level, care and attention to specific nutrients and a diversity of foods can ensure adequate intake and help prevent deficiency. There is abundant data to support the claim that people consuming plant-based diets can and do meet the recommended nutrient intakes. While it is true that some care may be required in order to ensure adequate intake of key nutrients and prevent deficiency, this is true regardless of the type of diet that is consumed.

HEALTH ADVANTAGES

In addition to being safe for growing children and meeting our nutritional requirements, appropriately planned plant-based diets offer many potential health advantages over other dietary approaches. As we stated at the beginning of this chapter, no single dietary approach guarantees a life free of disease, and many dietary approaches can allow for vibrant health. At the same time, however, we can look to population studies and clinical trials to better understand which dietary patterns are associated with positive health outcomes, both in terms of longevity and vitality.

One of the difficulties in studying nutrition at the population level is that it is a challenging and cumbersome thing to investigate. Unlike pharmaceutical trials where we can determine the effect of "x" on "y" (penicillin for a particular infection), the side effects of "x," and even drug "x" vs. drug "y," nutrition research is not as clear-cut. As we mentioned earlier, in addition to diet, many other factors such as socioeconomic status, environment, stress, sleep, and genetics can influence our overall health and well-being. Food and nutrient intake can be challenging to measure, follow, and control for. Additionally, what a person or population may eat on a given day or even over the span of several years can vary quite a bit. And finally, many of the outcomes that researchers track to determine the effect of diet on health (heart disease, cancer, and death) require extensive periods of follow-up, sometimes even decades. This does not mean that studying nutrition and its impact on health is not useful and relevant. Although it is unlikely that we will be able to say definitively that a particular diet will cause or prevent a particular disease, we can come to understand which diets, foods, and even nutrients are associated with a variety of health outcomes. Sometimes the requirement of definitive causation is not necessary for us to make well-informed recommendations and decisions. Remember, there is no randomized controlled trial that proves that smoking causes cancer, but we have enough reliable information to know that the association is incredibly strong and to make recommendations at both the individual and public health level. Although it can feel quite confusing when conflicting research, clickbait headlines, and the latest best-seller attempt to persuade us that the newest fad diet is the hidden key to health, the truth is that there is abundant evidence and general consensus amongst leading experts to know which dietary patterns are associated with health.

A 2014 paper published in the Annual Review of Public Health provides an overview of many of the significant dietary variants.[27] In it, the authors outline major dietary patterns (from low-carb and low-fat to Mediterranean and paleo), delineate the features of each, and review what the evidence shows with regards to diet and health. The authors conclude that "the literature strongly supports a common set of dietary principles for health promotion and the prevention, or management, of virtually all prevalent conditions in modern societies . . . both the scientific literature and consideration of indelible links between native diet and adaptation for all species including our own lead to the conclusion that a diet of foods mostly direct from nature and predominantly plants is supportive of health across the life span." A plant-based diet certainly meets this requirement.

LIVE LONG AND PROSPER

One of the broadest ways in which we can examine diet and its connection to health is to look at populations in terms of longevity. Dan Buettner and his team from National Geographic and the National Institute of Aging sought to uncover the specific aspects of lifestyle and environment that led to longevity.[28] They found five geographical areas with the highest concentration of centenarians. They labeled these regions the "Blue Zones" (named after the blue circles used to identify these regions on a map) and found that people living in these regions (including Loma Linda, California, USA; Nicoya, Costa Rica; Sardinia, Italy; Ikaria, Greece; Okinawa, Japan) had ten times the rate of people living to age one hundred as in the general United States population. The investigators identified shared lifestyle factors that might explain the longevity enjoyed by these communities. In addition to natural movement, living with a sense of purpose and belonging, and social connection, they found that a plant-centered diet (especially including beans, such as fava, black, soy, and lentils) was the cornerstone of most centenarian eating patterns. In the communities where meat was consumed, it comprised a very small part of the diet.

Numerous studies chronicle the health advantages of plant-based diets. Notably, two large, ongoing centers of research have studied the effects of vegetarian diets on health; they include the Oxford cohort of the European Prospective Investigation into Cancer and Nutrition study (EPIC-Oxford) and the Adventist Health Study in the United States. Although some findings from these studies seem to conflict, "the evidence from these studies has supported vegetarian diets as healthy dietary patterns associated with a reduction in several common disease risk factors and reduced risk of some chronic diseases of public health." The authors of a recent review of these studies propose that the differences in findings have less to do with whether or not plant-based diets promote health and more to do with the type of vegetarian diet that is followed, offering that, "one cannot assume that simply avoiding animal foods will necessarily produce such a healthy diet."[29] As we have mentioned previously, there is a diversity of vegetarian dietary patterns and this diversity likely impacts what the data shows.

In terms of overall mortality, many studies have found a protective effect of plant-based diets. As we mentioned earlier, the diets of the Seventh Day Adventists (representing one of the Blue Zones!) are of particular interest because they exhibit a variety of dietary habits (from non-vegetarian to vegan with close to half following some form of a vegetarian or semi-vegetarian diet) with a strong emphasis on health. This allows researchers to compare various dietary patterns, while controlling for known non-dietary confounders, such as alcohol and tobacco use. In a review published in *Nutrients* entitled *Beyond Meatless, the Health Effects of Vegan Diets: Findings from the Adventist Cohorts*, the authors reported on three large cohorts to assess the effect of vegetarian diets on disease and health outcome. The findings revealed, "in all three cohorts, vegetarians experienced a 10 percent to 20 percent decreased in all-cause mortality. Similarly, vegetarians had 26 percent to 68 percent lower risks of mortality from ischemic heart disease, cardiovascular disease, and cerebrovascular disease. Vegetarians experienced a 48 percent risk reduction in mortality from breast cancer, and modest risks reduction from other-cause total mortality."[30]

In general, plant-based diets have been found to be protective against a variety of health conditions. They are associated with improved cardiovascular health (coronary artery disease, blood pressure, blood lipid profiles), lower rates of diabetes, lower rates of certain cancers, and lower mortality rates. In addition, they have been shown to provide effective treatment for some chronic diseases, particularly heart disease and diabetes. Below is just a brief summary of some of the research that highlights the health advantages of plant-based diets:

Overall health and mortality:
- Several large studies have shown a consistent relationship with diet and BMI with a step-wise reduction in average BMI the more the diet trended toward being vegan.[31] In one study observing over 60,000 people following a generally health-conscious diet, those following a vegan diet were the only group with an average BMI that fell in the normal range of less than 25 (23.6 for vegans, 25.7 for lacto-ovo vegetarians, 26.3 for pesco-vegetarians, 27.3 for semi-vegetarians, and 28.8 for nonvegetarians).[32]

- A comprehensive review of evidence from the Adventist cohorts on the potential health effects for vegan and lacto-ovo-vegetarian diets on disease and mortality found that "the published studies of North American Adventists paint a consistent picture across all three study cohorts, associating vegetarian diets with lower body mass index, coronary heart disease, hypertension, type 2 diabetes, and metabolic syndrome. Similarly, vegetarians have lower risks for colon, gastrointestinal tract, prostate, and overall cancer. Among males, vegetarian diets seem to be protective against all-cause mortality and CVD mortality."[34]

Cardiovascular Health:

- Numerous studies have shown a protective effect of plant-based diets on cardiovascular health, with decreased rates of high blood pressure, improved blood lipid profiles, and reduced risk of death from ischemic heart disease and stroke.[33, 34, 35]

- Stroke is a leading cause of death and morbidity worldwide. It is estimated that 90 percent of the risk factors related to stroke are modifiable and include hypertension, diabetes, elevated cholesterol, physical activity, smoking, and diet. A prospective study examining the effect of a vegetarian diet on the incidence of stroke in Taiwan found that vegetarians had roughly half the risk of overall stroke.[36] However, a study of the EPIC-Oxford cohort in the United Kingdom mentioned previously reported that while vegetarians had lower rates of ischemic heart disease, they had higher rates of hemorrhagic stroke compared to meat eaters. The authors hypothesized that this could have been due to lower levels of certain nutrients (including vitamins B12 and D, and omega 3 fatty acids) and potential misclassification of strokes.[37] More research is needed to examine risks of sub-types of stroke and to determine whether dietary factors such as a low intake of vitamin B12 in vegetarians might have an adverse impact on risk of stroke.[38]

- High animal protein intake (especially red and processed meat) has been positively associated with cardiovascular mortality, whereas high plant protein intake has been shown to be protective against all-cause and cardiovascular mortality among individuals with at least one lifestyle risk factor.[39]

- A low-fat plant-based diet in combination with other healthy lifestyle changes (tobacco cessation, exercise, stress reduction) has been shown not only to slow down the progression of existing heart disease but actually to demonstrate regression (meaning reversal) of coronary atherosclerosis.[40,41]

Diabetes:

- Vegans and vegetarians have been found to have a lower risk of developing type 2 diabetes[42,43,44] A study following over 50,000 people found that vegan, lacto-ovo vegetarian, and semi-vegetarian diets were associated with a substantial reduction in risk of diabetes compared to non-vegetarian diets with vegans having over 60 percent reduction in risk of developing diabetes.[45,46]
- There is data to support the role of plant-based diets in the treatment and management of diabetes with one study showing improvements in certain areas over the American Diabetes Association diet.[47]

Cancer:

- The research on health outcomes for cancer (which includes a wide variety of diagnoses, including sex-specific cancers such as breast and prostate cancer) is not quite as robust. However, where an association between diet and cancer has been found, plant-based diets have been shown to be generally protective. While some studies show no difference in cancer rates between vegetarians and non-vegetarians, the ones that do, show a protective effect.[35,48,49,50,51,52]
- A comprehensive meta-analysis published in 2017 looking at the association between vegetarian and vegan diets and multiple health outcomes found an 8 percent reduction in total incidence of cancer among vegetarians compared to omnivores and a 15 percent reduction among vegans.[53]
- The two large prospective studies mentioned earlier both suggest that for all cancers combined, fish-eaters, lacto-ovo vegetarians, and vegans appear to have lower overall rates of cancer than nonvegetarians, with the lowest risk being for vegans in both studies.
- The International Agency for Research on Cancer (IARC), which is the cancer research agency for the World Health Organization, classified processed meat as a carcinogen and red meat as a probable carcinogen.[54]
- The American Cancer Society Guidelines on Nutrition and Physical Activity for Cancer Prevention recommends a healthy diet, with an emphasis on plant foods, including limiting the consumption of red and processed meats and including plenty of fruits, vegetables, lentils, and whole grains.[55]

- Evidence from epidemiological and laboratory studies suggest that diet and lifestyle may have a role in the development of prostate cancer. A study conducted at the University of California San Francisco found that intensive lifestyle changes may beneficially affect the progression of early, low grade prostate cancer in men.

Microbiome/Gut Health:

- Emerging research points to the gut microbiota (the trillions of microorganisms living in our guts) as having an important role in our overall health, from our immune system to gut and brain health as well as systemic conditions such as obesity, atherosclerosis, type 2 diabetes, cancer, Alzheimer's and Parkinson's disease, autism spectrum disorders, and atopy to name a few. Dietary patterns determine the composition of our gut microbiota, and research suggests that "a plant-based diet can be an effective way to promote a diverse ecosystem of beneficial microbes that support overall health" by supporting the development of a more diverse gut microbial system.[56]

Miscellaneous Health Conditions:

- Studies suggest a lower risk of diverticular disease of the colon among vegetarians (and especially vegans) due to both increased fiber intake among vegetarians as well as a possible alteration in the metabolism of bacteria in the colon from high meat intake.[57]

- Age-related cataracts are responsible for almost half of world blindness. The EPIC-Oxford cohort showed a strong association between diet group and risk of cataracts with a progressive decrease in cataract risk from high meat eaters to low meat eaters, fish eaters, vegetarians, and vegans, with vegans showing a 40 percent lower risk of developing cataracts.[58]

- A recent study found vegetarian diets to be protective against uncomplicated urinary tract infections in women.[59]

- Non-alcoholic Fatty Liver Disease (NAFLD) is the most common form of chronic liver disease worldwide, affecting of 20 to 30 percent of the global population. Currently there are no approved medications or procedures that can treat NAFLD, which is associated with metabolic syndrome and obesity. Diet and physical activity are the standard treatment. Vegetarian diets in which plant foods are substituted for animal foods (soy for meat), have been shown to be protective against the development of NAFLD.[60]

While much of this data is preliminary, what we do know is that the long-term health of vegetarians appears to be good and may be better than that of comparable non-vegetarians for some conditions.

PLANT-BASED DIETS AND KID'S HEALTH

A wealth of research supports the health benefits of plant-based diets.[34, 61, 62, 63, 64, 65] Chronic diseases such as diabetes, high blood pressure, and heart disease may make their most dramatic appearances in adulthood, but they often begin developing in youth. A landmark paper published in the *Journal of the American Medical Association* in 1953 described the high frequency of atherosclerotic lesions (ranging from fibrous thickening to large plaques) in the coronary arteries of soldiers that died in the Korean War. The average age of these soldiers was just twenty-two years.[66] The Pathobiological Determinants of Atherosclerosis in Youth (PDAY) study[67] documents the development of atherosclerosis at an early age based on autopsy findings of adolescents and young adults. The multi-center investigation concluded that "five decades of study of the natural history and pathogenesis of atherosclerosis have provided abundant evidence that atherosclerosis begins in childhood" and thus "true primary prevention of atherosclerosis must begin in childhood or early adolescence."[68]

A recent publication in *Nutrition Reviews* provides a constructive summary of plant-based diets for children as means of improving adult cardiometabolic health. The authors conclude that "vegan and vegetarian children have lower rates of overweight and obesity. Preliminary evidence suggests that they have lower cholesterol levels and higher antioxidant status in the blood. They consume more fruits and vegetables than their omnivore counterparts. Moreover, a recent trial showed that an intervention with low-fat vegan diet was more effective than the American Heart Association–recommended diet at reducing CVD risk factors in obese and hypercholesterolemic children aged 9–18 years old."[69, 70] Data in children for many of the other chronic diseases that we encounter is limited, but knowing what we know about the effects of diet on adult health outcomes, it would be reasonable to assume that beginning these dietary patterns in childhood, while ensuring adequate nutrient and caloric intake, could be protective from an early age. Additionally, we know that the longer a person suffers from chronic diseases, the earlier and more severe the complications can be (for instances, eye, kidney, and nerve damage with diabetes). This means that if children are diagnosed with diseases that typically arise in adulthood, they will begin experiencing complications at an earlier age.

In addition to helping to prevent diet-related chronic diseases, a healthy diet in childhood is associated with numerous positive health outcomes. Additionally, regular consumption of certain animal-based foods, especially dairy, has been linked to specific pediatric disorders.

- Both childhood constipation and infantile colic have been linked to cow's milk intolerance. For children with significant constipation or infantile colic, a trial off cow's milk (or in the case of an infant that is breastfed, elimination of dairy from mother's diet) is reasonable.[71, 72, 73]

- There has also been a link reported between the prevalence and severity of acne and consumption of dairy and foods with a high glycemic load (typically low fiber carbohydrates).[74]

- Emerging research on the gut-brain axis connects neurodevelopmental conditions such as autism to our microbiome. Researchers have proposed that "quality food and the use of pre/probiotics could be both a protective factor for autism spectrum disorders."[75, 76] Some investigators are even looking at the effectiveness of fecal microbiota transplant as a therapeutic tool.[77] Again, the research is limited, but it will be interesting to follow future developments on the influence of diet on our microbiota and in the development and treatment of neurodevelopmental disorders.

- One congenital condition worth mentioning when it comes to vegetarian diets is hypospadias, which is an abnormal or incomplete closure of the urethra at the underside of the penis. Though the cause is not known, it is believed that a combination of genetic and environmental factors plays a role. An earlier study published in 2000 reported a higher proportion of boys with hypospadias were born to mothers who were vegetarian during pregnancy.[78] However, subsequent studies have not supported this finding. In fact, one study reported that the lowest incidence of hypospadias occurred in children born to mothers who followed a "health conscious diet" that was rich in fresh fruit and vegetables, dried fruit, fresh or frozen fish, soy products, pulses, olive oil, and organic food. Based on these follow-up studies, it is reasonably safe to assume that there is not an increased risk of hypospadias in children born to vegetarian mothers.[79, 80] To our knowledge, appropriately planned plant-based diets have not been associated with any other negative health outcomes for children.

There are still many unanswered questions when it comes to the relationship between childhood diseases and plant-based diets. However, where a link has been found, plant-based diets tend to be protective. Perhaps the most significant protective effect of plant-based diets for children is the establishment of lifelong dietary habits that promote health beginning at a young age.

IS IT ALL OR NOTHING?

Research shows that shifting towards a plant-based diet can have a positive impact on health, but it is not an all or nothing proposition. The authors of a study published in the *American Journal of Clinical Nutrition* propose a "provegetarian" food pattern. Their findings "support a relative reduction in the risk of death from any cause of greater than 30 percent associated with only a modest decrease in the consumption of animal foods together with compensatory increases in plant-based foods. This modest change is realistic, affordable, and achievable…All of these reasons increase the translational potential of our results into health and nutrition policies."[81] In *Eat, Drink, and Be Healthy: The Harvard Medical School Guide to Healthy Eating*, the authors contend that, "many studies have supported the benefits of a primarily plant-based diet" and that, "even a partial shift away from a meat- and dairy-centered diet and toward more plant sources of protein is a big step in the direction of long-term good health for you and planet Earth."[82]

There is ample data to support the shift toward a plant-based diet for families. Earlier research focused on the presumed nutrient deficiencies of plant-based diets. With growing evidence of the protective benefits of diets centered around plants and increasing awareness around potential nutrients of concern, we have seen a paradigm shift in the risks and benefits of plant-based diets. Joan Sabaté, a physician and leading nutrition researcher, eloquently states that "an adequate diet, by definition, prevents nutrient deficiencies by providing sufficient nutrients and energy for human growth and reproduction. An optimal diet, in addition, promotes health and longevity, reducing the risk of diet-related chronic diseases. Although the composition of an adequate diet is basically known, the composition of an optimal diet is not. However, recent scientific findings are suggesting that diets largely based on plant foods, such as some vegetarian, Mediterranean, or Asian diets, could best prevent nutrient deficiencies as well as diet-related chronic diseases. These diets contain no or very little meat. If plant-based diets are generally healthier than meat-based diets, this constitutes an important departure from previous views on dietary recommendations to prevent disease conditions."[83] While all diets are associated with potential health benefits and risks, we can aim to optimize health with a well-balanced plant-based diet by reducing the risk of nutrition-related chronic diseases while also minimizing the risk of nutrient deficiency.

People eating plant-based diets do get heart disease, cancer, diabetes, Alzheimer's, and even the flu. Diet is just one aspect of health, but the evidence and scientific consensus overwhelmingly supports a diet centered around plants as the foundation of health. Even if you can't imagine yourself ever becoming 100 percent plant-based, consider aiming for a diet that is 80 to 90 percent plant-based (more on how to get there in the chapters to come), avoiding red and processed meats, and minimizing your consumption of highly processed foods, including sugar-added beverages. But just as diet is only one aspect of health, health is only one aspect of the impact of our food choices. The next two chapters address the consequences of our food choices beyond our individual health and reveal how the answer to the simple question of "what's for dinner?" may be far more consequential than we ever imagined.

Chapter 2

Home

"Changing how we eat will not be enough,
on its own, to save the planet, but we cannot save
the planet without changing how we eat."

—*Jonathan Safran Foer*

IS IT REALLY A CRISIS?

We are not climate scientists, and this is not a book about climate change. But talking about food without considering the environmental impacts of our choices and recommendations is no longer reasonable or responsible. In recent years we have seen the devastation of the effects of climate change. From the California wildfires, the burning of the Amazon, and the unprecedented bushfires in Australia, to Hurricanes Sandy, Maria, and Harvey, and the floods and droughts that have introduced the term "climate refugee" into our lexicon, there is no denying that the climate crisis is real and at our doorstep.

A 2018 report by the Intergovernmental Panel on Climate Change (IPCC), *Global Warming of 1.5° C,*[1] loudly and alarmingly asserted that the scientific evidence for warming of the climate system is unequivocal. The IPCC, which was assembled in 1988, is the United Nations body for assessing the science related to climate change. It is the world's foremost collection of climate scientists whose main objective is to provide governments at all levels with scientific information to develop climate policies. The reason for such widespread alarm following the dissemination of their 2018 report was because the report predicted that the impact of 1.5° C of warming (which experts fear we will reach in as little as ten years, and most certainly by the year 2050) will likely result in far greater than expected record-breaking storms, forest fires, droughts, coral bleaching, heat waves, and floods around the world. The IPCC further emphasized that the difference between the effects of warming to 1.5° C vs. 2° C were substantial and that limiting global warming to 1.5°C compared with 2°C would reduce challenging impacts on ecosystems, human health, and well-being. Such impacts include stronger storms, more erratic weather, dangerous heat waves, rising seas, and largescale disruption to infrastructure and migration patterns.[2] Limiting warming to less than 1.5° C seems prudent, limiting warming to less than 2° C seems critical.

While the report did not discuss the effects of a rise beyond 2° C, the outcomes are likely to be catastrophic to human survival. In his recent book, The *Uninhabitable Earth: Life After Warming*, David Wallace-Wells offers that "the research summarized in the report was not new, and the temperatures beyond 2 degrees were not even covered. But though it did not address any of the scarier possibilities for warming, the report did offer a new form of permission, of sanction, to the world's scientists. The thing that was new was the message: *It is okay, finally, to freak out.*"[3]

In addition to weather related disasters and the economic burden of addressing them, climate change will also lead to worsening air pollution, increasing fatalities and illnesses (from heat stress, cardiovascular disease, kidney disease, respiratory illnesses, and a new onslaught of insect-borne diseases), ocean acidification (leading to extinction of some marine species and damage to coral reefs), loss of species diversity and even species extinction, coastal erosion (and loss of coastal cites), land degradation, food insecurity, and water shortage.[4] While the causes and potential cures are complex, multifactorial, and yet to be fully understood, there is no doubt that "climate change represents an urgent and potentially irreversible threat to human societies and the planet."[5] Burning fossil fuels for heat and electricity account for nearly one third of greenhouse gas (GHG) emissions. Transportation, industry, deforestation (primarily for grazing and to raise crops for livestock), and of course agriculture are also significant contributors to climate change.[6]

At times the problem seems entirely overwhelming and a tangible solution feels beyond our reach. In fact, the Carbon Majors Report published by the Climate Accountability Institute in 2017 identified that 70 percent of the world's GHG emissions can be traced back to just one hundred companies.[7] This might lead one to believe that change at the individual, family, or even community level would be inconsequential. Addressing the climate crisis in a meaningful way will most certainly require a coordinated and robust effort involving policy change, international co-operation, corporate responsibility, and technological and agricultural advancement. Many argue convincingly that individual choice (perhaps responsibility is a more fitting word) should not be the focus of climate change policies as they can hardly make a dent in such a sizeable and complex problem.

However, in an interview, Richard Heede, the co-director of the Climate Accountability Institute, explained that, "they're (the corporations) producing the fossil fuels we all use . . . But to be clear, it's the consumers that actually burn and demand the fossil fuels that these companies provide. The companies may have some responsibility for their product—for lobbying in favor of the carbon economy, and for getting subsidies and arguing for subsidies—but some responsibility ought to fall on individuals, households, and corporations." He goes on to say that governments, corporations, and individuals all need to participate. In addition to voting to affect policy change, we can also make choices at the consumer level. Heede encourages us to consider that "there is some personal satisfaction in doing right by ourselves as well as our grandchildren. We can't solve the problem by ourselves, but it would be a morally better choice to attempt to do something and derive satisfaction by it, rather than saying, 'My carbon savings don't matter,' Because they do matter! They matter symbolically. They matter financially. They matter morally. They matter to your neighbors."[8] Since consumers drive demand, changing what and how we consume collectively, has tremendous potential.

In *We Are the Weather: Saving the Planet Begins at Breakfast*, Jonathan Safran Foer affirms this call to action by stating, "social change, much like climate change, is caused by multiple chain reactions that occur simultaneously. Both cause, and are caused by, feedback loops. No single factor can be credited for a hurricane, drought, or wildfire, just as no single factor can be credited for a decline in cigarette smoking—and yet in all cases, every factor is significant. When a radical change is needed, many argue that it is impossible for individual actions to incite it, so it's futile for anyone to try. This is exactly the opposite of the truth: the impotence of individual action is the reason for everyone to try."[9]

WHY FOOD MATTERS

We can do many things that matter. We can change what or if we drive, how much or if we fly, have fewer children, and of course, shift towards a plant-based diet.[10] Though many of these mitigating solutions seem impractical if not impossible, one is immediately available to us three or more times a day. Shifting towards a plant-based diet is one of the most immediate, practical, and meaningful ways we can help to protect our planet.

> Shifting towards a plant-based diet is one of the most immediate, practical, and meaningful ways we can help to protect our planet.

All of these actions are worth exploring and pursuing; calling for a shift in diet does not negate the impact of driving and flying less, reducing, reusing, and recyling, demanding corporate responsibility, and voting. We are all on the same team, and our efforts to combat climate change can be additive instead of competitive. Far too often we can resign ourselves to inaction because we fear our individual actions will not amount to much and will not be (perfect) enough. We can counter this fear by taking the approach offered by author, speaker, and vegan advocate, Collen Patrick-Goudreau: "Don't do nothing because you can't do everything. Do something. Anything." So, let's start by taking a look at how our food choices impact our climate.

It is estimated that the global food supply chain is responsible for nearly 30 percent of GHG emissions. Moving towards diets that limit animal products has "transformative potential" by reducing food's land use by 76 percent, food's GHG emissions by 49 percent, acidification by 50 percent, eutrophication (which causes algae blooms, ocean dead zones, and fish kills) by 49 percent, and scarcity-weighted freshwater withdrawals by 19 percent. "For the United States, where per capita meat consumption is three times the global average, dietary change has the potential for a far greater effect on food's different emissions, reducing them by 61 to 73 percent."[11] Some estimates report that

> Some estimates report that livestock is responsible for 18 percent of greenhouse gas emissions, which is more than the emissions from all transportation.

livestock is responsible for 18 percent of greenhouse gas emissions, which is more than the emissions from all transportation.[12]

The livestock sector is by far the single largest user of land. In all, livestock production accounts for 70 percent of all agricultural land and 30 percent of the land surface of the planet. Given how much land it takes to grow food to feed livestock, meat production is a leading cause of deforestation.[13] It is estimated that animal agriculture is responsible for over 90 percent of the Amazon forest destruction. The clearing and burning of forests releases billions of tons of greenhouse gases into the atmosphere and results in loss of biodiversity (largely because of habitat loss), soil degradation, and water pollution.[14]

> Given how much land it takes to grow food to feed livestock, meat production is a leading cause of deforestation.

Livestock contribute significantly to both water depletion and pollution. Approximately one third of the world's water consumption goes towards animal agriculture.[15] Livestock is also a major source of water pollution, emitting nutrients and organic matter, pathogens, and drug residues into rivers, lakes, and coastal seas.

The statistics around animal agriculture's disastrous effect on the health of our planet are mounting and alarming. Cattle (raised for both beef and milk) are responsible for the most emissions, representing about 65 percent of the livestock sector's emissions. Feed production and processing and enteric fermentation from ruminants are the two main sources of emissions, representing 45 and 39 percent of total emissions, respectively. Manure storage and processing represent 10 percent. The remainder is attributable to the processing and transportation of animal products.[16]

THE INEQUALITY OF CLIMATE CHANGE

The impacts of warming will not be equitable. A recent publication from the Department of Earth System Science at Stanford University found that "there is growing evidence that poorer countries or individuals are more negatively affected by a changing climate, either because they lack the resources for climate protection or because they tend to reside in warmer regions where additional warming would be detrimental to both productivity and health. Furthermore, given that wealthy countries have been responsible for the vast majority of historical GHG emissions, any clear evidence of inequality in the impacts of the associated climate change raises critical questions of international justice."[17]

The concept of climate justice becomes especially important when considering possible solutions to address this clear and present danger. Far too often privilege or the advantage of having the means to make certain choices is heralded as a reason not to press for change at the individual level—that to ask people to shop, eat, or live differently is a caustic burden that the privileged hurl upon those with fewer resources to do so. In fact, it is the responsibility of those who are able, to be held to greater accountability for the repair. Again, in *We Are the Weather,* Foer makes a poignant argument that "it's true that this is an issue of economic justice. We should talk about it as one, rather than using inequality as a way to avoid talking about inequality. The richest 10 percent of the global population is responsible for half the carbon emissions; the poorest half is responsible for 10 percent. And those who are the least responsible for global warming are often the ones most punished by it . . . So, no, it is not elitist to suggest that a cheaper, healthier, more environmentally sustainable diet is better. But what does strike me as elitist? When someone uses the existence of people without access to healthy food as an excuse not to change, rather than as a motivation to help those people."[9]

According to a report by the World Health Organization, currently, 821 million people (roughly 1 in 9) suffer from hunger and limited progress is being made in addressing the multiple forms of malnutrition, ranging from child stunting to adult obesity, putting the health of hundreds of millions of people at risk.[18] This is happening at the same time that roughly half the grains grown worldwide are fed to animals raised for meat, eggs, and dairy. Many experts believe that we could largely solve the problem of world hunger (by diverting resources to feed people instead of livestock) and significantly reduce our use of fossil fuels, land, and water by minimizing our consumption of animal-based foods and shifting more towards a plant-based diet.[19]

> Many experts believe that we could largely solve the problem of world hunger and significantly reduce our use of fossil fuels, land, and water by minimizing our consumption of animal-based foods and shifting more towards a plant-based diet.

EATING FOR OUR PLANET

According to a report published by the Food and Agriculture Organization (FAO) of the United Nations, "livestock activities have significant impact on virtually all aspects of the environment, including air and climate change, land and soil, water and biodiversity. The impact may be direct, through grazing for example, or indirect, such as the expansion of soybean production for feed replacing forests in South America. Livestock's impact on the environment is already huge, and it is growing and rapidly changing. Global demand for meat, milk and eggs is fast increasing, driven by rising incomes, growing populations and urbanization."[20] The FAO further emphasized that in addition to looking at diet as a way to promote and optimize health, we need to also consider how a sustainable diet can be part of the solution to our current climate crisis. They define sustainable diets as those diets with low environmental impacts that contribute to food and nutrition security and to healthy life for present and future generations. Sustainable diets are protective and respectful of biodiversity and ecosystems, culturally acceptable, accessible, economically fair and affordable; nutritionally adequate, safe and healthy; while optimizing natural and human resources.

Plant-based diets have consistently been found to offer the greatest environmental protection and meet the UN's definition of sustainable diets. While it is true that different foods will have varying environmental impacts in terms of land and water use as well as emissions, as a whole, vegan diets have been shown to have the least environmental impact. Even with diets that include animal products, a positive effect can be seen by reducing their intake substantially.[21]

> As a whole, vegan diets have been shown to have the least environmental impact. Even with diets that include animal products, a positive effect can be seen by reducing their intake substantially.

An expanding global population, estimated to grow to nearly 10 billion by the year 2050, and rising global income (with subsequent greater demand for animal-based food products), will place greater environmental pressure on our food system. Climate scientists assert that "GHG emissions cannot be sufficiently mitigated without dietary changes towards more plant-based diets (and that) .... an important first step would be to align national food-based dietary guidelines with the present evidence on healthy eating and the environmental impacts of diets."[22]

In fact, over the last several years, this is precisely what has occurred. We have already discussed many of the health advantages of plant-based diets, and increasingly we are seeing dietary recommendations that emphasize sustainability and environmental protection. In its 2016 position statement on vegetarian diets, the Academy of Nutrition and Dietetics not only underscored the healthfulness and nutritional adequacy of plant-based diets, but emphasized that such diets are more environmentally sustainable than diets rich in animal products because they use fewer natural resources and are associated with much less environmental damage. In a similar way, Canada's 2019 highly praised Food Guide urges people to consider a plant-leaning planetary diet that favors plant foods, minimizes animal foods, and designates water as the beverage of choice (downplaying the need for dairy).[23] Even the Dietary Guidelines Advisory Committee, which is responsible for providing scientific support in developing the Dietary Guidelines for America, asserts that "consistent evidence indicates that, in general, a dietary pattern that is higher in plant-based foods, such as vegetables, fruits, whole grains, legumes, nuts, and seeds, and lower in animal-based foods is more health promoting and is associated with lesser environmental impact (GHG emissions and energy, land, and water use) than is the current average U.S. diet."[24]

Perhaps one of the most compelling reports connecting human health to planetary health is the recent publication of the EAT–Lancet Commission on Healthy Diets from Sustainable Food Systems.[25] The commission included experts in various fields from human health, agriculture, political sciences, and environmental sustainability and worked to develop global scientific targets based on the best evidence available for healthy diets and sustainable food production. The members of the commission sought to integrate human health and environmental sustainability into a common global agenda to achieve planetary health diets (healthy diets from sustainable food systems) for nearly 10 billion people by 2050.

Key points from the report include:

- Food is the single strongest lever to optimize human health and environmental sustainability on Earth. However, food is currently threatening both people and planet.
- Without action, the world risks failing to meet the UN Sustainable Development Goals (SDGs) and the Paris Agreement.

- Unhealthy diets now pose a greater risk to morbidity and mortality than unsafe sex, alcohol, drug, and tobacco use combined. Global food production threatens climate stability and ecosystem resilience and constitutes the single largest driver of environmental degradation and transgression of planetary boundaries.

- Diets rich in plant-based foods and with fewer animal source foods confer both improved health and environmental benefits. Overall, the literature indicates that such diets are "win-win" in that they are good for both people and planet.

- The commission calls for a "great food transformation" which will require dramatic reductions in food losses and waste, major improvements in food production practices, and substantial shifts toward mostly plant-based dietary patterns.

Perhaps the most vivid intersection of human health, environmental health, and sociopolitical considerations is the COVID-19 pandemic that brought the world to a halt in 2020. It is believed that the novel coronavirus emanated from the wet markets in China, but as reported by Vox News, for years, leading health organizations like the World Health Organization (WHO) and the Centers for Disease Control (CDC) have been "warning that most emerging infectious diseases come from animals and that our industrialized farming practices are ratcheting up the risk. Livestock health is the weakest link in our global health chain."[26] Similar reporting in the *New York Times* by Jonathan Safran Foer takes it a step further by insisting that protecting against future pandemics will require us to look more closely at our food choices because while the wet markets draw great attention, factory farming may be a more significant breeding ground for pandemics. He offers that, in part, due to the climate crisis, we have been inching our way away from diets that rely heavily on animal foods and that "our hand has been reaching for the doorknob for the last few years. COVID-19 has kicked open the door... With the horror of pandemic pressing from behind, and the new questioning of what is essential, we can now see the door that was always there. As in a dream where our homes have rooms unknown to our waking selves, we can sense there is a better way of eating, a life closer to our values. On the other side is not something new, but something that calls from the past—a world in which farmers were not myths, tortured bodies were not food and the planet was not the bill at the end of the meal...One meal in front of the other, it's time to cross the threshold. On the other side is home."[27]

The climate crisis is real. There is no single cause and no single cure. Yet, it is undeniable that animal agriculture is a significant contributor. It may not be within our individual capacity to assemble a government that acknowledges and prioritizes the environment, influence corporations, or innovate new forms of transportation, energy, and technology. All of those things will be necessary. Innovation and political change require time, persistence, and a strong collective will. Just as for health, shifting the way we eat to care for our planet may seem intellectually reasonable but personally more complex and challenging. There is enough to worry about in the world without adding to the list of what we aren't doing well enough. Moving towards a plant-based diet is not a trivial step, but we can be a part of the larger global solution in both small and big ways. The fewer animal products we consume, the less will be the demand. We do not have to become vegan overnight. We can start by making simple changes and expanding. Small things done on a large scale can have enormous influence. Who knew a veggie burger could change the world?

Plant-based diets are good for us and they are good for the planet. So far, it is indeed a *win-win*. One last stop before we get to all of the details you are likely eagerly awaiting.

Chapter 3

Heart

"Non-violence is not a garment to be put on and off at will.
Its seat is in the heart, and it must be an
inseparable part of our being."

—*Mahatma Gandhi*

We know what compassion feels like. It is seeing the suffering of another and the deep wish that it was not present. We experience it in our everyday lives with family, friends, and even strangers. The child that gets left out, a loved one that falls ill, or a beloved family pet that has died all evoke a sense of pain and loss. We can also know it in stories far away—a refugee crisis, sweeping hurricanes, and horrific acts of animal violence such as the annual Yulin dog meat festival in China , the Festival of the Ox in Brazil, or the Day of the Geese in Lekeitio, Spain (it hardly seems like a day for the geese when they are drenched in oil, hung from a rope in the harbor, and a winner is declared when the goose is effectively decapitated by someone hanging on its neck)—that elicit a sense of sorrow, grief, and perhaps even a call to action. These are all moments when our compassion can become activated.

We can feel such tenderness and love towards fellow humans and certain animals in certain spaces. We have come to believe (at least in the United States) that dogs and cats deserve special status as our companion animals. They are loved and cared for as members of the family. They are cute, cuddly, and showered with affection. Even farm animals in some settings are cherished. We visit them, pet them, and even create wild animated stories to personify them. Yet somehow, we are able to separate ourselves from them when it comes to mealtime. There is a heavy gap between the adorable piglet running and squealing about and the bacon cheeseburger being served for lunch. How is it that we have allowed this gap to grow so large that we can swiftly and completely separate the two?

If you have ever witnessed the graphic images of slaughter that are hard to even watch, you know that these animals experience fear and pain. Whether it is the torture of confinement for factory farmed animals, the cries as babies are torn away from mothers, or the gruesome slaughter of every animal raised for food, there is no denying that these animals endure unspeakable suffering.

This is perhaps the most challenging topic that will be covered in this book. It's painful, delicate, and incredibly uncomfortable. Such conversations often make us feel judged and defensive. Our goal in bringing this topic to center stage is not to cause discomfort and certainly not to pass judgment. Rather, we aim to bring understanding and hope to the conversation by broadening our capacity for compassion in recognizing that these farm animals are sentient beings—they think, feel, and suffer. As such, they are worthy of our mercy. It is a hopeful conversation because actionable steps are within reach.

Although myriad health and environmental benefits come with a plant-based diet, one of the truly unique aspects of being vegan is the incorporation of kindness and compassion into our dietary choices. We talk about compassion in order to address one of the most fundamental "whys" when it comes to adopting a plant-based approach to feeding your family. The health and environmental advantages could alone support the recommendation to adopt a plant-based diet for all, but perhaps one of the most compelling reasons to favor plants is the call to mitigate animal suffering. While some may argue that such ethical concerns have no place in the conversation about dietary recommendations, we assert that excluding them from our view is absurdly myopic. Not taking into account the environmental impacts, misuse of resources (antibiotics and food diverted away from the hungry), and unthinkable animal suffering, is an act of willful neglect. If we concede that a variety of diets can promote health, it becomes difficult to simply ignore the horrific acts of violence bestowed upon countless innocent animals each and every day. How can that not matter?

Humans across the world enjoy a variety of diets based on cultural and geographical differences, personal beliefs, preferences, and issues of food access. No one precise way of eating guarantees a life free of disease, and in fact, people eating a variety of diets can lead full, healthy lives. If we can agree, that there exist a variety of diets that can reduce our risk of certain diseases (heart disease, diabetes, cancer, and even Alzheimer disease) and allow us to optimize our health while at the same time provide for connection and enjoyment when it comes to food, it becomes obvious why compassion counts. Given two equally convenient, appetizing, satisfying, and healthful choices, we no doubt would choose the more compassionate option.

As former meat eaters ourselves, we understand the cognitive dissonance that allows us to eat animals without consideration of their suffering. As Melanie Joy eloquently explains in her works, we are able to take cover under the umbrella of the three N's—the normal, natural, and necessary defenses of meat eating.[1] The idea that consuming meat is normal, natural, and necessary for human health binds us to the untenable tradition of eating animals.

As we have outlined in Chapter 1, countless studies reveal that the consumption of animal foods is not necessary for human health. One need only look to the Blue Zones, to discover how some of the longest-lived populations on the planet have not only survived but thrived on diets centered around plants. If consuming animal foods is not required to optimize health, then we must ask ourselves, why is it such an accepted practice?

Normal and natural are cultural constructs that society determines. For instance, as Joy points out, in some cultures eating dogs may be considered to be "normal and natural" while in others it would be considered to be sociopathic. As society evolves, the notions of normal and natural do as well. Moving away from old ideas of what normal and natural look like, however, come at a considerable cost. No meaningful shift happens without sacrifice.

Matthieu Ricard, a Buddhist monk, known as "the happiest man in the world" wrote an inspiring book, *A Plea for the Animals*, in which he argues against the practice of eating animals.[2] In it, he acknowledges that "standing up for the right thing might be painful, but that pain can, and should be, transmuted into determination and courage—the courage of compassion. As Elie Wiesel put it in his acceptance speech for the Nobel Peace Prize: 'Neutrality helps the oppressor, never the victim. Silence encourages the tormentor, never the tormented.' It's all completely up to us."[2]

Whether it means sticking out from the herd, giving up certain comforts such as a favorite holiday meal, the ease of eating out without worry, feeling like an outsider, or perhaps even being the object of disdain, being vegan is certainly not the norm in today's world. It is no small task to abandon the practice of eating animals. The willingness to contemplate animal suffering is understandably difficult. The reality is harsh and quite painful to stomach. Again, in his book *A Plea for the Animals*, Ricard shares an excerpt from a talk given by renowned anthropologist, Jane Goodall:

> *What shocks me the most is that people seem to become almost schizophrenic the moment you bring up the terrible conditions that prevail in intensive breeding operations, the cruel heaping up of sentient beings in tiny spaces—conditions so horrible that you have to constantly give them antibiotics to keep them alive, otherwise they'll just let themselves die. I often describe the nightmare of transport. If they fall during transport, they are yanked up by one leg, which breaks. And the slaughterhouses, where so many of the animals are not even rendered unconscious before being skinned alive or plunged into boiling water. It's obviously excruciatingly painful. When I start talking to people about all that they often reply: "Oh please don't talk to me about that I'm too sensitive and I adore animals." And I say to myself has this person lost it all together?*[2]

By nature, we are sympathetic, humane beings. A poll conducted by the American Society for the Prevention of Cruelty to Animals (ASPCA) found that 94 percent of Americans agreed that animals raised for food deserved to live a life free from cruelty and abuse.[3] This is incongruent with the reality that 72 billion animals worldwide are slaughtered for food each year and over 99 percent of the 10 billion farm animals raised in the U.S. for food each year are raised in concentrated animal feeding operations (CAFOs), otherwise known as factory farms. The term "factory farm" has come to represent what many of us recognize as the large animal agriculture operations that

Over 99 percent of the 10 billion farm animals raised in the U.S. for food each year are raised in concentrated animal feeding operations (CAFOs), otherwise known as factory farms.

serve to maximize output in the form of meat, dairy, and eggs, while minimizing cost inputs. This leads to overcrowding of animals, unthinkable mutilations, torturous slaughter, and the rampant use of pharmaceuticals to enhance growth and production as well as combat the numerous infections that are inevitable under such unsanitary conditions.

The meat and dairy industries are so invested in hiding the many nefarious acts that occur under factory farming that they have gone to extreme measures to lobby for legislation that would punish photographers, videographers, and animal protection agencies from documenting and disseminating factual information about the conditions and cruelties of factory farming.[4] It's quite shocking that in the United States there exists the Animal Enterprise Terrorism Act (popularly known as ag-gag laws) that serve to fight against so-called "terror" acts against factory farming industries by protecting them from individuals and organizations that work to reveal the true conditions endured by animals and employees at these facilities. Specifically, the government serves to "provide the Department of Justice the necessary authority to apprehend, prosecute, and convict individuals committing animal enterprise terror."[5] The pharmaceutical, fur, and farming industries lobbied Congress aggressively to pass such legislation. "Under its terms, anyone who damages the property or the profit line of an animal business and who uses 'interstate commerce' such as a cellphone or the internet to carry out the action can be convicted of terrorism even though no violence is involved."[6] These so-called acts of terror are in reality only measures to protect the profits of industry while failing to protect against the true terror that these animals endure.

It's unthinkable that we have prioritized potential profits over the pain, suffering, and death of billions of farm animals. They are stuffed in overcrowded cages. They are unable to roam or sit, are forced to endure prolonged and extreme confinement, are deprived of sunlight, plagued with poor air quality, and are unable to establish their natural sense of hierarchy and social order. Additionally, the animals are bred to grow unnaturally large and fast to maximize meat, egg, and milk production. Their bodies cannot support this rapid rate of growth, and the animals suffer in painful and debilitating ways. These brutal conditions contribute not only to obvious physical problems but also mental and behavioral

It's unthinkable that we have prioritized potential profits over the pain, suffering, and death of billions of farm animals.

issues such that the animals show obvious signs of stress and unusual aggression, prompting farms to mutilate (such as beak trimming and tail docking) animals without any form of anesthetic. In theory, these "procedures" are supposed to prevent the animals from pecking, scratching, and chewing one another's tails. These behaviors are, however, a reaction to the abominable conditions in which they are forced to live.

In many industrialized countries such as the United States, there seems to be quite an enormous disconnect between these torture-filled acts and what we experience as "food" on our plates. As Matthieu Ricard explains, "the various ways in which animals are mistreated still are most often ignored, tolerated, or even approved. Why are they ignored? Because the overwhelming majority of these abusive practices are inflicted on animals far from public view, in the industrial breeding facilities and in slaughterhouses. And the agro-industrial and food processing industries exercise tacit but very tight censorship, making sure that no shocking images are allowed to get beyond the walls of their torture chambers. Today in the rich countries, the animals one sees are not the animals one eats." Ricard summarizes the flaws of animal agriculture by explaining "we are responsible for an ongoing massacre of animals on a scale unequaled in the history of humankind. Every year sixty billion land animals and a thousand billion marine animals are killed for our consumption…(this is) madness on a global scale. It perpetuates hunger in the world, increases the world's ecological imbalances, and is even harmful to human health…Why do we blind ourselves, now at the beginning of the twenty-first century, to the immeasurable suffering that we inflict on animals, knowing that a great part of the pain that we cause them is neither necessary or unavoidable?"[2]

> Every year sixty billion land animals and a thousand billion marine animals are killed for our consumption…(this is) madness on a global scale. It perpetuates hunger in the world, increases the world's ecological imbalances, and is even harmful to human health…

While organic, cage-free, and grass-fed labels seem more humane by claiming to provide the animals with natural pasture to graze upon, the reality is that these labels can be misleading. A great amount of suffering may still be endured by the animals in these environments. Farm Sanctuary, a leading farm animal rescue and protection organization in the United States, outlines some of the real truths with regards to many of the labels that we see on our supermarket shelves.[7]

- Producers of cage-free eggs often purchase hens from hatcheries that routinely kill male chicks at birth because they will not produce eggs. Over 260 million baby chicks per year are killed in this way.
- The beaks of even cage-free hens are amputated without pain relief.
- Poultry animals are excluded from the federal Humane Slaughter Act. As a result, packing plants that receive cage-free laying hens are not required to render these animals unconscious prior to slaughter.
- Though "cage-free" hens are not confined to battery cages, they may still be packed by the thousands into poorly ventilated, windowless warehouses. Undercover investigations have revealed "cage-free" hens commonly living indoors, packed so tightly that they can barely move or spread their wings.
- USDA regulations do not specify the amount, duration, or quality of outdoor access provided to "free-range" animals. This means that a warehouse with thousands of "free-range" hens could have a single door leading to a small, enclosed outdoor area that hens would have to struggle to access.
- "Grass-fed" labels indicate that animals receive a majority of their nutrients from grass throughout their life, but USDA grass-fed stipulations do not limit the use of antibiotics, hormones, or pesticides, all of which are harmful to the environment and human health.
- Organic dairy may be free of antibiotics and hormones, but it is not free of cruelty. Because cows produce milk only when pregnant or nursing, all dairy farms subject their cows to a relentless cycle of impregnation and birth. Their babies are taken away immediately, so that the milk can be collected for human use. Male calves, since they are of no use to the dairy industry, are sold for beef or veal. When a cow's milk production declines at an average of less than five years, she too is slaughtered for meat (the average natural life span of cow could be as long as twenty-five years).
- Investigations have shown that some organic milk producers keep cows confined indoors much of the time. Because the requirements for the "organic" label prohibit the use of many medicines, producers frequently allow cows to languish with ailments that otherwise could easily be treated.

In his book, *Eating Animals*, Jonathan Safran Foer eloquently and succinctly maintains that "the free-range label is bullshit. It should provide no more peace of mind than 'all-natural,' 'fresh,' or 'magical.'"[8] Ultimately, no matter how humanely an animal was raised, it is eventually slaughtered for food. For most, the horrors of the slaughterhouse are so far removed from what we see at the market that it becomes quite easy to disassociate the two. "In general, we are ignorant of the abuse of living creatures that lies behind the food we eat. Our purchase is the culmination of a long process, of which all but the end product is delicately screened from our eyes,... There is no reason to associate [a neat plastic] package with a living, breathing, walking, suffering animal."[9]

Even if we could, in fact, ensure that animals were raised humanely—allowed to roam and live without suffering—the simple truth is that we do not have grasslands vast enough to raise animals in this way such that it would meet the current demand for meat.

We understand that this may be a difficult topic for many families to explore. There can be an urge to resist looking at the issue because of a fear of not being able to be "perfectly vegan enough." In his book, *How to Create a Vegan World*, Tobias Leenaert explains that "the term vegan and veganism were coined by Donald and Dorothy Watson...The Watsons defined veganism as 'a way of living which seeks to exclude, as far as possible and practical, all exploitation of animals.'"[10] This definition provides for some flexibility as each individual and family can determine what is reasonably possible and practical for them (and this may change over time). However, as Leenaert goes on to say, "many vegans expect of themselves and others complete abstention from animal products. Being vegan becomes like pregnancy: being 97 percent vegan is as impossible as being 97 percent pregnant. Under such logic, if you don't wholly avoid non-vegan foods and products, you cannot call yourself a vegan...This absolutism is unfortunate, because veganism as the total avoidance of animal products—always and everywhere—sets the bar unnecessarily high for non-vegans."[10] He argues that a stepwise approach may not only be reasonable, but in fact preferred. In truth, every small step we make, makes the next one a little easier and has the potential

to have great impact. Leenaert goes on to explain
that meat reducers (those simply cutting back on
their consumption of animal foods) are crucial to
the movement to limit animal suffering in five
key ways:

> In truth, every small step we make, makes the next one a little easier and has the potential to have great impact.

1. Together, they change the system faster than a few vegans. As a larger percentage of the population, they have a greater capacity to drive market demand and in this way are crucial for societal change (for instance, more vegan options at restaurants and grocery stores).
2. As a group they save more animals than vegetarians and vegans. In fact, "all the reducers together are responsible for avoiding more animals being killed than vegetarians and vegans combined."
3. Those people reducing their consumption of animal products are more likely to become vegetarian or vegan than regular meat eaters. "Asking people to make small steps (going a day without meat) and thus increasing the chance of an experience of success, is a crucial step for creating change."
4. Moving forward gradually leads to longer lasting change.
5. Because reducers are far more spread out in society, they have a greater capacity to influence other people and institutions.

As we stated in Chapter 1, definitions and labels should be embraced when they are useful and supportive towards your efforts. Leenaert talks about looking at veganism as more of a direction rather than a position or destination—"*vegan as a term is much more usefully and productively applied to dishes and products than people. It's easy to make a dish or product that's wholly vegan. It's much harder to be one hundred percent vegan.*"[10]

The road to compassion has many paths. The first step may simply be to allow yourself to be curious and aware. We hope that this conversation has opened the door for further consideration and dialogue for you and your family, one that is guided by compassion because, as so famously said by the Buddha himself, it goes without saying that our compassion is incomplete if we cannot extend that compassion to ourselves and those we care for.

At some level, it makes perfect sense that we turn our attention away from the daily animal atrocities that occur. To look straight ahead at them would simply break our hearts. Perhaps the best we can do, as is stated in the translator's preface to *A Plea for the Animals,* is to hope for our "compassion to be a little further awakened."

Part II

CARE

Navigating nutrition is no picnic. No matter where you turn, another study claims to set the record straight. For health pro-fessionals, it can be daunting; for the average consumer, it is often overwhelming. There are, however, a few nutrition nuggets experts agree on. First, the standard Western diet is akin to walking across Niagara Falls on a tightrope. For the vast majority of us, it is, shall we say, risky. Experts concur that most people would benefit by eating more whole plant foods, like fruits and vegetables, and fewer fast foods, sweet beverages, and other highly processed foods. Where health experts tend to diverge is on the subject of animal products. To be clear, most leading health authorities like the World Health Organization (WHO), the World Cancer Research Fund (WCRF), the Eat Lancet Commission, and the Food and Agriculture Organization (FAO) agree that diets should be largely plant-based. Even the Nutrition Guidelines for America and Canada's Food Guide lean quite clearly towards plant-based dietary patterns. However, none suggest a complete elimination of animal-based foods. Most advise the removal of processed meat, the reduction of red meat, and moderate consumption of other animal-based foods such as poultry, fish, and dairy. There is no question that human beings can survive and even thrive on a relatively wide range of diet patterns, assuming they are mostly unprocessed and reasonably rich in plant matter. So why would a family choose an entirely plant-based diet over a mostly plant-based diet? This choice is commonly driven by the ethical and environmental issues that were the subjects of Chapters 2 and 3. For the most part, the decision on how plant-based to go is a personal one. Rest assured whether you decide to be exclusively plant-based or predominantly plant-based, your family can be well nourished.

In the previous section we explored the boundless benefits of plant-based diets. In Part II: Care, we take a deeper dive into the nutrition piece and the practical aspects of feeding your family. We begin by exploring the three macronutrients—carbohydrates (plus fiber), protein, and fat, and then delve into the details of micronutrients, specifically the vitamins and minerals that may present a challenge to parents. After summarizing the key aspects of putting together a diet that is nutritionally sound and superbly protective, we follow with a walk through of the various ages and stages of growth—pregnancy, lactation, infancy, childhood, and adolescence.

Chapter 4

Managing Macronutrients and Fiber

"Good food is a right, not a privilege.
It brings children into a positive relationship with
their health, community, and environment."

—*Alice Waters*

Macronutrients are nutrients that people require in large amounts (macro = big). These nutrients are the ones that provide us with the energy (calories) we need to support growth, development, metabolism, and all other bodily functions. There are three energy-giving macronutrients—carbohydrate, protein, and fat. Fiber will also be part of our discussion, as it resides in the carbohydrate family. While, on the surface, macronutrients may seem like a rather lackluster topic, rest assured they are anything but. Macronutrients drive many of our most pressing nutrition controversies. The three biggest dietary trends of the decade—plant-based, paleo, and keto—are defined by macronutrients. Plant-based is a carbohydrate-rich protocol; paleo is protein dominant, and keto is fueled by fat. Over the decades, macronutrients have come and gone as dietary villains—fat was demonized in the eighties and nineties, and since then carbohydrates have taken a hit. Although protein has traditionally worn a health halo, specific protein sources are now falling from grace as links to chronic disease emerge.

Scientists have spent decades in discussions about the optimal quantity of macronutrients and the relative percentages of each nutrient that best support human health. The World Health Organization suggests 55 to 75 percent of calories come from carbohydrate, 10 to 15 percent from protein and 15 to 30 percent from fat.[1] The Institute of Medicine suggests 45 to 65 percent of calories from carbohydrate, 10 to 35 percent protein, and 20 to 35 percent fat.[2] It is very telling to look at macronutrient intake ranges in healthy populations such as those of the Blue Zones. They are inconsistent, especially where carbohydrate and fat are concerned. In Okinawa, macronutrient distribution is about 85 percent carbohydrate, 9 percent protein, and 6 percent fat, while in Ikaria, Greece, it is about 37 percent carbohydrate, 50 percent fat, and 13 percent protein. On average, Blue Zone populations get about 65 percent of their calories from carbohydrates, 20 percent from fats, and 15 percent from protein.[3] While macronutrient ranges matter, they may matter less than what we are led to believe. What matters most is the sources of those macronutrients and their quality. When macronutrients come from foods that are unprocessed or minimally processed and are rich in food components known to be protective to health—like fiber, antioxidants, phytochemicals, and micronutrients—they consistently support health. When macronutrients come from highly processed foods that have been stripped of these valuable dietary components and infused with fat, sugar, salt, additives, and preservatives, they consistently undermine health. If this seems somewhat simplistic, it is.

This chapter summarizes the science and provides practical guidelines to help you navigate the world of macronutrients with ease. Let's start with the macronutrient that predominates in plants—carbohydrate.

CARBOHYDRATES

Four-year-old Samantha's favorite foods were pasta, pizza, French fries, and toast. You could say they were her dietary staples. She might have opted for cake, cookies, and cinnamon buns, but alas, these are at her disposal less often then she relished. Samantha's parents, Charlotte and Michael, didn't worry too much about Samantha's starch-heavy diet—that is until they learned that refined carbohydrates provide no health advantage over the meat they were gradually replacing in their family's diet. Could it be that despite their best intentions, Charlotte and Michael were setting Samantha up for health challenges down the road?

What Are Carbohydrates and Why Are They Important?

Carbohydrates are vital packages of energy manufactured by plants, with the help of energy from the sun, water from rain, and carbon dioxide from air. They are generated through a beautiful miracle of nature called photosynthesis, which supports all life on Earth. Carbohydrates can be single sugars or monosaccharides (mono = one) or a series of sugars bound together. Disaccharides (di = two) are two units of sugar; oligosaccharides (oligo = few) are three to nine units of sugar, and polysaccharides (poly = many) are ten or more units of sugar. Polysaccharides include starches (the stored form of energy in plants) and fiber (the material that gives plants their structure). The final members of the carbohydrate family are polyols or sugar alcohols. Plants such as fruits and vegetables naturally contain small amounts of sugar alcohols, but most of the polyols in the food supply are produced from sugars and starches for use as low-calorie sweeteners and in "sugar-free" foods.

Carbohydrates are important for our health because they serve as the main source of energy (calories) for the body, and are the preferred fuel for the brain, red blood cells, and nervous system.[2] The only other sources of energy are protein, fat, and alcohol. Protein can be used for energy, but it is more of a back-up fuel. When we have sufficient carbohydrate, we spare protein, so it is available for critical roles like building and repairing tissues and making hormones, enzymes, and other body chemicals. Fat is used as a fuel, but it is not ideal either as some tissue such as liver cells and red blood cells can only use carbohydrates for energy. Alcohol is highly toxic to the body, especially the brain, liver, and pancreas, so is a very poor choice for our energy supply.

Carbohydrates and protein each supply approximately four calories per gram, while fat provides about nine calories per gram. In addition to serving as our major source of calories, carbohydrate-rich whole foods can help to reduce hunger, control blood glucose and insulin metabolism, and keep cholesterol and triglyceride levels in check. These foods also help us maintain a healthy gastrointestinal tract, protecting against constipation, and intestinal diseases and disorders.

Carbohydrate Conundrums

Carbohydrates have received a bad rap for good reason. While most carbohydrates are derived from whole plant foods, few are eaten as whole plant foods. The vast majority of carbohydrates consumed are refined. Refined carbohydrates are carbohydrate-rich foods that have been stripped of most of their beneficial components by food processing techniques before we eat them. There are two main categories of refined carbohydrates—sugars and starches. When we extract the sugars and starches from plants, we leave behind much of what is of value to human health. The most highly processed or ultra-processed refined carbohydrate foods are designed to be hyperpalatable. They are infused with just the right amount of sugar, fat, and salt to achieve a bliss point that keeps consumers coming back for more.

There is overwhelming evidence that excessive intakes of refined carbohydrates are linked to a laundry list of adverse health outcomes. These foods promote overeating and obesity,[4,5] elevate triglycerides,[6,7] increase blood pressure,[8,9] impair blood glucose control and insulin sensitivity,[10,11] increase risk of certain cancers,[12,13] contribute to gastrointestinal disturbances,[14,15] fuel inflammation and oxidative stress,[16,17] drive nonalcoholic fatty liver disease,[18] and promote poor dental health.[2] To be clear, carbohydrates, per say, are *not* the problem. In fact, throughout the world, people who eat unprocessed or minimally processed diets that are rich in whole food carbohydrates enjoy remarkably good health. Two cases in point are the Blue Zones where calories from carbohydrates average 65 percent, and the Tsimane of Bolivia where calories from carbohydrates average 72 percent. The Tsimane have the lowest reported rates of heart disease in the world.[19] Among the Tsimane, the principle sources of carbohydrates are plantains, rice, cassava, and corn. In Okinawa, one of the most famous Blue Zones, 67 percent of the calories in the traditional diet come from purple sweet potatoes and

15 percent come from grains. These two poignant examples are proof positive that high carbohydrate diets are consistent with health and longevity, when the carbohydrates are largely unprocessed. This evidence is further strengthened by a large 2018 meta-analysis that examined the link between carbohydrate intake and mortality; those eating the fewest carbohydrates experienced a 32 percent increase in mortality.[20]

Another argument in favor of carbohydrates is that they are the primary macronutrient in many of our most protective foods: vegetables, fruits, legumes, and whole grains[1, 21, 22, 23] Fruits average about 92 percent carbohydrate, starchy vegetables about 90 percent, grains and legumes about 70 to 75 percent, and non-starchy vegetables about 60 percent.[24] The bottom line is that carbohydrates only appear to be problematic when they are stripped of their protective components such as fiber, vitamins, minerals, antioxidants, and phytochemicals before we eat them.

You may be thinking, okay, I get it. Carbohydrates are best coming from whole plant foods rather than highly processed foods. But children are constantly bombarded with food products designed to appeal to them—like presweetened cereals, cookies, fish-shaped crackers, candies, cake, ice cream, and soda. The list is endless. How does a parent get a child to love carbohydrates that will love them back? Is it okay for children to have some refined carbohydrates? Let's explore the practical side of the carbohydrate story.

Correcting Carbohydrates

When it comes to carbohydrates, our goal is to gradually shift away from choices that are heavily processed and towards choices that feature carbohydrates as nature intended—packaged with protective components. This means relying more on vegetables, fruits, legumes, and whole grains for carbohydrates, and relying less on foods that are made from refined flours and sugars. For children, the early introduction to whole food carbohydrates makes it easier to ensure healthful carbohydrate choices for life. Chapter 6 provides tips and guidelines for instilling excellent eating habits in children of all ages.

Let's take a deeper dive into how we can incorporate more whole, plant sources of carbohydrates in place of the highly processed alternatives.

Added Sugars: Not so Sweet After All!

The US Dietary Guidelines Advisory Committee recommends that added sugar be limited to not more than 10 percent of total calories.[25] While the World Health Organization also recommends less than 10 percent of total calories from added sugars (12 teaspoons in a 2,000 calorie diet), they include a conditional recommendation to lower added sugars to not more than 5 percent of total calories (6 teaspoons in a 2,000 calorie diet) for greater health benefits. The American Heart Association suggests that adults limit sugar to no more than nine teaspoons per day for men and six teaspoons a day for women.[26] They recommend no added sugar for toddlers younger than two years of age, and a limit of six teaspoons a day for children over two years old.[27] Note that on a food label 4 grams of sugar equals approximately one teaspoon. Americans average about 14 percent of total calories[28] from added sugars or seventeen teaspoons in a 2,000 calorie diet, well above current recommended upper limits.

Sugar itself is not inherently harmful. Glucose is the preferred fuel for the human body, and we are well equipped to handle it when it is naturally present in the matrix of a whole food. It is excess sugar that is the issue, particularly when it comes from added sweeteners. Nearly half of the sugar in American diets comes from sweet beverages such as soda, energy drinks, sports beverages, sweetened coffee or tea beverages, fruit drinks, and sweet alcoholic beverages.[29] Intake of sugar-sweetened beverages is linked to mortality, weight gain, type 2 diabetes, coronary heart disease, hypertension, and non-alcoholic fatty liver disease.[30,31,32,33,34] In children, sugar consumption, especially from sugar-sweetened beverages, has been reported to adversely impact cognition, while fruit intake favorably affects cognition.[35]

Putting a Lid on Sugar: Practical Pointers

1. **Rewire your taste buds.** Train your taste buds to appreciate less intense sweetness by gradually reducing the sweeteners used in foods and beverages.

2. **Minimize beverages with added sugars.** Instead of soda and other sweet beverages, stick with water. For a fizzy drink, try soda water with lemon, lime, fruit, or a splash of antioxidant-rich juice such as blueberry or pomegranate.

3. **Think outside the box.** Sugar is a major component of many processed foods (in addition to all the familiar terms for sugar, words ending in "ose" are also added sugars). Reducing these foods will naturally reduce intake of added sugars. When you purchase prepared foods, select unsweetened or "no added sugar" products, such as nondairy milks, applesauce, nut butters, oatmeal, and canned fruit.

4. **Get cooking at home.** When you are cooking at home, you are in control of the amount and types of sugars added. In baking, cut sugar in half, select less refined sugars and, when possible, use fresh or dried fruits in place of sugar. Use vanilla bean or vanilla extract, citrus zest, or spices like allspice, cardamom, cinnamon, ginger, nutmeg, and star anise to bring out the natural sweetness in foods. Making foods from scratch provides a wonderful opportunity to create marvelous memories with kids in the kitchen.

5. **Make fruit your go-to sweet treat.** Fruit makes a nutritious, convenient sweet treat. To increase intake among children, teens, and adults alike, slice fruit on a plate and dish it up as a snack or dessert.

Refined Starches: The Great Grain Robbery

Refined starches are widely embraced comfort foods. Think macaroni and cheese, cinnamon buns, shortbread cookies, bagels and cream cheese, and potato chips. When these foods are mainstays, the quality of the diet can be diminished.

Processing wheat kernels into white flour, removes two of the three parts of the wheat kernels: the germ and the bran. The germ is the storehouse of nutrients for the kernel of wheat; it is where essential fatty acids, vitamins, minerals, and phytochemicals are concentrated. The bran is the outer husk, which protects the contents of the grain. While the bran provides nutrients and phytochemicals, its main claim to fame is fiber. The part of the grain that remains is called endosperm, which is mainly starch, some protein, and miniscule amounts of vitamins and minerals. In the process of refining wheat to make white flour, we lose approximately 70 to 90 percent of the vitamins, minerals, and fiber. To add insult to injury, a 200- to 300-fold loss in phytochemicals occurs.[36] Granted, some of the lost nutrients are added back. For example, when wheat or rice are refined, they are commonly enriched with four B vitamins—thiamin, riboflavin, niacin, and folic acid—and the mineral iron. However, other vitamins and minerals, including pantothenic acid, vitamin B6, vitamin E, boron, calcium, magnesium, manganese, potassium, selenium, and zinc are not added back. Nor are any of the phytochemicals, plant sterols, essential fatty·acids, or fiber. And, of course, no one eats a bowl of white flour. Before it is consumed, it is anointed with various combinations of salt, fat, sugar, artificial and natural flavors, colors, and preservatives. Then we eat the white flour in the form of bread, crackers, cookies, cakes, pies, and other processed foods. So, not only have we extracted most of the components that protect health, we have added a variety of components that may harm health.

To be fair, including small amounts of refined grains, especially those that are minimally processed, on occasion and in moderation is perfectly acceptable for healthy individuals. While we want most of our grains to be whole grains, going out for an Italian pasta dinner or an Asian meal with white rice is not a nutrition faux pas. Indeed, being somewhat flexible on a plant-based diet makes the experience more interesting, enjoyable, and inviting. Aim to use whole grains over refined grains for your daily fare, and don't stress too much about the rest.

Pushing Back Refined Starches

1. **Learn to read labels.** If a product contains "whole wheat four," the entire phrase will be spelled out in the ingredient list. Products that say "contains whole grains" or "made with whole grains" are typically mostly refined grains.

2. **Replace refined grains with whole grains.** For example, use brown rice instead of white rice or whole grain bread instead of white bread. The Dietary Guidelines for Americans suggests no more than half of your grain intake be refined. If your family isn't used to whole grains, consider adding fiber-rich ingredients (vegetables, beans, lentils) to your regular white rice or pasta dishes and gradually shift to the whole grain counterpart. When using processed grains, select those with the fewest ingredients.

3. **Minimize deep-fried salty snack foods.** Most of the deep-fried, salty starch-based snack foods are prepared with refined starches.

FIBER

It is universally accepted that fiber is good for you. Some people refer to it as "nature's broom" because it keeps things moving smoothly and efficiently through our intestinal tracts. It was not until the 1970s when Dr. Denis Burkitt discovered that people in rural Africa were free of Western diseases such as heart disease, diabetes, and obesity as well as intestinal disorders such as colon cancer and constipation that people began to realize that fiber is not just passing through, but performing some impressive feats along the way. More recently, it has been recognized that many of fiber's benefits are mediated by our gut microbiota.

Fiber is a type of carbohydrate that cannot be broken down by digestive enzymes in the small intestine of humans. However, certain types of fiber can be broken down by the microorganisms living in our intestinal tract, and, for them, it is premium fuel. There are many different types of fiber, each providing unique benefits. Fiber can be soluble or insoluble, depending on whether or not it dissolves in water; it can be viscous or non-viscous, depending on whether or not it becomes gel-like and gummy when mixed with water; it can be fermentable or nonfermentable, depending on whether or not bacteria can ferment it to extract energy. Fiber-rich, whole plant foods generally contain all of these fiber types, in varying amounts.

You may have heard of the term "resistant starch." This is a type of starch that acts like fiber because it is not digested, but rather arrives in the large intestine and is fermented by gut bacteria. Because it acts like fiber, it is often classified as part of total dietary fiber. The fermentation of resistant starch produces short-chain fatty acids which are protective to human health.[37] The production of one particularly beneficial short-chain fatty acid called butyrate is greater with resistant starches than with dietary fiber.[38] Examples of foods rich in resistant starch are underripe bananas, whole grains such as oats and barley, and legumes. It is also present in starchy foods such as potatoes or rice that have been cooked and cooled.

The Institute of Medicine recommends 14 grams of fiber per 1,000 calories for everyone over one year of age.[39] While Recommended Dietary Allowances have not been set for fiber, Adequate Intakes (AIs) were established in accordance with this fourteen-gram figure. The AIs, based on average energy intakes for various ages and genders, are provided in Table 4.1. Less than 5 percent of the population meets the recommended intakes for fiber,[40] and the percentage drops in children, with fewer than 1 percent of toddlers meeting the target.[41] In other words, only one in twenty people meet recommended intakes, and that drops to less than one in one hundred for young children.

Table 4.1: Dietary Reference Intakes (DRI) for Fiber

	AGE (years)	DIETARY FIBER DRI (g/day)
Children	1–3	19
	4–8	25
Females	9–13	26
	14–18	26
	19–50	25
	50+	21

Males	9–13	31
	14–18	38
	19–50	38
	50+	30

Source: [2]

So why all the hoopla about fiber? The evidence that fiber promotes health and prevents disease is impressive. Fiber reduces risk of heart disease, stroke, hypertension, gastrointestinal disorders, obesity, type 2 diabetes, and several cancers. When we eat a high fiber meal, we feel fuller, and stay satiated for longer periods of time. Fiber is critical to regular, healthy bowel movements, and that is important at every stage of life. Constipation is not much fun whether you are a toddler or a senior.

How do we ensure children meet their needs for fiber? It's uncomplicated—feed them plenty of plants. Here are some specific tips for boosting fiber intake for children—the tips work for adults too!

1. **Include fiber-rich foods at meal and snack times.** The most nutritious fiber-rich foods are whole plant foods. Table 4.2 provides the fiber content in a variety of common foods. If serving refined packaged foods, pair them with fiber-rich whole foods. For example, top ready-to-eat cereals with fresh fruit, berries, nuts, or seeds; add peas and broccoli to macaroni.

2. **Choose whole grains over their refined counterparts.** Pick whole grain breads, pasta, crackers, and pizza crust. Select brown, red, or black rather than white rice. Use whole grain flours instead of refined flours when baking muffins, cookies, or other treats.

3. **Add grains and legumes where possible.** Throw beans or lentils and whole grains (barley, quinoa) into soups, salads, stews, stir-fries, and burritos. Choose legume-based pastas.

4. **Load up on a wide variety of vegetables and fruits.** Include a variety of vegetables and/or fruits with meals and snacks. If hunger strikes before dinner, serve up a plate of veggies and dip.

5. **Pick fiber-rich treats.** Serve popcorn or kale chips instead of potato chips, frozen banana pops instead of ice cream bars, homemade granola bars using oats, dried fruits, nuts, and seeds instead of the sugary commercial bars.

Table 4.2: Fiber Content of Common Foods

AMOUNT OF FIBER PER SERVING	FOOD AND SERVING SIZE
Very high-fiber foods **10 or more grams**	Legumes (beans, lentils, and split peas), cooked, 1 cup Split peas, cooked, 1 cup Avocado (1 medium), 6.7 ounces High fiber bran cereals, ½ cup
High-fiber foods **5 to 9.9 grams**	Berries (raspberries, blackberries), fresh, 1 cup Fruit (pears, papayas), 1 medium Dried fruit (apricots, figs, pears, prunes, raisins, etc.) ½ cup Coconut, fresh, shredded, ½ cup Flaxseeds, 2 tablespoons Grains (most whole grains), cooked, 1 cup Potatoes, regular or sweet, baked, 1 medium Pasta, whole wheat, 1 cup Artichoke, 1 medium
Moderate-fiber foods **2 to 4.9 grams**	Berries (blueberries, strawberries), fresh, 1 cup Fruit (most varieties), 1 medium/2 small, or 1 cup Vegetables (most), raw, 2 cups; cooked 1 cup Nuts and seeds (most varieties), ¼ cup Grains (brown rice, millet, oats), cooked, 1 cup Whole grain breads, read label, 2 slices Pasta, white, 1 cup Popcorn, 3 cups
Lower-fiber foods **1.9 grams or less**	Melon, 1 cup Fruit *or* vegetable juice (all varieties), 1 cup Sprouts (grain, legume, or vegetable), 1 cup Lettuce, all types, 2 cups Cucumber, 1 medium (8-inch) Refined grains, most (white rice, cream of wheat) Refined cold cereals, 1 ounce

Source: [42]

Cautionary Notes

While it is unlikely that a person would get too much fiber from whole plant foods, it is possible. For small children, very high fiber intakes can make the diet too bulky, jeopardizing energy intakes and potentially leading to failure to thrive. If a child is underweight or not growing appropriately, add more calorie dense, lower fiber foods such as tofu, nut and seed butters, and some refined grains like pasta. Excessive fiber can be a problem if concentrated fiber sources such as wheat bran are used regularly. Wheat bran is very high in phytates and can inhibit the absorption of minerals, so it is best not used as a regular feature in the diet.

A Final Word on Carbohydrates

The highest quality carbohydrates come from whole plant foods—whole grains, legumes, vegetables, and fruits. Make these foods your dietary staples. If refined sugars and starches predominate in your diet or the diets of your loved ones, shift toward a more whole foods diet one meal and snack at a time. Make changes gradually. Celebrate every step along the way—even the baby steps.

FAT

Amelia was seven years old when the doctor told her parents that she had drifted into the fifteenth percentile for height and the fifth percentile for weight. Her parents hadn't worried about her small stature because she was happy, active, and did well in school. Still, with average sized parents, Dr. Jeng thought further assessment was warranted. When she asked about their diet, Dr. Jeng discovered that the whole family was following a low-fat plant-predominant diet. Their staples were whole grains, vegetables, fruits, and beans. Although they did include dairy products in the mix, they selected only fat-free options such as skim milk and non-fat yogurt. They also included enough flax and chia seeds to provide omega-3 fatty acids, but otherwise avoided oils, nuts, seeds, coconut, avocado, and other high fat plant foods. Dr. Jeng suggested some changes to Amelia's diet, specifically adding high fat foods, and small amounts of oil. They were stunned. Was the diet they were providing their daughter really too low in fat?

What Are Fats and Why Are They Important?

Fats are part of the lipid family, a group of organic compounds that do not generally dissolve in water. In addition to fatty acids from fats and oils, the family includes sterols (such as cholesterol and plant sterols), phospholipids (such as lecithin), and waxes. Fats supply essential fatty acids that the body cannot make on its own and must obtain from dietary sources. They are an essential part of cell membranes, are used to make hormones and hormone-like substances, and play critical roles in growth, immune function, nervous system development and maintenance, reproduction, and metabolism. Fats are needed for the absorption of fat-soluble vitamins such as vitamins A, D, E, and K, and phytochemicals. They provide insulation and physical padding, protecting our vital organs and increasing tolerance for temperature variations. The most common type of fat in food comes in the form of triglycerides—a glycerol backbone with three fatty acid tails attached. Fatty acids vary in size and structure, and those differences are associated with health outcomes. They are categorized according to the number of carbons in the molecule and the degree to which they are saturated with hydrogen. The three main types of fatty acids include saturated, monounsaturated, and polyunsaturated. Trans fatty acids represent a sub-category of unsaturated fats. In addition, cholesterol and plant sterols are present in whole foods in varying amounts—cholesterol in animal products and plant sterols in plant foods.

All whole foods contain a mix of fatty acids with variable amounts of each. There are three specific considerations when designing a diet that supports growth and development in children and the preservation of health throughout the life cycle:

1. What are the most healthful sources of fat?
2. How much fat should we eat?
3. How do we ensure sufficient omega-3 fatty acids?

For parents, the maze of opinions surrounding fat can be challenging to navigate. The pages that follow will help you through this quagmire, to a place of solid ground.

What Are the Most Healthful Sources of Fat?

Not all fat is bad. Indeed, fat is critical to the structure and function of the human body, and it helps to promote optimal lifelong health. However, some fats, especially when consumed in excess, can have significant deleterious effects. Dietary fats that are most strongly linked to adverse health consequences are trans fatty acids from processed foods, saturated fats from animal products and tropical oils, and damaged fats from fried foods. Fats that tend to be neutral or beneficial to health are monounsaturated fats and polyunsaturated fats, both of which are concentrated in plants. Let's briefly review the impact of various fatty acids on health, and the sources for each. Figure 4.1 provides a handy visual for quick reference.

Figure 4.1: Types of Fats and Fatty Acids

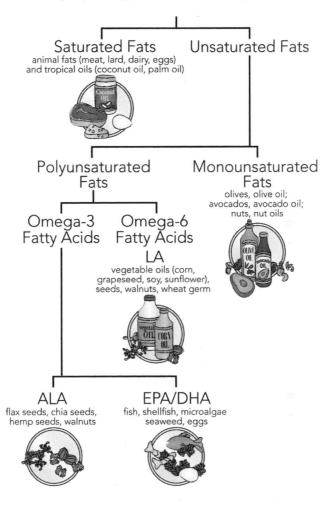

Saturated Fat

Saturated fatty acids are completely *saturated* with hydrogen and have no double bonds. Generally, the more solid a fat is at room temperature, the more saturated fat it contains. Saturated fat is found in all foods that contain fat, but it is most concentrated in animal products and tropical oils. About 11 to 12 percent of calories in Western diets, and at least 20 percent of calories in low carbohydrate diets are derived from saturated fat. The U.S. Dietary Guidelines recommends that saturated fat account for less than 10 percent of total calories for all individuals two years of age and older. The American College of Cardiology and the American Heart Association advise that people who are at risk for heart disease limit saturated fat to no more than 5 to 6 percent of total calories.[43] The evidence linking saturated fat to higher cholesterol and atherosclerosis is strong and consistent. Saturated fat is also associated with inflammation, insulin resistance, fatty liver, and several cancers.[44, 45, 46, 47, 48, 49, 50, 51] Many health advocates claim that children require high intakes of saturated fat for optimal growth and development, especially for their brains. However, a recent review and meta-analysis reported that in children and adolescents ages two to nineteen years of age, reducing saturated fat results in a significant reduction in LDL-cholesterol and blood pressure, without adverse effects on growth and development.[52] The authors advised that dietary guidelines for children and adolescents should continue to recommend diets low in saturated fat. To keep saturated fat under 10 percent of calories in a child's diet means an upper intake of 11 grams of saturated fat per 1,000 calories. So, for an average six-year-old eating 1,400 calories, the upper limit would be 15 grams. The numbers add up quickly—a cup of whole milk or an ounce of cheddar cheese delivers about 5 grams, while two slices of pepperoni pizza or a quarter pound cheeseburger weigh in at about 12 grams.

The richest dietary sources of saturated fats are full-fat dairy products such as butter, cheese, creams, full-fat milk, full-fat yogurt, ice cream, and prepared foods such as pizza, macaroni and cheese, and dairy desserts. Although tropical oils contain a higher percentage of calories from saturated fat than animal products, total intake from these oils has traditionally been much smaller than from animal products. This is changing with the rise in coconut products and tropical oils used in place of partially hydrogenated fats in processed foods. About 50 to 87 percent of the fat in tropical oils is saturated. This compares to over 60 percent in dairy, about 40 percent in red meat, 30 percent in chicken, and 20 to 30 percent in fish. The fat in most other plant foods (apart from tropical oils) ranges from about 10 to 20 percent saturated.

Monounsaturated Fat

Monounsaturated fatty acids have one spot in the carbon chain where hydrogen is missing (one point of unsaturation). Monounsaturated fats have been shown to have neutral or slightly beneficial effects on health, with modest favorable effects on blood cholesterol levels.[53] These fats are generally liquid at room temperature, but become cloudy and thick when refrigerated, as with olive oil. The

richest dietary sources of monounsaturated fat are olives, olive oil, canola oil, avocados, avocado oil, nuts (except for walnuts, butternuts, and pine nuts) and their
oils. Generally, about half of our dietary fat should be monounsaturated, unless
the diet is very low in fat, in which case polyunsaturated fat should predominate.

Polyunsaturated Fat

Polyunsaturated fatty acids have two or more spots in the carbon chain where
hydrogen is missing (two or more points of unsaturation). These fats are usually
liquid at room temperature and when refrigerated.

There are two distinct families of polyunsaturated fats—the omega-6 and
omega-3 families. It is within these families that our two essential fatty acids
reside. These are fatty acids that we need for survival but cannot make in the body
so must get from food. One is the omega-6 fatty acid, linoleic acid (LA), and the
other is the omega-3 fatty acid, alpha-linolenic acid (ALA). While we need both
LA and ALA, consumers typically get more than enough LA but fall short on ALA.
LA and ALA are called "parent" fatty acids because our body has the capacity to
convert them into bigger, more biologically active, long-chain polyunsaturated
fatty acids (LCPUFA). The LCPUFA are metabolized to hormone-like compounds
that have a significant impact on a variety of body functions, including blood
clotting, blood pressure, immune response, cell division, pain, and inflammation. Omega-3 LCPUFA favorably affect the composition and functioning of cell
membranes, enhancing intracellular signaling processes and gene expression.
They are used as raw materials for building the brain, nervous system, and cell
membranes; with DHA being especially abundant in the retina, brain, and semen.
There is evidence that LCPUFA play key roles in prevention and modulation of
specific disease processes, including cardiovascular disease, autoimmune diseases,
hypertension, rheumatoid arthritis, several cancers, and, although the evidence
is weaker, they may also protect against dementia, diabetes, and asthma.[54, 55, 56, 57,
58, 59, 60] While these LCPUFA are critical to health, they are considered either non-
essential because they can be produced by the body, or conditionally essential, in
cases where conversion is lacking or compromised.

The primary sources of the two essential fatty acids, linoleic acid (LA) and
alpha-linolenic acid (ALA) are plants from the land and in the sea. The most concentrated sources are seeds and walnuts. Other plant foods provide a mix of these
two polyunsaturated fats, with grains being higher in omega-6 fatty acids and

greens being higher in omega-3 fatty acids. LCPUFA are found mainly in animal foods, with long-chain omega-6 fatty acids predominating in meat, poultry, dairy, and eggs, and the long-chain omega-3 fatty acids predominating in fish, eggs, and plants from the sea.

Trans Fatty Acids

Trans fatty acids can be either mono- or polyunsaturated. These are fatty acids in which the position of one of the hydrogen atoms has been flipped, so the normally curved, flexible molecule becomes straight and rigid. Trans fatty acids are formed either through an industrial process called partial hydrogenation or via bio-hydrogenation in the guts of ruminant animals.

Industrially produced trans fatty acids were developed as a replacement for animal fats such as butter and lard. It was believed that because they are technically "unsaturated" they would be healthier choices. We now know that industrial trans-fatty acids (generally listed as partially hydrogenated oils) are more damaging to health than any other fats. As a result, they have been banned in several countries, including the United States and Canada, and there are international initiatives to reduce their presence in the global food supply.[61, 62, 63] While the jury is still out on trans fatty acids from ruminant animals, studies have reported adverse effects.[64, 65]

Sterols

Sterols occur naturally in plants, animals, and fungi. The most well recognized sterol is cholesterol. As an essential part of cell membranes, cholesterol is a precursor to vitamin D, bile acids, and steroid hormones. The primary food sources of cholesterol are eggs, shellfish, meat, poultry, fish, and dairy products. However, humans have no requirement for dietary cholesterol at any age because we are cholesterol-making machines—every tissue in the body is capable of making cholesterol. In fact, the Institute of Medicine (IOM) has set no Estimated Average Requirement (EAR) for cholesterol, no Adequate Intake (AI) and no Recommended Dietary Allowance (RDA) for this very reason.[2] The IOM recommends that people maintain their dietary cholesterol as low as possible, while consuming a diet that is nutritionally adequate in all required nutrients. Although dietary cholesterol does not raise blood cholesterol levels as strongly as saturated fat, it still raises blood cholesterol levels. The risk associated with dietary cholesterol appears greater for those with diabetes or at risk of heart failure. Of course, most cholesterol-rich foods come packaged with plenty of cholesterol so it is hard to ingest one without the other. While there are cholesterol proponents suggesting it provides health benefits, especially for children, the evidence does not support their contention. In the 2020 American Heart Association scientific advisory on dietary cholesterol (a very mainstream health organization) came out with guidelines recommending that consumers focus on overall dietary patterns that minimize intake of major sources of saturated fat (animal fats) and include liquid non-tropical oils. They advised individuals to choose plant-based protein sources to limit cholesterol intake and added that patients with elevated cholesterol should be cautious about consuming foods rich in cholesterol.[66]

Plant sterols are structurally similar to cholesterol, but unlike cholesterol, they support favorable health outcomes, lowering blood cholesterol levels by competing against cholesterol and blocking its absorption.[67] Sources of plant sterols are legumes (especially soybeans), seeds, nuts, and vegetable oils.

Highest Quality Fat

The highest quality fat is naturally present in nuts, seeds, avocados, olives, and other whole plant foods. If oils are extracted from these foods, protein, unrefined carbohydrates, fiber, vitamins, minerals, antioxidants, plant sterols, and a host of protective phytochemicals are left behind. Even unrefined, organic vegetable oils pale in comparison to the whole foods from which they were extracted. On the other hand, high quality oils can have a place in the diet. They can help to boost calories (when necessary) without increasing food volume. Fats and oils increase absorption of fat-soluble nutrients, provide vitamins E and K, contribute protective phytochemicals, and can enhance flavor.

Fats can become oxidized or otherwise damaged by heat, light, and oxygen. When fats are heated, especially above their smoke point, products of oxidation form that are associated with adverse health outcomes.[68, 69, 68, 70, 71] Whole foods come naturally packaged in hard shells to protect them from damaging light, heat, and oxygen, so they're less prone to the ravages of free radicals than oils. To preserve the quality of fats in foods, it's important to store them properly. Nuts and seeds will keep in their shells for up to a year or more if stored in the refrigerator (32–45 degrees F/0–7.2 degrees C). Most nuts will keep for up to four to six months in their shells at room temperature (although cooler temperatures will extend storage time). However, once their shells have been removed, nuts and seeds are best refrigerated or frozen.

The evidence supporting the health benefits of higher fat, whole plant foods is overwhelming. In fact, if you try to find data suggesting adverse effects of these foods, chances are you will come up empty-handed. Here's a quick run-down on how to ensure a good supply of healthy fats for kids.

Top 3 Tips: Adequate Healthy Fats for Kids

1. **Carefully select milks for infants and children.** Continue breastfeeding for at least twelve months, and preferably two years and beyond. If you are not breastfeeding, use a commercial infant formula for at least twelve months. After this time, infants can be introduced to full-fat fortified soy or pea milk or full-fat cow's milk (for those who include dairy products). For dairy consumers, health authorities suggest whole cow's milk from twelve to twenty-four months, after which time a gradual switch to lower fat options is advised. Note that full-fat soy or pea milk are lower in fat than whole or 2 percent cow's milk, so additional fat from nut and seed butters and creams, and avocado is recommended.

2. **Include a variety of high fat whole plant foods in the daily diet.** High fat whole plant foods are loaded with fiber, micronutrients, and plant sterols. To ensure adequate intakes:

   - Use nuts, seeds, their butters, creams, cheeses, and yogurts. Sprinkle nuts and/or seeds on cereal, salads, main dishes, and desserts; add to loaves, patties, smoothies, and baked goods. Spread nuts or seed butters on crackers, bread, muffins; use to stuff celery; blend into sauces, dressings, puddings, and smoothies.
   - Serve tofu, tempeh, edamame, and other soy products as regular features of the diet. Try tofu scramble for breakfast; add soft tofu to puddings and smoothies; add tofu or tempeh to stir-fries; serve boiled or steamed edamame as a snack (kids love to pop the beans out of the shells).
   - Spread avocado on toast or crackers; use in dipping sauces such as guacamole; blend into smoothies, add to salads, bowls, and sandwiches.

- Dish up fresh coconut; grate coconut into puddings, overnight oats and other cereals; use as a topping on main dishes and desserts; add coconut to trail mix, power balls or baked goods.

3. **Carefully select concentrated fats and oils.** Oils have about 120 calories per tablespoon, so they can add considerable calories to a dish without increasing food volume. While most of a child's fat should come from whole plant foods, including concentrated fats and oils can serve as a practical way to enhance flavor and boost calories, especially for slow growing children. Add high quality oils to salad dressings, vegetables, pasta, grains, or other dishes. Select less refined oils such as extra-virgin olive oil rather than solids fats such as coconut oil. Instead of a hard spread such as butter or margarine, spray olive, avocado, flax, or hempseed oil on popcorn; use with balsamic vinegar as a dip for bread. If using oil for cooking (such as with a stir-fry) select an oil with a high smoke point (e.g., avocado oil).

How Much Fat Should We Eat?

Percent of calories from fat varies wildly among even the healthiest populations around the world. Traditional diets of rural Asians commonly provide about 10 to 15 percent of calories from fat, while those of Mediterranean populations frequently exceed 35 percent of calories from fat.[72] While there is no question that fat matters, the percent of total calories from fat is not as critical for health and longevity as many believe.[73, 2]

This large variation in percent of calories from fat consumed by healthy populations, is mirrored within plant-based populations. Some come in under 10 percent of calories from fat, while others exceed 40 percent or more of calories from fat, with heavy use of coconut, avocado, nuts, and seeds. So, what makes sense for your garden-variety plant-based family? The answer is not one size fits all. What is best for a baby is not what is best for a senior who has diabetes or heart disease. Requirements vary with age, state of health, physical activity, metabolism, and genetics. In general terms, a relatively broad range of fat intake can be conducive to good health. There are two important caveats. First, we must not be overconsuming calories, and second, healthful sources of fat must be selected.

In North America, the Dietary Reference Intakes (DRIs) do not include a Recommended Dietary Allowance (RDA), Acceptable Intake (AI), or Upper Limit (UL) for total fat except during the first year of life. Instead, a criterion known as the Acceptable Macronutrient Distribution Range (AMDR) is applied.[2] For children, the AMDRs are based on a gradual transition from the high-fat diet of infancy (55 percent of calories during the first six months of life and 40 percent of calories from six to twelve months) to a more moderate fat diet in adulthood. The recommendations are provided in Table 4.3.

Table 4.3: AMDR for Fat at Various Ages

AGE GROUP	AMDR
Ages 1–3	30–40%
Ages 4–18	25–35%
Adults	20–35%

Individuals who are very physically active or require a lot of calories to maintain body weight may find it advantageous to aim towards the higher end of the range (25 to 35 percent of calories from fat). Those who are overweight, require few calories, or have a chronic disease such as heart disease, may prefer to aim towards the lower end of the range (20 percent of calories from fat or less). Fat intakes below 20 percent of total calories, while effective in the treatment and reversal of chronic disease, are not generally considered suitable for children or adolescents.

The evidence supporting the use of very low-fat plant-based diets (10 percent of calories or lower) as therapeutic treatment for chronic disease, particularly cardiovascular disease, is growing.[74, 75, 76, 77, 78] These diets exclude oils and minimize intake of high-fat whole foods such as nuts and avocados, whereas higher fat plant-based diets contain varying amounts of high fat plant foods such as avocados, nuts, seeds, coconut, tofu and other soy products and may or may not include concentrated fats and oils.

We have yet to put very low-fat diets to the test against whole food plant-based diets that contain more fat. Although very low-fat diets have proven effective in treating chronic diseases, we cannot assume that such diets are gold standard for everyone. In establishing appropriate guidelines for fat intake in healthy plant-based populations, many factors need to be considered. Optimal fat intakes must support excellent health at every stage of the life cycle, including periods of rapid growth and development, such as pregnancy, infancy, and childhood. They must ensure good essential fatty acid status, adequate absorption of fat-soluble nutrients and phytochemicals, and smooth functioning of all body systems.

Very low-fat diets can have significant shortcomings, particularly for pregnant and lactating women, and for growing children. These diets may provide insufficient energy, especially for infants and children.[79] When higher fat plant foods are excluded from the diet, essential fatty acids can also slip below Acceptable Intakes (AI) set by the Institute of Medicine (IOM). Another important consideration is that the intake and absorption of fat-soluble nutrients (e.g. vitamins A, D, E and K) and phytochemicals may be compromised on very low-fat diets compared to diets containing moderate amounts of dietary fat.[2, 80, 81] Very low-fat intakes have also been associated with suboptimal intakes of zinc and some B vitamins. As zinc is a nutrient of concern in plant-based diets, especially for children, this is another reason to keep fat intakes from dropping too low.[2] Until we know more, it seems prudent for children who eat plant-based to stay within the AMDR for fat.[79]

How Do We Ensure Sufficient Omega-3 Fatty Acids?

Omega-3 fatty acids are commonly associated with fish, so there is often concern about whether plant-based eaters will meet needs. To be clear, it *is* possible for plant-based eaters to get enough omega-3 fatty acids without eating fish. Plants are good sources of the parent omega-3 fatty acid, ALA, and some of this ALA is converted to EPA and DHA in our bodies. What comes as a surprise to many people is that most EPA and DHA are made by plants in the ocean, and these plants are the primary source of EPA and DHA for fish. Omega-3-rich microalgae can be cultured and the EPA and DHA extracted and used in foods and supplements. So, even the long-chain omega-3 fatty acids, EPA and DHA, can be acquired from plants.

Of course, for those who are pescovegetarian (plant-based fish eaters), omega-3 fatty acid intake could easily exceed usual intakes for omnivores. For lacto-ovo vegetarians, DHA intakes vary with egg consumption, and can be significant, particularly if omega-3-rich eggs are featured regularly in the diet. For plant-exclusive eaters, intakes of the long-chain omega-3s are often negligible. However, small amounts of EPA can be obtained from seaweed, and larger amounts of EPA and DHA can be supplied by microalgae in supplements and fortified foods. Not surprisingly, omega-3 status is reflected by dietary intakes. Typically, plasma, blood and tissue levels of long-chain omega-3 fatty acids are about 30 percent lower in lacto-ovo vegetarians compared with omnivores, while plant-exclusive eaters have levels that are about 40 to 50 percent lower.[82] Of course, the big question is, so what? Do we know for sure that the higher levels in omnivores provide a health advantage? The simple answer is no, we do not yet have a definitive answer, however, the weight of the evidence does suggest potential advantages to higher omega-3 status.[83] So how do we help to boost omega-3 status in plant-based eaters who exclude fish, and possibly eggs from their diets? Balancing essential fatty acids is achievable when the diet is based on whole foods and a rich source of omega-3 fatty acids is regularly featured. The following guidelines will help you to put together a diet that optimizes omega-3 status.

1. **Ensure a healthful, nutritionally adequate diet.** By consuming sufficient protein, vitamins, and minerals, you will maximize your ability to convert ALA to EPA and DHA. There is no question that maximizing conversion of ALA makes good sense for all those who do not consume fish or other sources of EPA and DHA. Avoid trans fatty acids and, for teens and adults, excess intakes of alcohol or caffeine. These can also reduce your capacity to convert ALA. Do not exceed the upper limit on total fat intake as high fat diets may reduce conversion.

2. **Include sufficient ALA (omega-3 fatty acids from plants) in your daily diet.** Adequate Intakes (AI) set by the IOM may not be sufficient for those who do not consume EPA and DHA directly. For these individuals, some experts suggest doubling the AI for ALA.[82,84] See Table 4.4 for recommended omega-3 intakes throughout the lifecycle. The best sources of ALA are flaxseeds, chia seeds, hempseeds, and walnuts. Flaxseeds are a rich and economical source of omega-3 fatty acids, but need to be ground to increase digestibility of the ALA. Chia seeds are also an excellent source of ALA, and while grinding may further enhance ALA absorption, these are more delicate seeds that break down more easily than flax, so grinding is not as important. Both hempseeds and walnuts provide a good balance of omega-6

to omega-3 fatty acids. If using omega-3-rich concentrated oils such as flax or hempseed oil, do not use them in cooking, as omega-3 fatty acids are easily oxidized. Instead, add to salad dressings, mashed potatoes, vegetables, or popcorn. Table 4.5 provides the omega-3 content of selected foods.

3. **Reduce intake of omega-6 fatty acids, if excessive.** Omega-6 fatty acids compete against omega-3 fatty acids for conversion to LCPUFA. Many plant-based eaters have high intakes of omega-6 fatty acids and this can reduce conversion of ALA to EPA and DHA by 40 to 50 percent.[85] The easiest way to reduce omega-6 intake is to minimize omega-6-rich cooking oils such as sunflower, safflower, corn, grapeseed, sesame, and soy and packaged foods made with these oils. Instead, select oils that are monounsaturated, such as extra-virgin olive oil, avocado oil, organic canola oil, or high-oleic sunflower or safflower oils (high mono). Omega-6-rich seeds and nuts (e.g., sunflower seeds, pumpkin seeds, sesame seeds, and pine nuts) are wonderfully nutritious additions to the diet, so continue to enjoy these whole foods.

4. **Consider direct sources of EPA and DHA.** For some individuals, it is not necessary to obtain direct sources of EPA and DHA, as ALA from plant foods such as flax and chia seeds is adequately converted. However, for others, the ability to generate EPA and DHA from ALA is highly inefficient due to genetic variability, smoking, advancing age, or chronic diseases such as hypertension, metabolic syndrome, diabetes, and non-alcoholic fatty liver disease.[86, 87, 88, 89] In some cases, such as during pregnancy and lactation, even though conversion is more efficient, EPA and DHA levels may still be below what is considered optimal. In these cases, a microalgae supplement may be warranted. Microalgae (tiny plants from the sea) are the only significant sources of both EPA and DHA. Although seaweed does contain smaller amounts of EPA (but no DHA), intakes are typically too small to make a significant contribution. Note that regular consumption of seaweed can lead to excessive iodine intake (see Chapter 5 for more information). Plant-based EPA and DHA supplements are widely available. Microalgae-based DHA is also being added to some infant formulas and soy milks, cold-pressed oils, juices, cereals, and other foods, in small amounts. Omega-3 status is not routinely assessed by physicians. However, a test called the omega-3 index (which is a measure of the EPA and DHA content of red cell membranes) has been used in certain clinical situations.

Table 4.4: Recommended Intakes of Omega-3 Fatty Acids

AGE GROUP	ADEQUATE INTAKE (AI) FOR ALA (g/day)	SUGGESTED ALA INTAKE FOR PLANT-EXCLUSIVE EATERS* (g/day)	SUGGESTED DHA/EPA IF USING SUPPLEMENTS** (mg/day)
Infants—newborn to 12 months	0.5***	0.5***	
1–3 years	0.7	1.4	70
4–8 years	0.9	1.8	90
Boys 9–13 years	1.2	2.4	120
Girls 9–13 years	1.0	2.0	100
Males 14 years+	1.6	3.2	160
Females 14 years+	1.1	2.2	110
Pregnancy	1.4	2.8	200–300
Lactation	1.3	2.6	200–300

*This amount is also appropriate for plant-based eaters who do not eat fish or DHA-rich eggs as part of their regular diet.

**For those using supplements, no increase in ALA over the AI is suggested. If only occasional supplements are used (e.g. once or twice weekly), aim for the suggested ALA intakes for plant-exclusive eaters.

***For infants, the AIs apply to total omega-3s (ALA, EPA, and DHA). The amount is based on intakes typical of healthy breastfed infants. For ages 1 year and older, the AIs apply only to ALA because ALA is the only omega-3 that is essential. The IOM did not establish specific intake recommendations for EPA or DHA.

Table 4.5: ALA Content of Common Foods

FOOD	SERVING SIZE	ALA CONTENT (g)
Flaxseed oil	1 tablespoon	7.3
Chia seeds	2 tablespoons	5
Flaxseeds, ground	2 tablespoons	3.2
Walnuts	1 ounce (3.2 tablespoons)	2.6
Hempseed oil	1 tablespoon	2.5
Hempseeds	2 tablespoons	2.0
Walnut oil	1 tablespoon	1.4
Canola oil	1 tablespoon	1.3
Tofu, firm	½ cup	0.7
Edamame, shelled	1 cup	0.6

Source:[42]

A Final Word on Fat

Higher-fat whole plant foods add immeasurably to both enjoyment of eating and to the nutritional quality of the diet. Fat is necessary for the optimal growth and development of our little ones. While very low-fat diets may be reasonable choices for adults with heart disease, they are not appropriate for growing children. Ensuring suitable amounts and types of fat at various stages of the life cycle can be achieved either by including sufficient higher fat whole plant foods or with a combination of higher fat whole plant foods and high-quality fats and oils.

> Fat is necessary for the optimal growth and development of our little ones. While very low-fat diets may be reasonable choices for adults with heart disease, they are not appropriate for growing children.

PROTEIN

When Mark's wife Sharon gave birth to their son, Riley, they were determined to raise him on a plant-exclusive diet. They had been following leaders of the plant-based world for many years, and the one thing they had become convinced of was that protein was a non-issue. They remembered a chart comparing 100 calories of broccoli with 100 calories of steak. They were amazed that the broccoli had more protein than the steak! They recalled a lecture where they learned that even if all you ate was rice, you would still get enough protein. So, they had no worries about protein for their son. The same could not be said for their families and friends. Oh, they had worries, all right. How could responsible parents even consider raising a child without a decent source of protein—which of course meant meat, poultry, fish, and eggs. Surely, he would end up failing to thrive, which could mean stunted growth and compromised brain development. When questioned about where Riley would get his protein, Sharon and Mark responded with a single word, "broccoli." They knew he would get protein from many foods, but it was fun to shock their family and friends with this answer, then show them the broccoli versus beef poster. They considered it an opportunity to educate people about the nutritional wonders of plants. While the poster was a surprise to the onlookers, their parents didn't buy it. To ease their minds, Mark and Sharon agreed to see a plant-friendly dietitian. What they learned was not what they had expected.

What Are Proteins and Why Are They Important?

Proteins are large, complex macronutrients that are part of every cell of the body. They are made up of various combinations of amino acids, some of which can be produced by the body and some of which cannot. Those that we are unable to manufacture are deemed "essential." Proteins are necessary for building and repairing muscles, bones, skin, hair, nails, cartilage, and other body tissues. They are a part of red blood cells that supply the body with oxygen and nutrients. The enzymes that digest our food are made of protein; certain hormones and several chemical messengers are predominantly protein. Proteins help to balance fluids, control body pH, boost immune function, transport and store nutrients, and provide energy. So, yes, protein is a critical nutrient, and yes, we need to make sure dietary sources are adequate.

There are two big issues that arise in any conversation about protein adequacy in plant-based diets. The first is the quantity question—can we get enough protein from plants? The second is the quality question—can we get all the essential amino acids we need from plants?

The Quantity Question: Can We Get Enough Protein from Plants?

In order to answer this question, we must examine our protein requirements. The recommended dietary allowance (RDA) for protein is 0.8 grams per kilogram (1 kg = 2.2 pounds) body weight for adults.[2] Additional protein is needed during times of growth, such as pregnancy, infancy, childhood, and adolescence, and possibly during the senior years when protein digestion is often reduced. Our actual needs vary based on our body size, composition, and metabolism. Even two males or females of identical body weights can have different protein needs. As a result, the RDA has a generous safety margin built in so that 97.5 percent of the population will be covered. In other words, for most of the population, needs would be less than the RDA.

The protein RDA for children is significantly higher per kilogram body weight than for adults. During the first year of life, infants require almost twice as much protein as adults, per kilogram of body weight. However, because the body is so small, actual needs are also small. For example, two- to six-month-old babies need about 9 grams of protein per day, while six- to twelve-month-old babies need about 11 grams per day. The amounts of protein required per kilogram body weight gradually declines until the child reaches adulthood.[2]

An important question that arises for plant-based eaters is whether or not intakes should be increased to compensate for the reduced digestibility of plant protein in high fiber foods. No increase is necessary for those who include some animal products such as dairy, eggs, or fish, in a plant-predominant diet, or for plant-exclusive eaters who regularly consume highly digestible protein-rich plant foods such as tofu, soy milk, veggie meats, and peanut butter. For those who do not include these sorts of highly digestible foods and eat mostly high fiber whole plant foods, an increase *may* be warranted. This is because in high fiber foods such as legumes, up to 10 percent of the protein is not effectively extracted during digestion and passes into the stools.[92] Table 4.6 lists the RDA for various ages and genders, with the last two columns showing suggested increases for plant-exclusive eaters who do not consume highly digestible products.

Table 4.6: Protein RDA At Various Ages and Stages

LIFE STAGE	PROTEIN RDA (g/kg/ day)	REFERENCE BODY WEIGHT LBS (kg)	RDA (grams/ day)	SUGGESTED INCREASE FOR HIGH FIBER PLANT-EXCLUSIVE	HIGH FIBER, PLANT-EXCLUSIVE (grams/day)
0–6 months	1.52 (AI*)	13 lbs (6 kg)	9.1	—	—
7–12 months	1.2	20 lbs (9 kg)	11	—	—
1–3 years	1.05	27 lbs (12 kg)	13	+30%	17
4–8 years	0.95	44 lbs (20 kg)	19	+20%	23
9–13 years	0.95	79 lbs (36 kg)	34	+15%	39
Females 14–18 years	0.85	119 lbs (54 kg)	46	+15%	53
Males 14–18 years	0.85	134 lbs (61 kg)	52	+15%	60
Females 19 years+	0.80	126 lbs (57 kg)	46	+10%	51
Males 19 years+	0.80	154 lbs (70 kg)	56	+10%	62
Pregnancy	1.1	—	71 (or +25 g)	+10%	78
Lactation	1.3	—	71 (or +25 g)	+10%	78

*AI = Acceptable Intake. For infants 0-6 months of age, AI rather than RDA is used for protein.
Sources:[2,93]

So, the answer to the question is yes, you can rest assured that people of all ages and activity levels can get enough protein from plants. (See Table 4.7 for amounts of protein in common foods). However, it is a mistake to assume that eating any combination of plant foods, or a single food like rice will provide all the protein and essential amino acids needed. If a woman who needs 1800 calories and 46 grams of protein ate 1800 calories worth of rice, she would get 37 grams of protein—decidedly shy of the target. Recall the chart that convinced Mark and Sharon that 100 calories of broccoli provided more protein than 100 calories of steak. It turns out that claim is a bit of a stretch. Even if broccoli was higher in protein (which it is not), 100 calories of steak is a more manageable amount of food for a child than 100 calories of broccoli. According to the USDA nutrient database, 100 calories of cooked broccoli, or about 2 cups, provides 7 grams of protein. A hundred calories of lean broiled steak, or 2 ounces, contains about 16 grams of protein.[42] When it comes to protein, steak beats broccoli. The good news is that it's easy to put together a plant-based diet with plenty of protein, just use common sense, and eat a wide variety of whole plant foods!

Do People Eating Plant-Based Get Enough Protein?

A recent review reported protein intakes in plant-exclusive eaters (vegans) ranging from 62 to 82 grams of protein per day—well above the RDA of 46 grams for women and 56 grams for men.[94] This compares to about 100 grams per day, on average, in the general omnivorous population of most industrialized nations—very close to double the RDA.[94] Studies assessing protein intakes of people with varying dietary patterns tend to show a stepwise reduction in protein intakes as we go from omnivorous to semi-vegetarian, pesco-vegetarian, lacto-ovo vegetarian, and vegan, all being well above recommended intakes. One exception was the Adventist Health Study-2 (AHS-2) with 71,751 participants—the largest study to date. In this report, there was very little difference in protein intakes among people in different dietary groups. Meat eaters averaged about 75 grams of protein per day, pesco-vegetarians about 73 grams per day, and both lacto-ovo vegetarians and vegans came in at about seventy-one grams per day.[95] The small differences seen in this population are likely due to the low meat intakes of individuals within this population, regardless of their dietary leanings. Even the meat eaters are predominantly plant-based, deriving about 60 percent of their protein from plants, compared to about 30 percent in most Western omnivores.

In addition, the generous protein intakes reported among the vegans were the result of diets with plenty of legumes, whole grains, nuts, and seeds.

What about protein intakes of children? In the Vegetarian and Vegan Children Diet Study (VeChi Diet Study), protein intakes and growth rates of 430, one to three-year-old children in Germany were assessed.[96] There were no significant differences in calorie intakes or height and weight of vegetarian, vegan, and omnivorous children. Protein intakes were highest in the omnivores, averaging 2.7 g/kg/day, compared to 2.3 g/kg/day for vegetarians, and 2.4 g/kg/day for vegan children. All dietary categories came in at more than double recommended intakes. Fat and sugar intakes were highest among omnivorous children and lowest among vegan children, while fiber intakes were highest among the vegan children and lowest among the omnivorous children. The authors concluded that a vegetarian or vegan diet in early childhood can provide similar amounts of energy and macronutrients and lead to normal growth compared to an omnivorous diet.

Other studies of vegetarian and vegan children have also reported protein intakes that exceed recommended intakes.[97, 98] According to the Analysis of the National Health and Nutrition Examination Survey, average intakes in U.S. toddlers two to three years of age is 55 grams—four times the RDA.[100] A study from Australia reported that protein intakes in children up to five years of age were close to triple that of age-appropriate recommendations.[101] While we might assume high protein intakes could only be a good thing, they have been associated with early rapid growth, overweight, and obesity in several studies.[101, 102, 103, 104]

> While we might assume high protein intakes could only be a good thing, they have been associated with early rapid growth, overweight, and obesity in several studies.

Of course, it is possible to consume insufficient protein. There are two distinct types of malnutrition that feature protein deficiency (mainly in young children)—marasmus and kwashiorkor. Marasmus is caused by starvation and severe protein and energy malnutrition. Kwashiorkor, is a severe protein deficiency with adequate energy intake—we have all seen the sad images of very thin children with distended stomachs. This occurs when the diet is highly restrictive, such as in a relief camp where people are fed a single low protein food such as rice. Severe forms of malnutrition are extremely rare in developed countries. However, we do see protein deficiencies in people with eating disorders such as anorexia nervosa and in those who do not get sufficient calories because of serious illness.

We also see milder protein insufficiencies in people eating mostly sugar and fat. For example, a teenager who replaces meat and milk with fries and soda may not get enough protein. Likewise, tea and toast seniors can fall short. It is also possible for people eating a fruitarian diet (a diet that derives at least 75 percent of calories from fruit) to fall short on protein, if greens, seeds, and other higher protein foods are avoided. The good news is that correcting protein inadequacies by adding protein-rich plant foods is a breeze. Table 4.7 provides the protein content of many common foods. It also provides values for lysine, the amino acid that is most commonly lacking in the diets of children.

Table 4.7: Protein and Lysine Content of Common Foods*

FOOD	SERVING SIZE	PROTEIN (grams)	LYSINE (mg)
Legumes and Veggie Meats			
Tofu, firm	½ cup	22	1,110
Bean or lentil pasta	1 cup	20	N/A
Soybeans, cooked	½ cup	16	955
Tempeh	½ cup	17	755
Veggie burger patty	1 patty	11	703
Veggie burger crumbles	¼ cup	11	703
Edamame	½ cup	9	580
Beans, lentils (except soybeans)	½ cup	7–9	500–625
Nuts and Seeds (1 ounce = 3–4 tablespoons)			
Hemp seeds	1 ounce	10	383
Pumpkin seeds	1 ounce	9	350
Peanuts	1 ounce	7	256
Sunflower seeds	1 ounce	6	280
Flaxseeds	1 ounce	6	260
Almonds	1 ounce	6	161
Chia seeds	1 ounce	5	275
Cashews	1 ounce	5	263
Brazil nuts	1 ounce	4	139

Walnuts	1 ounce	4	120
Pecans	1 ounce	3	81
Grains			
Kamut, spelt *or* wheat berries, cooked	½ cup	6	139
Amaranth, cooked	½ cup	5	276
Quinoa, cooked	½ cup	4	221
Pasta, whole wheat *or* white, cooked	½ cup	4	182
Bread, whole wheat	1 slice	4	112
Barley, cooked	½ cup	4	149
Brown rice, cooked	½ cup	2.6	99
Oatmeal, cooked	½ cup	2.5	103
Vegetables and Fruits			
Peas, cooked	½ cup	4	251
Other vegetables, cooked	½ cup	1–2	75–125
Fruits, fresh, most	1 medium *or* 1 cup	1 *or* less	20–60
Non-Dairy Milks			
Soy	1 cup	7–8	434–478
Hemp	1 cup	2–3	77–115
Oat	1 cup	1–4	80–120
Almond, cashew *or* rice	1 cup	1	25–50
Animal Products			
Beef, lean or chicken breast, baked	3 ounce	25	2,127
Fish, cod, baked	3 ounce	16	1,460
Cow's milk	1 cup	8	742
Cheddar Cheese	1 ounce	7	570
Eggs	1 large	6	418
Yogurt, plain	½ cup	5	464

N/A = Not Available
Source: [42]
For protein RDA, see page 83; for lysine RDA, see page 90.

Are Protein Powders Recommended?

The best place to get your protein is from food, and it is easy for most people to meet recommended intakes from food alone. Protein powders are rarely needed, and not generally recommended for children. However, they may prove useful for those who have difficulty meeting recommended intakes with food alone. Examples might be an elderly person who eats poorly and has muscle wasting or an athlete with particularly high requirements and insufficient dietary intake. If purchasing a protein powder, there are a few facts you need to know. First, protein powders can be significant sources of environmental contaminants. A report by the Clean Label Project examined 134 different types of protein powders, screening for over 130 environmental toxins.[105] The results were downright disturbing. Protein powders, including popular plant-based options were often contaminated with heavy metals such as lead, arsenic, and cadmium. Most of the formulas also had high levels of bisphenol A (BPA), a known carcinogen. Natural or artificial sweeteners were typically added to mask the offensive taste of the powders. Even the healthiest looking powders had starch fillers, preservatives, and thickeners. So, if you do believe a supplement is warranted, do your homework. Better still, boost the protein in your smoothies by adding protein-rich plant foods such as hemp seeds, almond butter, frozen peas, soft tofu, or soy milk.

The Quality Question:
Can We Get All the Essential Amino Acids We Need from Plants?

Even if you manage to convince family and friends that it is easy to get *enough* protein from plants, one last hard ball may be hurled your way. The pitch might sound something like this: Even if plants have enough protein, they don't have the right kind of protein. Growing children need "complete" protein from animal foods; plant protein is "incomplete." The theory of complete and incomplete protein, or high and low quality protein, has been around since the 1970s, but what many people do not realize is that it was largely disproven in the 1980s. All plant foods contain all nine essential amino acids. Essential amino acids are essential because animals do not make them—they are made by plants. So, the answer to the quality question is *yes*, we can get all the essential amino acids we need from plants—it's where they come from.

Protein quality is the product of two factors: protein digestibility and essential amino acid content. Digestibility refers to the extent to which protein is digested and absorbed, and it is reduced by fiber in plant cell walls. When fiber passes into the large intestine and out in our stools it carries a small percentage of the protein in food out with it. If plant cell walls are removed by refining, as is done when soybeans are turned into tofu, the protein digestibility ranks about the same as meat (which has no fiber). The digestibility of protein in beef, fish, dairy products, and eggs ranges from about 94 to 97 percent. Low fiber plant foods such as tofu, peanut butter, soy protein isolate, and white bread compare favorably with digestibility ranging from about 93 to 96 percent. On the other hand, higher fiber foods such as whole grains and legumes (beans and lentils) have a protein digestibility of about 72 to 89 percent. Protein digestibility in these foods can be enhanced by soaking, sprouting, cooking, fermenting, and blending.[106, 107, 108, 109, 110] You may wonder if it might be preferable to select white flour products over whole grain products because of the greater digestibility. While it is true that food processing can improve protein digestibility, it removes fiber, vitamins, minerals, phytochemicals, and antioxidants. The bottom line is that it makes more sense to increase protein intake slightly to compensate for the lower protein digestibility rather than sacrificing these important nutrients. Including small amounts of refined foods, such as pasta, can be useful, especially when trying to enhance caloric intakes of young children who are small eaters.

Amino acid content refers to the relative amounts of essential amino acids present in a food relative to human protein-manufacturing requirements. Humans, at various ages and stages of life have amino acid requirements based on their needs for building and rebuilding body tissues. The greatest needs per kilogram body weight are in the very young. Over the years, scientists have used different systems to rate the quality of protein in food, but for consumers, these tools are not necessary. If we meet recommended intakes for protein and consume a reasonable mix of plant foods over the course of the day, protein and individual amino acid needs will generally be easily met.[93] If a person barely gets the amount of protein they require (e.g., they need 46 grams and get 46 grams), the one amino acid that is most likely to fall short is lysine, which is an amino acid that is important for growth and maintenance.[111] Lysine is considered the "limiting amino acid" worldwide. Shortages of this amino acid are most common in food insecure regions that rely mainly on rice or wheat for calories, both of which are low in lysine. In food secure communities, most plant-based eaters include plenty of lysine-rich foods such as beans, lentils, and tofu along with the grains.

The RDA for lysine is 58 mg/kg/day for one to three-year-olds, 46 mg/kg/day for four to eight-year-olds, 43-46 mg/kg/day for nine to thirteen-year-olds, 40-43 mg/kg for fourteen to eighteen-year-olds, and 38 mg/kg/day for adults.[2] A five-year-old child who weighs 20 kg (44 pounds) would require a daily intake of 920 mg lysine. For the lysine content of common foods, see Table 4.7.

How Do We Ensure Adequate Protein Intake on Plant-Based Diets?

While getting the optimal quantity and quality of protein is easier than one might expect, there are several adjustments that can be made to boost intake of plant protein in the diet:

1. **Include legumes in the daily diet, preferably three times a day.** At breakfast, use soy milk, enjoy scrambled tofu, or add lentils to cooked grains for breakfast bowls. Add pea or bean soups to lunch or dinner meals; throw some beans, tempeh, tofu, or veggie meat into stir-fries, stews, pasta dishes, casseroles, wraps, sandwiches, and salads; use legume-based pasta. Offer firm beans such as edamame, kidney beans or chickpeas, or crispy tofu fingers or cubes for snacks. Pick dessert recipes that include legumes such as black bean brownies and chickpea peanut butter cookies.

2. **Select richer protein choices within various food groups.** For example, wheat, kamut, spelt, amaranth, and quinoa are higher in protein than most other grains. Hemp and pumpkin seeds are richer protein sources than other seeds and nuts.

3. **Add protein-rich options to dishes or snacks that typically fall short on protein.** Throw frozen peas, hempseeds, soft tofu, or soy milk into fruit or green smoothies; use nut or seed butters or cheeses on toast, in celery, or on crackers or apple pieces; add nuts and seeds to oatmeal, granola, energy balls, bars, and cookies.

4. **Ensure sufficient calories.** While not an issue for most, for those that are challenged with eating enough food, add lower fiber, higher protein options such as tofu, peanut butter, and veggie meats.

Plant vs. Animal Proteins: Is There a Difference?

For many years, animal protein was considered superior to plant protein because animal products are more concentrated protein sources, and they contain an excellent profile of essential amino acids. Plant protein was dismissed as being inferior and, as we mentioned previously, thought to be lacking in essential amino acids. We have already seen that plants can provide both the quantity and quality of protein people of all ages require. What many do not realize, however, is that there are some compelling reasons to favor plants over animals for protein. Research studies have shown that plant protein significantly reduces mortality and risk of chronic disease when it replaces meat.[90, 91] Table 4.8 provides a simple comparison of protein from legumes with protein from meat. As you will see, the dietary components we are trying to maximize (fiber, antioxidants) are generally high in legumes and low or absent in meat, while the dietary components we are trying to minimize (saturated fat, pro-inflammatory agents) are generally absent or low in plants and moderate to high in meat.

Table 4.8: Legumes vs. Animal Protein

DIETARY COMPONENT	LEGUMES	MEAT
Beneficial Components		
Fiber	Highest fiber foods	Zero
Phytochemicals	High	Zero
Antioxidants	High	Low
Plant Sterols	Moderate	Zero
Potentially Harmful Components		
Saturated Fat	Very Low	High
Cholesterol	Zero	Moderate
Heme Iron (pro-oxidant)	Zero	High
Added Hormones and Antibiotics	Zero	Variable
Neu5Gc*	Zero	High
TMAO production**	Zero	Moderate
Chemical Contaminants	Low	High
Endotoxins***	Zero	Low to high

*Neu5Gc—a molecule in red meat that promotes inflammation.

**TMAO production—TMAO is a chemical formed from eating carnitine and choline (mostly from meat) that increases risk of cardiovascular disease.

***Endotoxins—breakdown product of dead gram-negative bacteria that increase inflammation.

A Final Word on Protein

It is time to put an end to the myth that animal protein is essential for humans, and that plant protein cannot meet human protein requirements. Not only can we design a diet to provide plenty of plant protein, multiple studies have demonstrated increased longevity and reduced disease risk when protein comes from plants instead of animals.[90, 91] Children have higher protein needs based on the amount needed per kilogram body weight, but children in Western nations get two to four times more protein than they need. Instead of feeling obligated to ensure children are eating sufficient animal protein, there appears to be a long-term health advantage to providing predominantly plant-based protein at all stages of life.

Take Home Message on Macronutrients

Macronutrients are the source of much controversy among authorities on nutrition. However, evidence suggests that the percent of calories from each macronutrient matters less than the sources of those macronutrients, just so long as our requirements for each are met. Aim for about 10 to 15 percent of calories from protein; keep fat consumption within current recommended intakes for each stage of the life cycle, and beyond that the balance of carbohydrates, fat, and protein can vary with your cultural traditions, your personal preferences, your state of health, and your access to food choices. Don't stress too much about the numbers. Eat a wide variety of whole plant foods as the foundation of the diet, and the numbers will take care of themselves.

Chapter 5

Micronutrients

"One farmer says to me, 'You cannot live on vegetable food solely, for it furnishes nothing to make the bones with;' and so he religiously devotes a part of his day to supplying himself with the raw material of bones; walking all the while he talks behind his oxen, which, with vegetable-made bones, jerk him and his lumbering plow along in spite of every obstacle."

—*Henry David Thoreau*

As you recall, there are three macronutrients: carbohydrate, fat, and protein. These are the nutrients that supply energy (calories) and structural material for the body. They are called *macro* because we need them in relatively large amounts—many grams per day. In this chapter, we shift our focus to the micronutrients—vitamins, and minerals. These nutrients are called *micro* because we need them in relatively small amounts—just milligrams or micrograms per day. Micronutrients do not provide energy or structure, but they are needed for the functioning of the body. There are thirteen vitamins and at least fifteen minerals that are essential for humans, plus several that are considered possibly essential for humans. The one thing we can be sure of is that over time, the number of nutrients confirmed essential will rise.

In this chapter, we begin with a brief look at research examining nutrient intakes in people eating largely or completely plant-based diets compared to similar, health-conscious omnivores. We identify nutrients that tend to be higher in omnivorous diets, those that tend to be higher in plant-predominant or plant-exclusive diets, and those that deserve special consideration for those shifting to plant-predominant or plant-exclusive diets.

In each of the vitamin and mineral sections, we delve into the finer details of the nutrients that are of special interest to those eating mostly or exclusively plant foods. Then, we conclude with a table that summarizes the critical information on each nutrient—recommended intakes, functions, dietary sources, and considerations for people eating plant-based diets.

MICRONUTRIENTS IN VARYING DIETARY PATTERNS

When it comes to micronutrients, how do plant-based eaters do relative to omnivores? Several studies have examined this question and there are some micronutrients that are consistently higher in plant-based diets, while others are consistently lower. This does not mean that one can't meet nutrient requirements on a variety of dietary patterns, but rather that there are some nutrients that we need to pay more attention to if we are leaning toward more plant-based diets and others we need to pay more attention to if we are leaning towards omnivorous eating patterns.

The two largest studies looking at micronutrient intakes in people consuming a variety of diets, were EPIC-Oxford with 30,251 participants and the Adventist Health Study-2 with 71,751 participants.[1,2] In EPIC-Oxford, meat-eaters had the highest intakes of vitamin B2, vitamin D, zinc, selenium, and iodine, while vegans had the highest intakes of vitamin C, vitamin E, folate, magnesium, iron, and copper. Lacto-ovo vegetarians had the highest intakes of calcium. Meat eaters had the lowest intakes of vitamin E, while vegans had the lowest intakes of vitamin B12 and iodine.[1] The authors concluded that compliance with dietary goals was high and prevalence of inadequate intakes low among all dietary groups, however, vegans need to use fortified foods or supplements to ensure adequate vitamin B12 and iodine. In the Adventist Health Study-2, meat eaters had the highest intakes of vitamin D, zinc, and sodium, while the vegans had the highest intakes of vitamin C, iron, potassium and magnesium.[2] Semi-vegetarians had the highest intakes of calcium, followed by lacto-ovo vegetarians. No dietary group had nutritional shortfalls, with the exception of vitamin D, which was low in all dietary groups. The reason that vitamin B12 and iodine were not a problem among the Adventists plant-based eaters is because of the availability of fortified foods and their use of supplements. Other smaller studies have reported similar findings.[3, 4, 5] Researchers generally agree that despite substantial differences in dietary intakes between plant-based eaters and omnivores, meeting requirements for micronutrients is not a problem when the diets are well planned and when appropriate fortified foods or supplements are included.

> Researchers generally agree that despite substantial differences in dietary intakes between plant-based eaters and omnivores, meeting requirements for micronutrients is not a problem when the diets are well planned and when appropriate fortified foods or supplements are included.

VITAMINS

Vitamins are organic (carbon-containing) molecules that are required for survival in miniscule amounts—about a half a gram per day—the weight of a single raisin. Some vitamins can be produced by the body, such as vitamin D from sunshine, vitamin K and biotin from gut bacteria, and niacin from the amino acid tryptophan. However, production often falls short of needs. The remainder of essential vitamins cannot be manufactured by the body and must be obtained from the diet. Every one of the thirteen vitamins humans require were discovered between 1913 and 1948. Yet, prior to this time, people knew that some foods had the power to heal serious diseases like scurvy; they just didn't realize it was a tiny molecule in the food that was responsible for the recoveries.

Vitamins are divided into two categories, fat-soluble and water-soluble. Vitamins A, D, E and K are fat-soluble, while the B vitamins and vitamin C are water-soluble. Some vitamins act like hormones that have far-reaching effects in the body, with vitamin A governing certain aspects of growth and vitamin D regulating mineral metabolism. Many vitamins are coenzymes that help enzymes do their jobs. Vitamins are impressive team players in several arenas, working together to protect us from free radical damage (vitamins A, C, and E) and to transform the carbohydrates, fat, and protein from foods into useable

However, there are two key vitamins that deserve special attention for those who are eating plant-predominant or plant-exclusive diets— vitamins B12 and D.

energy (the B vitamins). Plant-based diets deliver most vitamins in abundance. However, there are two key vitamins that deserve special attention for those who are eating plant-predominant or plant-exclusive diets—vitamins B12 and D. Let's explore the finer details of these two nutrients, and how plant-based eaters can be sure that their bases are covered. At the end of the vitamin section, Table 5.2 provides a brief summary of the key information, including recommended intakes, function, considerations for plant-based eaters, deficiencies and excess, and sources for each of the thirteen vitamins that we depend on for our survival.

VITAMIN B12

Julie and Larry decided to go 100 percent plant-based about three years before starting their family. Even though they enjoyed great health, when they told their doctor about their diet, she cautioned them about potential deficiencies, especially vitamin B12. When Julie became pregnant, despite the fact that she was careful about taking her prenatal vitamins, the doctor suggested adding some fatty fish, dairy, and eggs just to be on the safe side. The doctor made Julie feel as though she would be harming the baby if she did not include some animal products. It was discouraging, but Julie and Larry were unwavering in their convictions. They knew several families who had raised vibrant, brilliant, plant-based children, and they were confident that they could get this right. After the baby was born, they were reluctant to mention to the pediatrician their intention to raise the baby on a plant-exclusive diet. However, when he started asking questions about breastfeeding, their plans for introduction to solid foods, and supplements for mom and baby, they decided to spill the beans. The pediatrician's response was both unexpected and refreshing. As it turned out, he was completely supportive and plant-based himself. He took the time to address their concerns, and to provide practical, evidence-based guidelines that were so helpful—especially for vitamin B12. They left the office feeling relieved and excited about the journey ahead.

What Is Vitamin B12 and Why Is It Important?

Vitamin B12, or cobalamin, represents a group of compounds that contain the mineral cobalt. It has the largest and most complex molecular structure of any vitamin and was the last vitamin to be discovered in 1948. Critical for the healthy functioning of the nervous system, vitamin B12 is involved in production and maintenance of the protective myelin sheath around nerve fibers. It is necessary for the synthesis of DNA, and thus is crucial during times of growth when cells reproduce rapidly. Cobalamin is required for the formation of red blood cells and is part of a team of vitamins that converts macronutrients into useable energy. Vitamin B12 also helps to keep homocysteine levels in check.[6, 7] High homocysteine may increase the risk of cardiovascular diseases, pregnancy complications, and neural tube defects.[8, 9, 10]

There are several forms of vitamin B12 including cyanocobalamin, methylcobalamin, adenosylcobalamin, and hydroxycobalamin. Cyanocobalamin is the manufactured form of the vitamin, and, once absorbed, it is converted into the two biologically active forms, methylcobalamin and adenosylcobalamin. Hydroxycobalamin is a form of the vitamin that is often used for injections. Some foods contain inactive analogs that look like vitamin B12 but cannot perform the functions of active B12. These inactive analogs can attach to vitamin B12 receptor sites, take the place of active B12, and potentially contribute to a B12 deficiency.[6, 11]

Are Plant-Based Eaters at Greater Risk for Vitamin B12 Deficiency?

In a word, yes. This is because plant foods are not reliable B12 sources. In studies assessing B12 status of people consuming different dietary patterns, omnivores are at the lowest risk of deficiency, followed by semi-vegetarians, pescovegetarians, and lacto-ovo vegetarians. The highest rates of vitamin B12 deficiency occur in people eating 100 percent plant-based (vegans) who do not use vitamin B12 supplements or consume B12-fortified foods.[1, 12, 13] Others at increased risk for vitamin B12 deficiency are adults over the age of 50, those with gastrointestinal disorders such as celiac disease or Crohn's disease, those who have had gastrointestinal surgery such as gastric bypass, and people on certain medications.[14]

Vitamin B12 intake varies quite dramatically among exclusively plant-based eaters, depending on access to B12-fortified foods and the use of B12 supplements. For example, in North America, the largest study assessing B12 intakes in people eating different dietary patterns reported median intakes ranging from a low of 6.3 mcg in vegans to a high of 8.5 mcg in pescovegetarians.[2] Intakes were adequate

among all dietary groups. The vegans, in this case, used supplements and fortified foods to ensure adequate intakes. By contrast, in the largest European study
assessing B12 intakes among people eating different dietary patterns, reported
average intakes ranging from a low of 0.75 mcg among vegans to a high of 8.24
mcg among meat-eaters.[1] The vegans in this group were less likely to consume
B12-fortified foods or take B12 supplements. Not surprisingly, vitamin B12
status using lab measures are reflected by the large gap in intakes. Deficiency
rates among vegetarians and vegans range from 0 to 86.5 percent among adults,
up to 45 percent in infants, 0 to 33.3 percent among
children and adolescents, and 17 to 39 percent among
pregnant women.[13] The bottom line is that the use of
supplements and fortified food dramatically diminishes
the risk of deficiency.

> The bottom line is that the use of supplements and fortified food dramatically diminishes the risk of deficiency.

What Causes Vitamin B12 Deficiency?

Vitamin B12 deficiency is generally the result of one of two factors: inadequate dietary B12 or insufficient B12 absorption. Inadequate dietary B12 can
result from plant-based diets that do not include B12 fortified foods or supplements. Insufficient absorption may be due to a lack of intrinsic factor, atrophic
gastritis (inflammation of gastric mucosa), gastrointestinal diseases such as
celiac or Crohn's disease, gastric surgeries, or prolonged use of medications such
as Metformin or acid-blockers.[7] People who do not produce sufficient intrinsic
factor develop pernicious anemia, as they cannot produce enough red blood
cells. Pernicious anemia can be easily treated with B12 injections, although high
oral doses can be effective as about 1 percent can be absorbed passively without
intrinsic factor.[7, 15]

What Does Vitamin B12 Deficiency Look and Feel Like?

Vitamin B12 deficiency can present as anemia with weakness, fatigue, irritability, shortness of breath, and paleness; nerve damage with numbness and tin-
gling in the extremities, and as it progresses, nervousness, depression, insomnia,
inability to concentrate, confusion, and paranoia; gastrointestinal disturbances
like sore tongue, reduced appetite, indigestion, and diarrhea; reproductive failure
like loss of menstruation or infertility, and elevated homocysteine levels that

increase our risk for cardiovascular disease, pregnancy complications, and neural tube defects.[6, 7, 16]

Vitamin B12 deficiency is easily reversed in the early stages, but if left unchecked, symptoms can become irreversible. In adults, deficiency can take years to manifest as B12 stores are generally substantial, while in infants it can happen in a matter of months. This is because infants have minimal B12 stores, while adults tend to have stores that can last for months or even years. Common symptoms of B12 deficiency in infants include weakness, irritability, anemia, lethargy, low muscle tone, developmental delays, and failure to thrive. Eventually, permanent brain damage can occur.[17]

> The take-home message is that getting adequate vitamin B12 is not an option, it is an imperative.

The take-home message is that getting adequate vitamin B12 is not an option, it is an imperative. Ensure reliable sources throughout the life cycle; if deficiency symptoms appear, seek medical attention as malabsorption may be responsible.

What Are the Most Reliable Sources of Vitamin B12?

The most reliable sources of vitamin B12 are supplements, vitamin B12-fortified foods, and animal products (for those ≤50 years). While plant foods may contain small amounts of B12, they are not typically reliable sources. It is interesting to note that while plants do not make B12, neither do animals. The presence of vitamin B12 in meat, milk, and other animal products is due either to a symbiotic relationship with B12-producing bacteria that reside inside their stomachs (e.g., in ruminant animals such as goats, sheep, and cattle), to the ingestion of B12 produced by bacteria in phytoplankton, soil clinging to the surfaces of plants or fungus, or from supplements provided to the animals.[18]

Products that are commonly fortified with vitamin B12 include non-dairy milks, veggie "meats," and cereals. Some nutritional yeast is grown on a B12 medium, so it can also be a good source. Check labels for the amount of B12 per serving. If a label states 100 percent of the DV (Daily Value), that means it contains 2.4 mcg of vitamin B12.*[19] Vitamin B12 in fortified foods is generally well absorbed.

---

*Note: The DV for vitamin B12 was changed from 6 mcg to 2.4 mcg in January of 2020, however, smaller companies have until January 2021 to make the necessary food label changes.

While animal products are the primary natural food sources of vitamin B12, the B12 content varies widely. A 3-ounce serving of meat, poultry, or fish averages about 2 mcg B12, with the range being about 0.3 mcg in chicken breast to about 4.8 mcg in salmon. Organ meats and shellfish can be much higher with beef liver providing about 70 mcg in a 3-ounce serving. A cup of cow's milk or two large eggs provide about 1.2 mcg vitamin B12.[20] It is important to note that in order to absorb the B12 from animal foods, it must first be cleaved off the protein it is bound to. The ability to successfully complete this task diminishes as we age due to reduced stomach acid (hydrochloric acid) and enzymes (gastric proteases). As a result, the Institute of Medicine recommends that everyone above the age of fifty years obtain most of their vitamin B12 from supplements or fortified foods, regardless of their dietary pattern.[6] In other words, once you reach your fifties, animal foods are no longer reliable sources of vitamin B12.[21, 19]

There are many claims made about plant foods with vitamin B12. Unfortunately, the vast majority of these claims have not been scientifically validated. Foods that are often touted as reliable B12 sources include seaweed and algae, organic produce, mushrooms, fermented foods, duckweed, and some teas. While small amounts of useable B12 are present in some of these foods, others contain inactive analogs. In the case of seaweed, active B12 can be converted to inactive analogs when the seaweed is dried. Until further research is released, it is best not to rely on these foods as your primary sources of B12.[11, 22, 23]

Some claims are made that internal production of B12 is sufficient for humans if the diet is high quality and our microbiota is robust. While it is theoretically possible to produce B12 in the small intestine (where it is absorbed) and in the oral cavity (if oral hygiene is lacking), the amounts produced are not generally sufficient to meet daily needs. Most internal vitamin B12 production occurs in the large intestine and is excreted in the feces.

How Much B12 Is Enough?

The RDA for vitamin B12 in those 14 years or more is 2.4 mcg. It is slightly lower in younger children, and slightly higher in those who are pregnant or lactating. See Table 5.2 for recommended intakes throughout the lifecycle. Factored into B12 recommendations is the assumption that only about 50 percent of vitamin

B12 will be absorbed from foods.[24] What this means is that we need to absorb 1.2 mcg, but must eat foods providing 2.4 mcg to get the necessary amount. The RDA is currently being challenged, as some evidence suggests that B12 status (and homocysteine levels) are better managed with intakes of 4 to 7 mcg per day in healthy adults ages nineteen to fifty years.[25] This suggests that we would need to *absorb* about 2 to 3.5 mcg of B12 per day from foods or supplements. For assurance of adequacy, it may be prudent to consume double the RDA for everyone beyond twelve months of age. Higher intakes may be required for older individuals or those with compromised absorption.[26]

Table 5.1 provides a summary of suggested intakes for vitamin B12 from fortified foods and/or supplements for those not consuming animal products. The safest way to ensure adequate B12 status is to take a B12 supplement daily or twice weekly. Taking a supplement once a week is also an option, though less frequent intake may also be less effective. Because intake of fortified foods is often inconsistent, it is advisable to include some B12 in supplement form as well (e.g. as part of a multivitamin or a weekly supplement). It is best to err on the side of more than less with vitamin B12.

You may be wondering why the recommended doses of supplements are so large compared to the tiny amounts of B12 necessary to ensure good B12 status. The reason is that the higher the amount in the supplement, the smaller the percentage that is absorbed. The following rates of absorption for vitamin B12 have been reported: [24, 27, 28]

- 5 mcg—28 percent
- 10 mcg—16 percent
- 25 mcg—5 percent
- 50 mcg—3 percent
- 500 mcg—2 percent
- 1,000 mcg—1.3 percent

So, for example, if you take 1,000 mcg of vitamin B12, you will absorb approximately 13 mcg.

Table 5.1: Suggested Intakes for Vitamin B12 from Fortified Foods or Supplements

AGE	2x DAILY FROM FOOD (mcg B12/ serving)	DAILY SUPPLEMENT (mcg)	2x PER WEEK SUPPLEMENT (mcg)	WEEKLY SUPPLEMENT (mcg)
1–3 y	1	10	250	n/a
4–8 y	1.5	25	500	1,000
9–13 y	2	50	750	1,500
14–64 y	2.5	100*	1,000	2,000
65+ y	2.5	500–1,000	n/a	n/a
Pregnancy and Lactation	3	100*	1,000	n/a

Note: N/A indicates that the less frequent supplementation is not recommended for this category.

*Preliminary evidence suggests 50 mcg daily may be sufficient to maintain adequate status,[29] however, based on estimated rates of absorption, we are suggesting 100 mcg to err on the side of caution.

Can I Get Too Much B12?

The Institute of Medicine has not established an Upper Limit (UL) for vitamin B12 because no significant adverse effects have been associated with excess vitamin B12 in healthy people.[6] Vitamin B12 is a water-soluble vitamin, so excess is excreted in the urine. What this means in practical terms is that it is no big deal if you take more than what is suggested in Table 5.1. For example, if you need 100 mcg per day and you take 200 mcg, it's all good. Although some people report acne and rosacea with hefty doses of B12, this is an uncommon side effect.[30, 31]

What Form of Vitamin B12 is Best?

There is considerable debate about what form of vitamin B12 is best. Some experts suggest cyanocobalamin because it is more stable, inexpensive, and effective in treating B12 deficiency.[12] Others suggest methyl- and/or adenosyl-cobalamin as these are the active forms of the vitamin in humans, they do not contain cyanide, so may be safer.[32] The issue is confusing for consumers and health professionals alike. Based on evidence to date, it does not appear that there are significant advantages to taking the active forms of B12 over cyanocobalamin for most individuals.[33] The active forms are more expensive and less stable. Although concern is often expressed about the cyanide portion of cyanocobalamin, amounts are not physiologically significant (higher amounts are often present in many common foods such as almonds, flaxseeds, lima beans, fruits, and vegetables) for most people. However, for those with inborn errors of cobalamin metabolism or chronic kidney disease, cyanocobalamin is not recommended. With inborn errors of metabolism, hydroxycobalamin is the preferred form.[33] Evidence does not suggest superior absorption from sublingual versus oral forms.[19] The bottom line is that what matters more than the form of B12 you take is that you are getting a consistent, reliable source.

VITAMIN D

In 1822, a Polish physician observed that infants and children living in rural areas where they had daily outdoor exposure, escaped the seemingly unstoppable scourge of rickets (a severe bone-deforming disease) that had become epidemic among infants and children living in the crowded industrial cities of northern Europe and North America. Near the close of the nineteenth century, autopsies showed that 80 to 90 percent of children in Boston and Leiden (a large city in the Netherlands) had rickets. In the 1930s, with educational initiatives encouraging sunshine exposure, and the fortification of cow's milk, the disease was largely eradicated.[34] One might imagine that would be the end of the story, but it is not. Over the past two decades, there has been a rather remarkable resurgence in rickets. One recent US study (Olmsted County, Minnesota) reported the incidence of nutritional rickets per 100,000 children (under three years) shot up from 0 in 1970, to 2.2 in 1980, 3.7 in 1990, and 24.1 in 2000.[35]

What Is Vitamin D and Why Is It Important?

The only vitamin that is a steroid hormone in its active form, vitamin D, is also the only vitamin that can be obtained without food sources given sufficient exposure to warm sunshine. Vitamin D (calciferol) is made in the skin after exposure to UVB light or consumption of food sources of vitamin D2 (ergocalciferol) or vitamin D3 (cholecalciferol). It gets transported to the liver and then the kidney for further conversions to produce an important hormone called 1,25-dihyroxyvitamin D, calcitriol or "active" vitamin D.[36]

Vitamin D enhances calcium and phosphorus absorption, enabling bone growth, bone remodeling, and bone mineralization. A lack of vitamin D can result in rickets in children, and osteomalacia (soft bones) or osteoporosis (brittle bones) in children and adults. Vitamin D is also needed for growth and maturation of cells and for neuromuscular and immune system function. There are multiple reports of relationships between vitamin D and chronic diseases, although the strengths of the relationships are not firmly established. Research suggests that vitamin D may play a role in the prevention of colon, prostate, and breast cancers. There may also be a role for vitamin D in the prevention and treatment of diabetes, hypertension, and multiple sclerosis.[37, 38]

In recent years, there has been an escalation in both vitamin D insufficiency, and frank deficiency throughout the world. Strong recommendations from national and international health authorities to avoid direct sun exposure in an effort to reduce rates of skin cancer may have inadvertently increased risk. Other contributing factors include rising rates of obesity, failure to provide a vitamin D source during breastfeeding, scanty vitamin D food sources (or food fortification initiatives), inadequate public education about the necessity of vitamin D, aging, working and playing indoors, wearing clothing that covers the whole body, and living in the north with little or no vitamin D production for at least half the year (especially people with darker skin).[39]

How Much Vitamin D Do We Need?

There are three sources of vitamin D—sunshine, food, and supplements. With ample sunshine, we have no requirement for dietary vitamin D (UVB light turns 7-dehydroxcholesterol in the skin into vitamin D). It is estimated that 50 to 90 percent of our vitamin D comes from sunshine.[40] How much sunshine is enough to produce sufficient vitamin D depends on latitude (as we move away from the equator we receive less UVB rays), temperature (warm summer sun is needed for vitamin D production), time of day (greatest production is between 10 AM and 3 PM), cloud, fog or smog cover (reduces UVB radiation 50 to 60 percent), glass barriers (UVB rays don't penetrate glass so there is no production through windows), area of skin exposure (the more skin that is exposed, the greater the production), sunscreen (SFP of 8 or more blocks production), age (production at age seventy is only about 25 percent of what it was at age twenty), smoking (reduces production), body fatness (excess body fatness reduces production), and melanin content of the skin (as melanin increases and skin tone deepens, less vitamin D is produced).[39, 36, 41] Skin color is a function of exposure to ultraviolet radiation—the first humans were amply pigmented (e.g., dark skin with high melanin content) so they could handle the extreme levels of ultraviolet radiation near the equator. As humans migrated north, depigmentation occurred (e.g., lighter skin with lower melanin content) as a means of maximizing vitamin D production in the face of limited UV radiation exposure. Taking all of these factors into consideration, exposing the arms, legs, or back to warm sunshine (without sunscreen) between 10 AM and 3 PM for 5 to 30 minutes two or more times a week may be enough to produce adequate vitamin D in many individuals, with higher exposure needed for those with darker skin tone.[42] For those living at latitudes above 33° N (e.g., Phoenix, Arizona) or below 33° S (e.g., Valparaiso, Chili), very little vitamin D can be produced from sunshine during the winter months.[39]

The other two sources of vitamin D are foods and supplements. As you can see from Table 5.2, requirements for vitamin D range from 400 IU (10 mcg) during infancy to 800 IU (20 mcg) during our senior years. There are very few foods that are naturally rich sources of vitamin D, so needs are rarely met by these sources alone. The most concentrated natural food sources are fatty fish, such as salmon, swordfish, tuna, and mackerel, but even these foods only provide about 100 to 400 IU (2.5–10 mcg) per serving. Smaller amounts can be found in egg yolks, beef liver, and mushrooms that are exposed to ultraviolet light. Vitamin D is commonly added to foods such as cow's milk, plant-based milks, and select ready-to-eat cereals. The Daily Value (DV) on food labels is 800 IU (20 mcg), so if one serving of food has 50 percent of the DV, it would provide 400 IU (10 mcg) vitamin D. For those who do not consume sufficient vitamin D from food, and do not receive sufficient sun exposure, a vitamin D supplement is recommended. While supplementing at levels consistent with the RDA (see Table 5.2) would seem reasonable, some researchers suggest that daily intakes of 1,000–2,000 IU are needed to achieve optimal vitamin D status. Recommendations by some governments include a guideline for sunshine and a guideline for vitamin D from food or supplements if insufficient sun exposure is achieved.

Is Sunshine a Friend or a Foe?

Our mothers encouraged us to eat our veggies, get a good night's sleep, and to go outside for fresh air and sunshine. We all know mom was right about the veggies and sleep, and while sunshine has been a little more controversial, it seems mom was right about that too. Sunshine provides vitamin D, and research has shown that it does a whole lot more. While vitamin D status (vitamin D in the bloodstream) is associated with reduced risk of chronic diseases such as heart disease, stroke, and some cancers, vitamin D supplementation doesn't seem to afford the expected protection.[43] Perhaps it is because the benefits of sunshine extend beyond vitamin D. Sunshine triggers the release of several beneficial compounds such as nitric oxide (a potent vasodilator), which has been shown to relax the inner muscles of the blood vessels so they widen, increasing blood flow, reducing blood pressure, and boosting serotonin, which plays key roles in emotional wellbeing, appetite and many other body functions. The result is a reduction in all-cause mortality, blood pressure, inflammation, and autoimmune disease.[44, 45, 46, 39] Sunshine also appears to improve our circadian rhythm and mood.

What about skin cancer? There is no question that excessive sun exposure, and particularly sunburns, increases risk of skin cancer. However, there are many studies that have reported a protective effect of UV exposure against many other cancers, and reduced overall cancer mortality.[47, 48, 49, 50, 51, 52, 53, 54] Rather than avoiding sunshine, we need to be sensible about sunshine. This means enjoying the great outdoors, without burning our skin. Once you have enjoyed sufficient sunshine, protect yourself with a hat, clothing, sunscreen, and shade!

Are People Eating Plant-Based Diets at Increased Risk of Vitamin D Deficiency?

People eating plant-based diets may be at higher risk, depending on how plant-based their diet is. For those who include fish and dairy products, vitamin D intakes from food could be higher than that of the general population. For plant-exclusive eaters, vitamin D intakes from food will almost always be lower than it is among omnivores.[1, 2, 55] However, vitamin D intake from foods is only one factor affecting risk. For individuals who get sufficient sun exposure and/or take vitamin D supplements, dietary intake is not a deciding factor. An interesting study involving 428 individuals from the Adventist Health Study 2 assessed vitamin D intake relative to vitamin D status (serum vitamin D levels).

The researchers reported no significant differences in serum vitamin D levels between the dietary groups, despite the higher dietary vitamin D intake among nonvegetarians. They concluded that other factors, such as use of vitamin D supplements, sun exposure, and skin pigmentation had greater influence on vitamin D status than dietary intake.[56]

Vitamin D deficiency is a global public health problem in people of all ages. One thorough review of the literature reported low serum vitamin D (levels below 50 nmol/l or 20 ng/ml) in 46 percent of black and 10 percent of white Americans, 69 percent of Germans, 40 percent of Australians, 71 percent of Pakistanis, 99 percent of East Indians, and at least 90 percent of those from several Middle Eastern countries.[57] The bottom line is everyone needs to ensure reliable vitamin D sources.

Table 5.2: Summary Chart—Vitamins

Key:

RDA = Recommended Dietary Allowances   RAE = Retinol Activity Equivalents

AI = Acceptable Intakes   NE = Niacin Equivalents

UL = Upper Limit   P = Pregnancy; L = Lactation

Micro-nutrient	RDA or AI (daily)	Primary Functions	Considerations for Plant-Based Eaters	Deficiencies/ Excesses	Richest Food Sources
Vitamin A	RDA Units—RAE 0–6 m—400 7–12 m—500 1–3 y—300 4–8 y—400 9–13 y—600 14+ y (F)—900 14+ (M)—700 P—770 L—1300	Normal vision Gene expression Reproduction Growth and development Immune function Healthy skin and mucous membranes Antioxidant (only provitamin A carotenoids from plant foods, not preformed vitamin A from animal products)	Plant-based eaters eating abundant vegetables and fruits meet or exceed the RDA. Carotenoid absorption is enhanced with cooking, fat, and juicing or blending. If concerned about conversion*, consume generous amounts of carotenoid-rich foods, or consider taking a vitamin supplement with preformed vitamin A (stay below UL).	*Deficiency:* xerophthalmia—night blindness leading to total blindness; increased infections. *Excess: Preformed vitamin A*—toxic in high doses—liver damage, birth defects, joint and bone pain, fractures; can be fatal. Do not exceed the UL of 3,000 mcg/day for adults (lower UL for children, teens) *Pro-vitamin A carotenoids*—no toxicity—can cause skin to become yellow-orange (harmless).	*Plant Sources (Provitamin A carotenoids)*— orange, yellow, red and green vegetables, fruits (e.g. sweet potatoes, kale, squash, carrots, mango, papaya, cantaloupe) *Animal sources (Preformed Vitamin A):*—liver, fish, milk, eggs

Table 5.2: Summary Chart—Vitamins *(continued)*

Micro-nutrient	RDA or AI (daily)	Primary Functions	Considerations for Plant-Based Eaters	Deficiencies/ Excesses	Richest Food Sources
Vitamin B1–Thiamin	RDA Units—mg 0–6 m—0.2 7–12 m—0.3 1–3 y—0.5 4–8 y—0.6 9–13 y—0.9 14–18 y (F)—1.0 18+ y (F)—1.1 14+ (M)—1.2 P or L—1.4	Energy release from carbohydrates and some amino acids RNA and DNA production Nervous system function	Plant-based eaters easily exceed the RDA. Added to enriched grains (most refined grains).	*Deficiency:* beriberi— peripheral neuropathy and wasting. Early signs —weight loss, lack of appetite, confusion, memory loss, muscle weakness, enlarged heart. Risk of deficiency high among alcoholics. *Excess:* no UL, as excess is excreted in the urine.	*Plant sources:* whole and enriched grains, legumes, nuts, seeds, nutritional yeast, some vegetables, fruits *Animal sources:* pork, fish
Vitamin B2– Riboflavin	RDA Units—mg 0–6 m—0.3 7–12 m—0.4 1–3 y—0.5 4–8 y—0.6 9–13 y—0.9 14–18 y (F)—1.0 19+ y (F)—1.1 14+ (M)—1.3 P—1.4 L—1.6	Energy release from macronutrients Assists B3 and B6 in their function	Generally adequate in varied plant-based diets, but limited diets may fall short. Bacteria in the large intestine produce absorbable riboflavin. Destroyed by light. Added to enriched grains (most refined grains).	*Deficiency:* ariboflavinosis—skin disorders, lesions in the corners of the mouth, swollen, cracked lips, hair loss, red, itchy eyes, damage to liver and nervous system. *Excess:* no UL; avoid very high dose supplements.	*Plant sources:* nutritional yeast, soy foods, enriched grains, fortified cereals, whole grains, some nuts, mushrooms, vegetables, fruits *Animal sources:* dairy products, liver, meat, eggs
Vitamin B3–Niacin	RDA Units—NE mg 0–6 m—2 7–12 m—4 1–3 y—6 4–8 y—8 9–13 y—12 14+ y (F)—14 14+ (M)—16 P—18 L—17	Metabolism of carbohydrate, fat and alcohol. Skin, digestive tract and nervous system health	Plant-based eaters generally meet the RDA. Both niacin and the amino acid tryptophan count towards overall intake; tryptophan can be converted to niacin (60 mg tryptophan = 1 mg niacin). Added to enriched grains (most refined grains).	*Deficiency:* pellagra— characterized by 4 D's— dermatitis, dementia, diarrhea, and death. Occurs mostly in limited diets of impoverished people. *Excess:* none from food; high dose supplements cause flushing, reddish skin tone, burning, tingling, and itching. Do not exceed UL of 35 mg/day for adults (lower UL for children, teens) unless medically indicated.	*Plant sources:* legumes, soy products, peanuts, nuts, whole and enriched grains, mushrooms, nutritional yeast, vegetables, fruits *Animal sources:* meat, dairy products, eggs

Vitamin B4–Choline	AI Units—mg 0–6 m—125 7–12 m—150 1–3 y—200 4–8 y—250 9–13 y—375 14–18 y (F)—400 19+ y (F)—425 14+ (M)—550 P—450 L—550	Structural integrity of cell membranes Cell membrane signaling Genetic expression Early brain development Metabolism, fat transport	Plants are less concentrated sources, but varied plant-based diets generally meet the AI. Declared an essential nutrient by the Institute of Medicine in 1998. Humans produce choline, but internal production is insufficient to meet needs. Not added to enriched grains.	*Deficiency:* muscle and liver damage, nonalcoholic fatty liver disease. Frank deficiency is uncommon, likely because of internal production. *Excess:* fishy body odor, vomiting, sweating, low blood pressure, liver damage. Do not exceed the UL of 3,500 mg/day for adults (lower UL for children, teens).	*Plant sources:* shitake mushrooms, soy milk and other soyfoods, wheat germ, legumes, quinoa, cruciferous vegetables, peanuts, peas, almonds, oatmeal, walnuts, potatoes *Animal sources:* liver, eggs, beef, chicken, fish, dairy products
Vitamin B5– Pantothenic acid	AI Units—mg 0–6 m—1.7 7–12 m—1.8 1–3 y—2 4–8 y—3 9–13 y—4 14+ y—5 P—6 L—7	Energy release from macronutrients Synthesis of amino acids, fatty acids, ketones, cholesterol, antibodies and other essential compounds	Plant-based eaters generally meet or exceed the RDA. Not added to enriched grains.	*Deficiency:* numbness and burning in hands and feet, headache, fatigue, irritability, heartburn, diarrhea, nausea, stomach pain. Rare in developed countries. *Excess:* no UL; no reports of toxicity. Very high intakes may cause mild diarrhea and stomach upset.	*Plant sources:* mushrooms, avocados, potatoes, peanuts, whole grains, legumes, some vegetables *Animal sources:* liver, eggs, fish, meat, poultry
Vitamin B6– Pyridoxine	RDA Units—mg 0–6 m—0.1 7–12 m—0.3 1–3 y—0.5 4–8 y—0.6 9–13 y—1.0 14–18 y (F)—1.2 14–18 y (M)—1.3 19–50 y—1.3 50+ y (F)—1.5 50+ y (M)—1.7 P—1.9 L—2.0	Energy release from amino acids Synthesis of amino acids, fatty acids and neuro- transmitters	Plant-based eaters generally exceed the RDA. Easily destroyed by cooking, freezing, canning, soaking. Not added to enriched grains.	*Deficiency:* anemia, itchy rashes, cracker in corners of mouth, swollen tongue, depression, confusion, reduce immune function. *Excess:* no excess from food, but high intakes from supplements for a year or more can cause serious nerve damage. Do not exceed the UL of 100 mg/day for adults (lower UL for children and teens).	*Plant sources:* Avocados, bananas and other fruits, seeds, nuts, vegetables, whole grains, fortified cereals *Animal sources:* liver, fish, meat, poultry

Table 5.2: Summary Chart—Vitamins *(continued)*

Micro-nutrient	RDA or AI (daily)	Primary Functions	Considerations for Plant-Based Eaters	Deficiencies/Excesses	Richest Food Sources
Vitamin B7 Biotin	AI Units—mcg 0–6 m—5 7–12 m—6 1–3 y—8 4–8 y—12 9–13 y—20 14–18 y—25 19+ y—30 P—30 L—35	Energy release from macronutrients Fatty acid synthesis	Plant-based eaters generally meet the RDA. Manufactured by bacteria in the intestinal tract, adding to dietary supply. Not added to enriched grains.	*Deficiency:* hair loss, scaly red rash around body orifices, pinkeye, high acid in blood and urine, seizures, nervous system disorders. Extremely rare in developed countries. *Excess:* Not an issue from foods. High amounts from supplements may cause false lab results, especially hormone measures.	*Plant sources:* Nuts, seeds, peanuts, bananas and other fruits vegetables, legumes, whole grains, nutritional yeast *Animal sources:* liver, eggs, fish, meat, poultry
Vitamin B9 Folate	RDA Units—mcg 0–6 m—65 7–12 m—80 1–3 y—150 4–8 y—200 9–13 y—300 14+ y (F)—400 14+ (M)—400 P—600 L—500	Metabolism of amino acids Production of DNA and amino acids Normal cell division Red blood cell production Elimination of homocysteine	Plant-based eaters generally meet or exceed the RDA. Sprouting can double folate in foods. Folic acid can mask a B12 deficiency. Folic acid is added to enriched grains.	*Deficiency:* anemia, neural tube defects in babies, low birth weight babies, open sores on tongue and inside mouth, change in skin, hair, and nails. *Excess:* none from food folate. Folic acid (supplements and fortified foods) decreases neural tube defects; may increase risk of some cancers. Do not exceed UL of 1,000 mcg/day for adults (lower UL for children, teens)	*Plant sources:* leafy greens, vegetables, avocado, legumes, fruits, nuts, seeds, enriched grain products *Animal sources:* liver, seafood, fish
Vitamin B12 Cobalamin	RDA Units—mcg 0–6 m—0.4 7–12 m—0.5 1–3 y—0.9 4–8 y—1.2 9–13 y—1.8 14+—2.4 P—2.6 L—2.8	Energy release from macronutrients DNA synthesis Maintains myelin sheaths around nerve fibers Red blood cell formation Elimination of homocysteine	Plant foods are NOT reliable sources. Plant-based eaters require supplements and/or fortified foods to meet the RDA. Animal products may not be reliable sources for those over 50 yrs.	*Deficiency:* megaloblastic anemia (weakness, fatigue, loss of appetite), numbness and tingling in fingers and feet, depression, confusion, dementia; failure to thrive and developmental delays in infants. *Excess:* no UL as low potential for toxicity. In rare cases, excess intakes from supplements may induce acne or rash.	*Plant sources:* fortified cereals, milks, meat analogs; some nutritional yeasts; mushrooms, some seaweeds *Animal sources:* meat, poultry, fish, eggs, dairy

Vitamin C	RDA Units—mg 0–6 m—40 7–12 m—50 1–3 y—15 4–8 y—25 9–13 y—45 14–18 y (F)—65 14–18 y (M)—75 18+ y (F)—75 18+ y (M)—90 Pregnancy—85 Lactation—120	Production of collagen, L-carnitine, and some neurotransmitters Protein metabolism Immune function Antioxidant and regeneration of other antioxidants Improves iron absorption	Plant-based eaters generally meet or exceed the RDA. Easily lost with cooking and prolonged storage.	*Deficiency:* scurvy—inflamed, swollen, bleeding gums, loss of teeth, red or purple spots on skin, fatigue, joint pain, poor wound healing, corkscrew hairs, anemia. *Excess:* Nausea, diarrhea, stomach cramps. May cause excess iron absorption in those with hemochromatosis. Avoid exceeding the UL of 2,000 mg/day for adults (lower UL for children, teens)	*Plant sources:* fruits and vegetables, especially red sweet peppers, citrus fruits, kiwi, broccoli, strawberries, cantaloupe, Brussels sprouts, cabbage, mango, tomatoes, potatoes, pineapples *Animal sources:* small amounts in liver, oysters, organ meats
Vitamin D	RDA Units–IU 0–6 m—400 7–12 m—400 1–70 y—600 >70 y—800 P + L—600	Bone health Calcium and phosphorus absorption and serum concentrations Growth and maturation of cells Immune function Neuromuscular function Control of inflammation	Dietary intakes are low in all dietary patterns; lowest among plant-exclusive eaters. Most of the vitamin D in the diet comes from fortified foods. Vitamin D needs can also be met through warm sun exposure (see page 106 for details).	*Deficiency:* rickets in children; osteomalacia (soft bones) in children and adults. *Excess:* Supplements toxic in excess. Can cause nausea, vomiting, decreased appetite, frequent urination, weakness, constipation, confusion, disorientation, calcification of blood vessels, damage to heart and kidneys, irregular heart rhythm. Only from supplements—not sunshine or food. Do not exceed to UL of 4,000 IU/day for everyone 9 years+ (lower UL for younger children).	*Plant sources:* vitamin D fortified foods such as non-dairy milks, juices, cereals and margarine; mushrooms exposed to UVB rays *Animal sources:* fish, liver, egg yolks, fortified foods such as milk

Table 5.2: Summary Chart—Vitamins *(continued)*

Micro-nutrient	RDA or AI (daily)	Primary Functions	Considerations for Plant-Based Eaters	Deficiencies/ Excesses	Richest Food Sources
Vitamin E	RDA Units—mg 0–6 m—4 7–12 m—5 1–3 y—6 4–8 y—7 9–13 y—11 14+ y—15 P + L—19	Antioxidant— protect cells against free radical damage Immune function Prevent blood clotting	Plant-based eaters generally meet or exceed the RDA and have higher intakes than omnivores. Intakes can be low in those eating very low-fat plant-based diets. Eight different chemical forms of vitamin E, but alpha tocopherol appears the most important for human nutrition.	*Deficiency:* nerve and muscle damage, loss of feeling in arms and legs, loss of muscle control, muscle weakness, vision problems, poor immune response. *Excess:* No excess from food. High doses from supplements may increase risk of bleeding, and hemorrhagic stroke. Do not exceed the UL of 1,000 mg/day (this equals 1,500 IU natural vitamin E or 1,100 IU synthetic).	*Plant sources:* Nuts and seeds (especially sunflower seeds, almonds, peanuts), wheat germ, vegetable oils, avocados, fruits and vegetables *Animal sources:* small amounts in fish, oysters, butter, cheese, eggs
Vitamin K	AI—Units—mcg 0–6 m—2 7–12 m—2.5 1–3 y—30 4–8 y—55 9–13 y—60 14–18 y—60 19+ y (F)—90 19+ (M)—120 P + L—90	Synthesis of proteins needed for blood clotting Bone metabolism Blood calcium regulation	Plant-based eaters generally meet or exceed the RDA. Plant foods are the main dietary sources; animal products have much lower amounts. K2 (in natto and animal products) is the active form; K1 (from plant foods) is converted to K2 by intestinal bacteria. K2 from natto or supplements may be warranted after antibiotic therapy.	*Deficiency:* Bruising, bleeding, hemorrhage (in severe cases), reduced bone strength, and increased risk of osteoporosis. Risk higher in the early infancy and in adults with malabsorption disorders. *Excess:* Not generally, although high intakes can interfere with anticoagulant medications such as warfarin.	*Plant sources (as K1):* leafy green vegetables, other vegetables and fruits, seaweed, lentils, peas, soy foods, natto (K2), vegetable oils *Animal sources (as K2):* Poultry, seafoods, fish, meat

Sources: [21, 37, 58, 59, 60]

Recent research suggests that carotenoid absorption is affected by our genes. In some individuals, this means a reduced ability to convert pro-vitamin A carotenoids into vitamin A.[61, 62] This has raised concerns that plant-exclusive diets could be lacking in vitamin A and that some individuals need animal products for preformed vitamin A. This is not the case. Those with reduced conversion ability still convert, though at a reduced rate. Eating more carotenoid-rich foods, including vitamin A-fortified foods such as non-dairy milks, or taking a multivitamin with small amounts of preformed vitamin A are reasonable solutions.

VITAMINS ... A FINAL WORD

In summary, the shift to a more whole food, plant-based way of eating is generally associated with increased intakes of vitamin C, folate, vitamin E, and vitamin K compared with mixed, omnivorous diets. Intakes of vitamin A and most B vitamins are usually within the recommended range, and similar to intakes on a mixed diet, while intakes of vitamin B12 and vitamin D can fall below intakes of omnivores. For vitamin B12, we need to rely on fortified foods and/or supplements. For vitamin D, if we lack access to sunshine, we need to rely on a supplement, as fortified foods rarely provide enough. It is important to note that both of these nutrients are commonly low in omnivorous diets as well. Older individuals (50+ years) cannot rely on any animal products for vitamin B12 as their ability to extract B12 from animal foods is often limited. Almost everyone is short on vitamin D, especially if living in regions with cooler climates. Where vitamins are concerned, varied plant-based diets have you covered, when reliable sources of vitamins B12 and D are included.

Where vitamins are concerned, varied plant-based diets have you covered, when reliable sources of vitamins B12 and D are included.

MINERALS

In human nutrition, minerals are inorganic (non-carbon containing) chemical elements that our bodies cannot make, but require for survival, so must be consumed. These chemicals are critical to the workings of the multiple dynamic systems that support and sustain our bodies. For example, they play significant roles in the formation of bones and teeth, manufacturing enzymes, hormones, and neurotransmitters, sending messages to nerve cells, forming red blood cells, destroying foreign proteins, building and rebuilding body tissues, fighting inflammation, curbing free radical reactions, maintaining electrolyte and acid/base balance, and extracting energy from foods.

Minerals are released from decaying matter into the soil with the help of bacteria and fungi, then absorbed into plants. Without exception, plants can provide every mineral humans need for their survival. Minerals are virtually indestructible. Even if we burn food so all that remains is a pile of ashes, those ashes are minerals from the food that could not be destroyed.

Minerals fall into one of two categories: major or macrominerals and trace elements or trace minerals. Major minerals are those needed by the body in relatively large amounts (at least 100 mg to hundreds of grams) and they include calcium, chloride, magnesium, phosphorus, potassium, sodium, and sulfur. Trace minerals are those we need in tiny amounts (milligrams or micrograms) and these include chromium, cobalt, copper, fluoride, iodine, iron, manganese, molybdenum, selenium, and zinc. There are also ultratrace elements that are considered possibly essential, but this is not yet confirmed. Examples include arsenic, boron, bromine, lithium, nickel, strontium, silicon, and vanadium. Plant-based diets deliver most minerals in abundance. However, a few minerals do invite special attention, including calcium, iodine, iron, and zinc. The balance of this chapter will explore the finer details of these minerals and discuss strategies for meeting needs.

> Plant-based diets deliver most minerals in abundance. However, a few minerals do invite special attention, including calcium, iodine, iron, and zinc.

Table 5.6 provides a brief summary of the key information on the minerals that have Recommended Dietary Allowances (RDA) or adequate intakes (AI) associated with them.

CALCIUM

Brenda (co-author) had been fully plant-based for twenty years when she went in for her annual physical exam. Her doctor asked her about her family health history and the question of osteoporosis came up. Brenda's mother had been diagnosed with osteoporosis at fifty years of age, and Brenda was forty-nine at that time. Considering her family history, her race (Caucasian) and stature (slim), and the fact that she had been dairy-free for twenty years, he was concerned. He ordered a DEXA scan, the gold standard test for osteoporosis, which measured bone density in the spine and femur. When she went to get her results two weeks later, the doctor opened her file and his jaw dropped. He had fully expected to see reduced bone density, but what he saw made him question much of what he had learned about diet and osteoporosis. Brenda's lumbar spine T-score (bone density) was 2.5 standard deviations above expected, and right femur T-score (bone density) was almost 2 standard deviations above expected. Osteoporosis is defined as a T-score of -2.5 or 2.5 standard deviations below expected—Brenda was at the opposite end of the spectrum. Admittedly bewildered, the doctor said, "I don't know what you are doing, but keep doing it." She shared two things that she believed were responsible—the first was daily, intense exercise, and the second was a well-designed plant-based diet, with plenty of calcium and other bone-building nutrients, including vitamin D, vitamin K, potassium and magnesium. The doctor asked her how she got calcium without milk, and she told him about fortified, nondairy milks, tofu made with calcium, low oxalate greens, beans, nuts, and seeds. For him, it was all a bit of a revelation.

What Is Calcium and Why Is It Important?

Calcium is the fifth most abundant element on earth, and the most plentiful mineral in the human body. About 99 percent of the calcium in the body is stored in the bones and teeth, while about 1 percent is reserved for critical nonstructural functions, like every beat of your heart! Calcium is essential for the contraction and dilation of blood vessels, muscle relaxation, nerve cell transmission, blood coagulation, and the regulation of cell metabolism. Our blood levels of calcium are tightly regulated because if they dip too low, the consequences can be catastrophic. When our blood levels start to fall, the parathyroid glands release parathyroid hormone (PTH) into the bloodstream to rapidly restore calcium levels—calcium absorption from the intestines is ramped up, calcium is reclaimed from the kidneys, and calcium is extracted from the bones.

Does Milk Really Do the Body Good?

Most of us were conditioned to believe that *"milk does the body good,"* but the science to support this contention is weak. In 2020, Harvard researchers released a comprehensive review on milk and health. They looked at the current evidence as it relates to growth and development, bone health and fracture risk, body weight and obesity, blood pressure and cardiovascular disease, diabetes, cancer, allergies and intolerance, and total mortality. Overall, dairy compared favorably with processed and red meat, but not so favorably with plant-protein sources such as nuts.[63]

There is no question that cow's milk is a concentrated source of calcium, with about 300 mg per cup of milk. Cow's milk is high in calcium because it is designed to promote the growth of big bones in short order. However, declaring the milk of one species of mammal essential for the health of another species defies rationality. Humans have no more requirement for cow's milk than they have for moose milk, which incidentally, is about twice as concentrated in calcium as cow's milk. So, why does the American government recommend three 8-ounce glasses a day for all those nine years of age or older, and two to two and a half cups for younger children?[64] The primary justification is that milk and milk products will help meet needs for calcium, and that by doing so, it will contribute to bone health and reduced risk of bone fractures. Cow's milk can help boost calcium intakes, though recommended intakes are highly variable among nations. Needs are affected by a multitude of factors, such as diet and lifestyle choices, health status, medications, age, and genetics.

Prior to the advent of animal husbandry, humans averaged an estimated 1,000 to 1,500 mg calcium without a single drop of cow's milk.[65] Even today, it is possible to obtain sufficient calcium without cow's milk, as people manage to do in cultures that consume little or no dairy. As for bone health, dairy intake does not seem to be a very reliable predictor of osteoporosis or bone fractures.[63] In fact, some of the highest rates of hip fractures occur in countries with the highest dairy intakes, while some of the lowest rates are found in countries with the lowest dairy intakes. While this does not prove that dairy causes osteoporosis, it is a pretty good indication that dairy is not necessary for strong bones.

While dairy consumption is common among many healthy populations, including several of the Blue Zones, there are potential downsides of dairy consumption. Approximately 70 percent of the global population is lactose-intolerant, with the highest rates occurring in people of African, Asian, and South American decent.[66] Lactose intolerance can cause abdominal pain, bloating, gas, diarrhea, and nausea. International comparisons suggest dairy consumption is correlated with prostate, breast, and other cancers, which may be driven by Insulin Growth Factor -1 (IGF-1).[63] The strength of the evidence is strongest for prostate cancer, particularly more aggressive forms.[67,68] Although the evidence is mixed for breast cancer, a recent AHS-2 report of 61,000 woman found that intake of milk was associated with a 41 percent increased risk of breast cancer when comparing those in the 90th to 10th percentiles of intake. When cow's milk was substituted for soy milk, risk was reduced by 34 percent.[69]

How Do Plant-Based Eaters Do?

Calcium intakes in plant-predominant eaters who include dairy (e.g., lacto-ovo vegetarians) are similar to or higher than that of omnivores, with amounts generally being close to or above the RDA.[70,71] In contrast, calcium intakes of plant-exclusive eaters are typically lower than for dairy consumers, ranging from less than 400 mg among Buddhist nuns[72,73] to over 900 mg among North American vegans.[2] However, bone mineral density and fracture risk do appear somewhat higher among plant-based eaters who do not consume adequate calcium with plant-exclusive eaters being at the highest risk.[74] Differences in bone mineral density appear to be largely explained by the lower BMIs of plant-based eaters,[75] although in some cases, lower calcium and vitamin D intakes may be contributing factors. For example, an EPIC-Oxford study including almost 35,000 participants reported a 30 percent increase in fracture risk for vegans compared to omnivores.[76] However, when vegans consuming less than 525 mg calcium per day were excluded, fracture risk was identical to that of omnivores. The authors concluded that higher calcium intakes were protective and that vegans should strive to consume at least 525 mg calcium per day. The take-home message is that while a plant-exclusive diet doesn't guarantee strong bones, neither does it preclude them.

> While a plant-exclusive diet doesn't guarantee strong bones, neither does it preclude them.

Can We Get Enough Calcium Without Dairy?

The short answer is yes, without a doubt. However, we cannot assume that all plant-based diets provide enough calcium. Plant-based diets need to be designed to include adequate calcium sources, especially for children who have high needs while they are growing. However calcium intake is not the only factor affecting the body's calcium balance—calcium absorption and excretion (what is lost in mainly in urine and feces) also come into play. Calcium absorption can be reduced by oxalates in plants, for example, and excretion can be increased by excess sodium.

Let's assume we are aiming for 1,000 mg of calcium per day from plant foods (the amount needed for 4- to 8-year-old children, women to age 50, and men to age 70—see Table 5.6 for the RDA at other ages and stages). Step one is to get familiar with plant foods that provide reasonable amounts of absorbable calcium. Low-oxalate, dark, leafy greens like broccoli, bok choy, Chinese greens, kale, Napa cabbage, watercress, mustard greens, and turnip greens are wonderful choices. Fortified non-dairy milks, and other calcium-fortified foods, tofu set with calcium, many legumes, nuts, seeds, and blackstrap molasses are also significant contributors of available calcium. From low-oxalate greens, we absorb about 40 to 60 percent of the calcium present. Absorption of calcium is about 30 to 32 percent in tofu and nondairy milks, which is comparable to cow's milk. We absorb an estimated 50 percent of the calcium in fortified orange juice, and around 20 percent from almonds, tahini, beans, and sweet potatoes. See Table 5.3 for the calcium content of common foods. Step two is to recognize foods that contain quite a bit of calcium, but due to the presence of oxalates (a key inhibitor of calcium absorption), the calcium is largely unavailable. Oxalates are tightly bound combinations of oxalic acid and minerals (e.g. calcium) that resist breakdown during food preparation and digestion. Spinach is a good example of a high oxalate green. It provides 243 mg calcium per cup of cooked spinach, however, because of its high-oxalate content, we only absorb about 5 percent of what is present. The story is similar for other high oxalate greens such as beet greens and Swiss chard. Some greens such as collard and dandelion greens have medium oxalate content, so we absorb intermediate amounts of calcium. If you use a higher-oxalate green such as spinach in a salad, it does not interfere with the absorption of calcium from lower oxalate greens such as kale. Boiling high-oxalate greens can reduce oxalate content by 30 to 87 percent, depending on the boiling time. Steaming is less effective (5 to 53 percent reduction), and dry-heat cooking appears to have little impact on oxalate content.[77]

Table 5.3: Calcium Content of Common Foods

FOOD	PORTION SIZE	CALCIUM (mg)
Fortified non-dairy milk	1 cup	300–450
Yogurt, plain	1 cup	296
Cow's milk, 2%	1 cup	293
Spinach, cooked*	1 cup	243
Tofu, raw (made with calcium sulfate)	½ cup	200–860 (check label—highly variable)
Blackstrap molasses	2 tablespoons	200–400 (check label)
Cheddar cheese	1 ounce	200
Broccoli raab, cooked	1 cup	199
Soybeans, cooked	1 cup	184

Kale, cooked	1 cup	177
Sesame seeds	2 tablespoons	176
Bok choy, cooked	1 cup	168
Beet greens*	1 cup	163
White beans, cooked	1 cup	161
Chia seeds	2 tablespoons	133
Tahini	2 tablespoons	128
Navy beans, cooked	1 cup	126
Okra, cooked	1 cup	124
Edamame, shelled	1 cup	122
Kale, raw, chopped	1 cup	120
Almond butter	2 tablespoons	112
Black turtle beans	1 cup	102
Swiss chard, cooked*	1 cup	102
Almonds	¼ cup	96
Pinto beans	1 cup	92
Parsley**	1 cup	83
Chickpeas	1 cup	80
Orange	1 large	74
Broccoli, steamed	1 cup	62
Sweet potato	1 medium	43
Flaxseeds, ground	2 tablespoons	40

Source: [20]

*Very high oxalate content; minimal calcium absorption[78]

**Very high oxalate content, but due to very high calcium content, and low oxalate:calcium ratio, calcium appears available.[78]

Note: The DV for calcium is 1000 mg, so 10% of the DV is 100 mg.

As you see, it can be challenging to get calcium to 1,000 mg a day, especially for a four- to eight-year-old child. The following tips can help you reach the goal:

1. Add 1 to 3 cups of fortified non-dairy milk (or other fortified foods) each day. Each cup of fortified nondairy milk provides about 300 to 450 mg calcium or more. Consider other calcium-fortified foods such as cold cereals and orange juice, if necessary.

2. Use calcium-set tofu. The amount of calcium is quite variable so check the label.

3. Make low-oxalate greens a part of the daily diet. Include them at least twice a day. Get kids involved in growing, selecting, and preparing greens. Add them to salads, rolls, smoothies, stir fries, soups, stews, side dishes, sandwiches, and veggie and dip trays. Find recipes your family loves.

4. Include calcium-rich choices within each food group.
    a. Vegetables—low-oxalate greens, broccoli, okra, yams
    b. Legumes—black turtle beans, edamame, great Northern beans, navy beans, soybeans, white beans
    c. Nuts and seeds—almonds and almond butter, chia seeds, tahini
    d. Fruits—oranges, figs
    e. Grains—amaranth, tortillas (with added calcium)

5. Use blackstrap molasses in place of other sweeteners, when possible. Use in power balls, cookies, and muffins, along with other calcium stars such as tahini, almonds or almond butter, and figs.

Can I Get Too Much Calcium?

Yes, it is possible to get too much calcium, although this is more of a concern with calcium supplements than with calcium from foods. It is preferable to get calcium from foods, when possible. Excessive calcium can contribute to constipation, calcification of soft tissues and blood vessels, and kidney damage. It may also interfere with the absorption of iron and zinc. There is some evidence that high intakes could increase the risk of prostate cancer and heart disease. The daily Upper Limit (UL) for calcium is 2,500 mg for children one to eight years, 3,000 mg for those nine to eighteen years, 2,500 mg for adults nineteen to fifty years, and 2,000 mg for those above fifty years.[37]

Are There Additional Steps I Can Take to Ensure Bone Health for Myself and My Children?

Absolutely, osteoporosis is not a dairy-deficiency disease. It is a multifactorial disease, and getting sufficient calcium, mainly from foods, is just one of the many steps you can take to help build and maintain strong bones for life. Here are some others:

- Work your bones—exercise is critical to building and maintaining strong bones—aim for sixty minutes each day. Include a mix of weight-bearing, cardio, and strength exercises.
- Ensure a reliable source of vitamin D—sunshine, fortified foods, or supplements.
- Include adequate protein. Studies have demonstrated that getting sufficient protein protects bones (while very high intakes, especially without adequate calcium, can be detrimental).[79, 80, 81]
- Avoid being underweight or obese, as both can increase risk of poor bone health in children and adults.[82, 83, 84]
- Eat more fruits and vegetables, as intake improves bone health.
- Go lightly on salt as it can increase calcium losses in the urine.
- Ensure a sufficient intake of bone-friendly vitamins, such as vitamin K, vitamin C, and folate (see Table 5.2 for dietary sources).
- Ensure sufficient bone-building minerals such as potassium, magnesium, and boron. (see Table 5.6 for dietary sources; the richest sources of boron are flaxseeds, prune juice, avocados, raisins, peanuts and peanut butter, fruits, vegetables, and legumes).
- Avoid smoking and excess alcohol.[85, 86, 87]

IODINE

Marylynn was a very conscious mother of three children, ages nine, six, and four years. They were energetic little bundles of joy, and she was determined to keep them healthy. She followed an almost exclusively, dairy- and meat-free plant-based diet. Marylynn favored less processed choices, with short ingredient lists and was big on preparing foods from scratch. After reading an article about the perils of iodized table salt, she switched to a natural salt. The salt she chose boasted eighty-four trace minerals and elements and no aluminum-laden anti-caking agents. When Marylynn mentioned her find to a plant-based friend, she was surprised by her response. Her friend asked her how she was replacing the iodine that the table salt provided. Marylynn had assumed there was enough iodine in the soil and her family would get ample from plants. With some internet digging, she learned that iodine in plant foods varied tremendously with soil, and that needs are seldom met from these foods alone. Common dietary sources include fish, seafood, dairy products, and eggs, but for plant-exclusive eaters, the main natural source is seaweed. The only time her family ate seaweed was when they had veggie sushi, which was only once every three or four months. She found an excellent article that examined differences in salts and learned that the contribution of minerals from natural salts is miniscule. In addition, among the eighty-four minerals and elements listed in her natural salts were tiny amounts of lead, mercury, arsenic, cadmium, and uranium. She discovered that the anti-caking agents used in table salt did not always contain aluminum (as sodium aluminosilicate on the label)—some are calcium or magnesium-based, and the amounts are so small that they are considered safe. Still Marylynn preferred to avoid the anti-caking agents, so she settled for an iodized sea salt and a little more seaweed.

What Is Iodine and Why Is It Important?

Iodine is a trace element that is necessary for the production of thyroid hormones that regulate many body functions, including protein synthesis, enzyme activity, metabolism, and nervous system development of the fetus and infant. Iodine also plays a role in our immune response and appears to reduce risk of fibrocystic breast disease. Iodine deficiency affects our ability to produce thyroid hormones, often causing hypothyroidism. Common symptoms include weight gain, elevated blood cholesterol, fatigue, weakness, hair loss, dry, flaky skin, intolerance to cold, depression, poor memory, heavy periods, and constipation. During pregnancy, chronic iodine deficiency can spell tragedy for the unborn baby, causing growth and cognitive losses, and, in some cases, miscarriage or stillbirth. In its most severe form, iodine deficiency can cause congenital hypothyroidism in the infant—a condition marked by intellectual disability, compromised physical growth and development, enlarged tongue, protruding abdomen, hair loss, and infertility. Even marginal iodine deficiency in infants and children can compromise brain function, leading to lower than average IQ.[59, 88] This is a massive public health concern, as it has been reported that more than 50 percent of woman of childbearing age have iodine levels below what the World Health Organization deems adequate. The situation is especially concerning in developing countries where salt is not iodized.[89]

Are People Eating Plant-Based Diets at Higher Risk for Iodine Deficiency?

People eating exclusively plant-based may be at greater risk for iodine deficiency, although there are just a handful of studies that have addressed this question. A study in the Boston area reported on urinary iodine levels (we excrete over 90 percent of the iodine we consume) in vegans and lacto-ovo vegetarians.[90] Average urinary iodine in vegans fell below the threshold of adequacy, while lacto-ovo vegetarians were within the normal range. Studies from Europe also suggest low intakes in plant-exclusive eaters, particularly those who avoid iodized salt and seaweed.[4,91,92]

What Foods Supply Iodine?

Natural iodine sources are relatively limited in the food supply. Iodine is most concentrated in seaweed, fish and shellfish, dairy products, and eggs. It is interesting to note that dairy products are not naturally rich in iodine. In dairy products, iodine comes from animal feed that is fortified with iodine and iodine-containing sanitizing agents used by the dairy industry.[88] Plants grown in iodine-rich soil can also be significant sources. Because iodine deficiency affects about 2 billion people worldwide, iodizing salt proved a very cost-effective solution, and many governments around the world made it mandatory. In the United States, although iodization is voluntary, about 70 percent of the table salt available is iodized. One half teaspoon of salt provides close to the RDA for adults. It is important to note that salt used in processed foods is not usually iodized, nor are salty seasonings like soy sauce or tamari. Table 5.4 provides the iodine content of common foods.

Table 5.4: Iodine in Common Foods

FOOD	SERVING SIZE	IODINE (mcg)
Kelp granules*	½ teaspoon	1,200
Dulce granules*	½ teaspoon	150
Iodized sea salt	½ teaspoon	142
Cod	3 ounces	99
Wakame*	½ teaspoon	67
Yogurt, plain	1 cup	75
Nori*	1 sheet	57
Cow's milk	1 cup	56
Shrimp	3 ounces	35
Egg	1 large	24

Prunes, dried	5 medium	13
Lima beans, cooked	½ cup	8
Banana	1 medium	3

Sources: [93, 88, 94]

*iodine content varies widely depending on source

How to Boost Iodine in a Plant-Based Diet

Babies seven to twelve months need 130 mcg iodine per day, those one to eight years need 90 mcg per day, nine to thirteen year olds need 120 mcg per day, and teens and adults ages fourteen or more need 150 mcg iodine per day (see Table 5.6 for recommended intakes at other ages and stages). Plant-predominant eaters who include iodine-rich animal products (e.g. fish, seafood, dairy, eggs) will likely get plenty of iodine even if intake from iodized salt is low. Plant-exclusive eaters need to rely mostly on iodized salt, seaweed, or supplements, as land plants rarely provide enough.

Although salt iodization has long been viewed as an important public health triumph, there are concerns that too much salt contributes to hypertension, heart disease, and premature death.[89] However, as most people do use some added salt, it is wise to select an iodized salt or iodized sea salt for the added salt we do use. If you are using iodized salt as the main source of iodine, you will need about one quarter teaspoon for children ages one to eight years, one third of a teaspoon for children nine to thirteen years, and one half teaspoon for those fourteen years or more. One quarter teaspoon supplies about 582 mg sodium and one third teaspoon provides about 777 mg sodium. The Institute of Medicine suggests a cut off for sodium called the Chronic Disease Risk Reduction Intake (CDRR) which is 1,200 mg for toddlers one to three years of age, 1,500 mg for children ages four to eight years, 1,800 mg for those nine to thirteen years, and 2,300 mg for those 14 years or more. Intakes should be reduced if they exceed the CDRR.[95]

For those who prefer, seaweed can be used as the primary iodine source, although it is important to be aware that the iodine content of seaweed is highly variable, and intakes can easily be excessive. Hijiki should be avoided completely due to arsenic contamination. If you and your family don't enjoy seaweed, a tiny sprinkle of kelp powder in soup or on salad is virtually undetectable (¹⁄₁₆ of a tsp provides about 150 mcg iodine—the RDA for an adult). Be very cautious about serving size, as iodine concentrations in kelp are very high, so the upper limit can be reached with less than one-half teaspoon kelp powder. If you are pregnant or lactating, make sure your prenatal supplement contains iodine (many do not)—the RDA is 220 mcg during pregnancy and 290 mcg during lactation.

Should I Avoid Goitrogens from Foods?

Goitrogens are substances that can interfere with iodine uptake in the thyroid gland and depress thyroid hormone production. Foods with significant goitrogen content include nutritious dietary staples such as cassava, cruciferous vegetables (e.g., broccoli, Brussels sprouts, cabbage, cauliflower, collards, kale, kohlrabi, and turnips), flaxseeds, lima beans, millet, peaches, peanuts, soybeans, strawberries, sweet potatoes, and teas (e.g., green, white and black). Cooking or fermenting can reduce goitrogens in some of these foods.[96] There are also goitrogens present in the environment, such as perchlorates in polluted water, chemicals in fertilizers, pesticides, and cigarette smoke.[89] Goitrogens do not need to be avoided in healthy individuals who are consuming sufficient iodine. For people with thyroid disorders, goitrogens can worsen thyroid function so it is best to consult with your endocrinologist.[97]

Can I Get Too Much Iodine?

Yes, high intakes of iodine can inhibit thyroid hormone production, thereby causing similar symptoms to inadequate intakes. In some individuals, excessive intakes can trigger hyperthyroidism which can lead to heat intolerance, excessive sweating, increased appetite, weight loss, anxiety, rapid or irregular heartbeat, difficulty sleeping, and more frequent bowel movements. Most often, excess comes from supplements, but it can also come from seaweed. The daily Upper Limit (UL) is 200 mcg for toddlers one to three years, 300 mcg for children four to eight years, 600 mcg for children nine to thirteen years, 900 mcg for teens fourteen to eighteen years, and 1,100 mcg for adults nineteen years or more.[59, 88]

IRON

Ben was a healthy, happy full-term baby. His mother, Claire, breastfed him for eleven months, and started him on solids at six months. As Claire was weaning Ben, she offered whole cow's milk in a bottle, so by one year of age, Ben was drinking about 28 ounces of milk each day. The family followed a plant-predominant diet, with some fish, dairy products, and eggs. Apart from milk, Ben's favorite foods were macaroni and cheese and grilled cheese sandwiches. He was happy to eat bits of other foods, but his appetite was small. By fourteen months of age, Claire began to notice that Ben was not as energetic as he used to be, and he was pale and fussy. When she took him to the doctor, blood tests confirmed that Ben had low iron levels. The doctor explained that high intakes of cow's milk and dairy products can contribute to iron deficiency in infants and toddlers. She suggested that Ben's milk be reduced to 16 ounces a day, that iron rich foods such as infant cereal and legumes be served regularly, and that a supplement with iron be provided. Within a couple of weeks, Claire observed improvements in Ben's energy and mood, and she was greatly reassured that the simple modifications were working their magic.

What Is Iron and Why Is It Important?

Iron is a mineral that is vital to health. The body uses iron in its production of hemoglobin and myoglobin, proteins that bind and transport oxygen. Hemoglobin is the component of red blood cells that binds and carries oxygen from the lungs to the rest of the body. Myoglobin takes oxygen from red blood cells, carries it to muscle tissues, and stores it so oxygen can be available as needed for working muscles. Iron is required to support physical growth and brain development. It plays a role in many enzyme systems, the immune system, and hormone production.

Iron deficiency is the most common nutritional deficiency in the world, and the most common cause of anemia, which affects an estimated 25 percent of the global population and approximately 50 percent of preschool children.[98, 99] The most common causes are insufficient dietary iron (due to limited diets in poverty stricken areas or to high milk intake), blood loss (due to cancer, ulcers, parasites, etc.), and disorders of nutrient absorption.[98] Infants and toddlers are at increased risk, especially if they are born premature. Eighty percent of iron stores are accumulated during the last trimester of pregnancy, so premature infants have limited reserves and typically require supplementation.[100]

Common symptoms of iron deficiency include weakness, fatigue, reduced mental performance, shortness of breath, cold intolerance, paleness, dry skin and hair, dizziness, restless leg syndrome, and pica (compulsion to eat non-food material such as dirt). In children, we also see behavior and mood shifts, loss of appetite, recurrent infections, and failure to thrive. Infants and children have very high iron needs relative to adults (see Table 5.6). For example, the RDA is 11 mg for a 7- to 12-month-old baby, 7 mg for a 1- to 3-year-old child, 10 mg for a 4- to 8-year-old child, and 8 mg for an adult man. So, meeting needs is a greater challenge for our little ones.

Are Plant-Based Eaters at Higher Risk for Iron Deficiency?

The results of studies assessing the iron status of plant-based adults are highly variable, although iron stores (serum ferritin levels) are consistently lower among plant-based eaters than among omnivores.[101, 102] Interestingly, this may turn out to be an advantage as high iron stores are associated with increased risk of developing metabolic syndrome,[103] diabetes,[104] cardiovascular diseases[105] and some forms of cancer.[106, 107] Within vegetarian populations, there is tremendous variability in status, with the average markers of iron status being in the normal range.[108] On the other hand, some plant-based eaters, particularly premenopausal women, may be at increased risk.[102] Iron status in children may also be somewhat lower among vegetarians compared to omnivores, although inadequate iron status is common among all dietary groups.[108]

Iron intakes of people eating plant-based are typically similar to or higher than that of omnivores.[1, 2] The reasons why vegetarians may experience somewhat higher levels of iron deficiency are that the iron in plant foods is less bioavailable than it is in animal products and plant foods contain a number of compounds that can inhibit iron absorption. Fortunately, both of these factors are easily mitigated.

How Can I Maximize Iron Intake and Absorption from Food?

There are two types of iron in foods—heme and non-heme iron. Heme iron is the type of iron in blood and muscle tissue, so is only present in animal flesh like meat, poultry, and fish. Heme iron is rapidly and relatively efficiently absorbed at a rate of about 15 to 35 percent.[109] Non-heme iron is present in both plant and animal foods, and it is absorbed less efficiently, at an estimated rate of 1 to 34 percent.[110] The rate of absorption of non-heme iron is dependent on the iron status of the individual (the lower your iron levels, the more you absorb), dietary iron inhibitors, and enhancers of iron absorption. Nonheme iron absorption can increase ten-fold in iron deficient individuals compared with those who have normal iron levels.[111, 112]

The key inhibitors of iron absorption are phytates (concentrated in bran, whole grains, and legumes), polyphenolic compounds (in tea, cocoa, spinach, and some other plant foods), and calcium (in dairy products and plant foods). Wheat bran is the most concentrated source of phytates so avoid sprinkling it on foods, or relying regularly on concentrated bran cereals. Phytates are reduced by sprouting, soaking, cooking, fermenting, and leavening.[113, 114] It is best to drink tea separately from meals to reduce impact on iron absorption, especially if iron status is low. Contrary to popular opinion, oxalates have not been shown to be significant inhibitors of iron absorption.[115] The iron absorption from spinach is low because of the high polyphenol content, not the high oxalate content. If using dairy products, keep intake to three servings per day or less, and serve milk between, instead of with, iron-rich meals.

The most impressive enhancers of iron absorption are foods rich in vitamin C and organic acids such as peppers, tomatoes, citrus fruits, and other fruits and vegetables. Other foods that appear to enhance iron absorption are allium vegetables such as garlic and onion, beta-carotene rich foods such as carrots, and spices such as pepper, turmeric, and ginger.[113]

In 2001, the Institute of Medicine recommended vegetarians consume 1.8 times more iron than nonvegetarians due to the lower digestibility of iron from plant foods.[59] However, this recommendation was based on limited data assuming maximum intake of iron absorption inhibitors and minimal intake of absorption enhancers. As this is not typical of vegetarian intakes, and more current evidence suggests adaptation to lower intakes over time, this is no longer considered necessary.[112] Nonetheless, a small increase in intake over the RDAs may be helpful for some individuals.

The richest plant sources of iron are legumes, tofu, nuts, seeds, some vegetables, and fortified foods such as breakfast cereals and meat analogs. The richest animal sources are organ meats, red meat, and shellfish. Table 5.5 provides a list of common food sources of iron.

Table 5.5: Iron Content of Common Foods

FOOD	PORTION SIZE	IRON (mg)
Fortified breakfast cereal containing 100% of the DV*	1 ounce	18
Cream of wheat, cooked	1 cup	12
Infant cereal, fortified, dry**	¼ cup	8.6
White beans, canned	1 cup	7.8
Blackstrap molasses	2 tablespoons	7.2
Chocolate, 70–85%	2 ounces	6.7
Lentils, cooked	1 cup	6.6
Spinach, cooked***	1 cup	6.4
Oysters, cooked	3 ounces	6
Black turtle beans	1 cup	5.3
Beef liver, cooked	3 ounces	5.2
Kidney beans	1 cup	5
Navy beans, cooked	1 cup	4.9
Chickpeas	1 cup	4.7
Adzuki beans, cooked	1 cup	4.6
Asparagus, cooked	1 cup	4.4
Lima beans	1 cup	4.2
Edamame, shelled	1 cup	4
Hempseeds	¼ cup	3.6
Tofu, firm	½ cup	3.4
Chia seeds	¼ cup	3.1
Kamut berries	1 cup	3
Quinoa, cooked	1 cup	2.8
Pumpkin seeds	¼ cup	2.4
Green peas, cooked	1 cup	2.4
Sunflower seeds	¼ cup	2.3
Beef, lean only, broiled	3 ounces	2
Bok choy, cooked	1 cup	1.8
Veggie patty	1	1.7

Prune juice	4 ounces	1.5
Whole wheat bread	2 slices	1.4
Cashews	¼ cup	1.4
Tahini	2 tablespoons	1.3
Almonds	¼ cup	1.3
Almond butter	2 tablespoons	1.1
Sweet potato	1 medium	1.1
Soy milk	1 cup	1.1
Kale, cooked	1 cup	1
Chicken breast, baked	3 ounces	0.9
Fish (cod), poached	3 ounces	0.2
Cow's milk, whole	1 cup	0.07

Source: [20]

*The DV for iron is 18 mg, so 100% of the DV is 18 mg and 50% would be 9 mg, etc. Many ready-to-eat cereals are very high in iron—read the labels.

**Amounts vary—read labels.

***Bioavailability low due to polyphenolic compounds.

What Can I Do to Protect My Infant or Toddler from Iron Deficiency?

Preventing iron deficiency during infancy is absolutely critical to healthy growth and development. Here are some basic guidelines to protect your infants and young children.

Preterm Infant: Breastfed preterm infants typically require an iron supplement at the rate of 2 mg/kg per day beginning at one month of age through twelve months of age. Those on iron-fortified formula may not need additional iron, but some may, depending on their iron status. Preterm iron status is highly variable depending gestational age, postnatal growth rate, blood transfusions, and other factors, so follow your pediatrician's recommendations.[100]

Full-term Infant: For breastfed infants, select iron-rich foods as the first solids, and talk to your pediatrician about whether your baby may need an iron supplement from four months until she consumes enough iron-rich solid foods to meet the RDA (e.g., two servings of iron-fortified infant cereal). For formula-fed infants, iron-fortified formula is recommended until twelve months.[100]

All Infants and Toddlers:

- Cow's milk is not recommended before one year of age as it can cause iron deficiency.[100] Cow's milk is low in iron, inhibits the absorption of iron, and, in infants under a year of age, it can invoke substantial blood loss (and iron loss) in the stools.[100, 116]
- Between ages one and five, do not provide more than 3 cups (24 ounces) of cow's milk a day.[117]
- Go lightly on other dairy products such as cottage cheese, cheese, and yogurt, particularly if your child consumes 2 or more cups of milk a day.
- Include a variety of iron-rich foods. The first solid foods should be iron-rich choices, such as iron-fortified infant cereal. Iron-fortified infant cereal can be continued during the toddler years—add to other cereals, pancakes, muffins, and cookies (use about ⅔ flour, ⅓ iron-fortified infant cereal—see recipes on pages 380 and 381). If you are predominantly or fully plant-based, include plenty of iron-rich foods such as lentils, beans, and tofu in the diet. Meat, poultry, and fish provide highly absorbable iron for those who include these products.
- Serve iron-rich plant foods with foods that help enhance absorption, such as those rich in vitamin C. For example, when serving Rustic Lentil Soup (page 350), add a squeeze of fresh lemon before serving.
- Limit foods that reduce iron absorption, such as concentrated wheat bran.

Can I Get Too Much Iron?

Yes, absolutely! Excessive iron can be harmful. For most people, iron from dietary sources is not an issue, unless you have hemochromatosis, a disorder associated with iron buildup in the body. For those with hemochromatosis, a plant-based diet is helpful as it eliminates the highly absorbable heme iron. Also, affected individuals are advised to avoid supplements with iron or vitamin C (which enhances iron absorption). For healthy individuals, iron excess is usually the result of supplements.[118] Accidental ingestion of concentrated iron supplements can be lethal for children. One study reported that 30 percent of accidental poisoning deaths in children were due to accidental ingestion of iron supplements.[119]

ZINC

In the first half of the twentieth century, there was good evidence that zinc was essential for some plants, poultry, rodents, and pigs. However, it was not until the early 1960s that Dr. Ananda Prasad made the connection between a syndrome marked by extreme growth retardation and hypogonadism (small genitals) in villagers near Shiraz, Iran, and zinc status.[120, 121] Affected individuals were subsisting on unleavened bread with few other foods. Unleavened breads are high in phytates that impair the absorption of the limited zinc that is present (leavening, by contrast, breaks down phytates making the zinc more absorbable). His team found a similar situation in Egypt, where zinc supplementation in affected individuals resulted in normalization of genitalia within three to six months, and a 5- to 6-inch increase in height within a year. The idea that zinc might be essential to humans remained controversial for about a decade, until these findings were corroborated, and multiple additional functions were discovered. In 1974, the US National Academy of Sciences declared zinc an essential element for humans and set a recommended dietary allowance (RDA).

What Is Zinc and Why Is It Important?

Zinc is an essential mineral that is critical for normal growth and development during pregnancy, infancy, childhood, and adolescence. It is necessary for immune function, wound healing, protein synthesis, cell division, cognitive function, taste and smell, as well as serving as an anti-inflammatory agent. Zinc is required by over 300 enzymes and over 1000 transcription factors (proteins needed for genetic information to be transcribed from DNA to RNA). Daily intake is important as we store little zinc in the body.[59, 121, 122]

Zinc deficiency can lead to growth retardation, depressed immune function, skin rashes, diarrhea, poor wound healing, and lack of appetite. In severe cases, it can cause dwarfism, hair loss, delayed sexual maturation, hypogonadism in males, and eye and skin lesions. Severe deficiency is uncommon in developed countries, unless a genetic disorder of zinc absorption is present. However, low intakes leading to mild deficiency are more prevalent than most people realize. It is estimated that 2 billion people in the developing world consume inadequate zinc. Premature and low-birth weight babies are at increased risk, as are those who are poorly nourished due to eating disorders, illness, or alcoholism.[59, 121, 122]

Are Plant-Based Eaters at Higher Risk for Zinc Deficiency?

Plant-based eaters may be at somewhat higher risk for reduced zinc status. Zinc is found in lower amounts in plant foods compared to animal products, and it is less bioavailable, especially in plant foods that are rich in phytates. Zinc intakes of adult vegetarians have been shown to be similar to or slightly lower than that of omnivores. In addition, serum zinc concentrations tend to be lower, but within normal limits.[123, 124] No adverse effects are apparent, possibly because the body adapts to lower intakes by enhancing absorption.[112] It appears as though zinc deficiency, while common in impoverished nations with limited access to a healthy range of foods, is far less of an issue in developed nations with an ample, varied food supply.[125] A meta-analysis of zinc status in vegetarians during pregnancy reported that although pregnant vegetarians have lower zinc intakes than omnivores, there is no difference in zinc status (zinc in serum, plasma, hair or urine) or in pregnancy outcomes.[126] Although data on zinc status of children eating plant-based diets is limited, there appears to be little difference in serum zinc or growth in vegetarian children on adequate, varied diets compared to omnivorous children.[127]

What Foods Are the Richest Dietary Sources of Zinc?

Zinc is typically most concentrated in protein-rich foods such as seeds, legumes, shellfish, meat, whole grains, and nuts. Table 5.5 provides the zinc content of common foods. Zinc absorption is less efficient from plant foods than from animal products, particularly from plant foods that are high in phytates. Vegetarian diets can increase zinc requirements as much as 50 percent, when phytates are excessive. This means, that a nine- to thirteen-year-old child or a female adult could need as much as 12 mg zinc instead of the 8 mg recommended for these groups (see Table 5.6 for the RDA in other groups). Food preparation methods such as fermenting, soaking (of nuts, seeds, legumes, and grains), sprouting, and leavening (of bread) can be used to reduce phytates and increase zinc absorption.[113] While yeast fermentation of bread reduces phytates and enhances zinc absorption, phytate breakdown is significantly greater in sourdough.[128, 129]

Table 5.5: Zinc Content of Common Foods

FOOD	PORTION SIZE	ZINC (mg)
Hempseeds	¼ cup	5
Adzuki beans, cooked	1 cup	4.1
Crab	3 ounces	4.0
Beef, lean, roasted	3 ounces	3.8
Kamut berries, cooked	1 cup	3.2
White beans, canned	1 cup	2.9
Ready-to-eat cereal with 25% of the DV*	1 serving	2.8
Pumpkin seeds	¼ cup	2.6
Chickpeas	1 cup	2.5
Lentils, cooked	1 cup	2.4
Cashews	¼ cup	2.2
Quinoa, cooked	1 cup	2
Dark chocolate, 70–85%	2 ounces	2
Tofu, firm	½ cup	2
Navy beans, cooked	1 cup	1.9
Kidney beans	1 cup	1.8
Chia seeds	¼ cup	1.8
Sunflower seeds	¼ cup	1.8
Infant cereal, oats	¼ cup	1.6
Brown rice, cooked	1 cup	1.4
Black turtle beans	1 cup	1.4
Oatmeal, cooked	1 cup	1.4
Tahini	2 tablespoons	1.4
Barley, cooked	1 cup	1.3
Green peas, cooked	1 cup	1.1
Almonds	¼ cup	1.1
Almond butter	2 tablespoons	1.1
Cow's milk, low-fat	1 cup	1
Chicken, boneless, breast	3 ounces	0.9
Peanut butter	2 tablespoons	0.8
Salmon	3 ounces	0.7
Eggs	1 large	0.6
Soy milk	1 cup	0.6

*The Daily Value (DV) is 11 mg for adults and children 4 years or older.
Source: [20]

Optimizing Zinc in Plant-Based Diets

Here are three simple steps you and your family can take to achieve and maintain adequate zinc status.

1. Think zinc when planning meals and snacks

   a. *Breakfast*—add quinoa, kamut berries, and other whole grains, nuts, and seeds to breakfast bowls; blend hemp seeds with non-dairy milk; spread cashew, almond, or other nut or seed butter on toast; select zinc-fortified cereals.

   b. *Lunch and dinner*—include beans, lentils, and split peas in soups, spreads, loaves, patties, stews, burritos, and dips; use tofu on sandwiches, on salads, in stir fries, and as a meat replacement in main dishes; throw pumpkin seeds on salads, and use cashews in sauces and dressings.

   c. *Snacks and treats*—add beans, nuts, seeds, and their butters to baked treats; snack on nuts and seeds, add a little dark chocolate; spread nut or seed butters on celery or apple slices; give toddlers large beans as finger foods; add nuts, seeds, frozen peas and tofu or soy milk to smoothies.

2. Prepare foods using techniques known to reduce phytates and improve zinc absorption.

   a. Soak beans and grains prior to cooking.

   b. Sprout grains, legumes, and seeds. Cook sprouted legumes (except peas and lentils) before eating.

   d. Add fermented foods such as tempeh and fermented nut cheeses.

   c. Opt for sourdough or leavened breads if breads are staples.

3. During pregnancy and lactation, use a prenatal supplement that includes zinc. For others, sufficient zinc can be obtained from a varied plant-based diet. However, providing a multi-vitamin mineral supplement with zinc can provide extra assurance that intake is adequate, especially for picky eaters.

Can I Get Too Much Zinc?

Yes, zinc can be toxic in excess, however this is typically only an issue with the chronic intake of supplements containing excessive amounts. Too much zinc can negatively affect copper and iron status and impair immune function. The daily Upper Limit (UL) for zinc is 7 mg for toddlers one to three years, 12 mg for children four to eight years, 23 mg for children nine to thirteen years, 34 mg for teens fourteen to eighteen years, and 40 mg for adults nineteen years or more. As you can see, the UL does not allow for very high intakes, so it is generally not advised to take a single nutrient zinc supplement unless medically indicated. Be cautious with use of cold nasal sprays, lozenges, and other over-the-counter cold medications with added zinc. Regular use has been associated with adverse effects, such as nausea. The FDA has warned against the use of nasal sprays due to multiple reports of loss of smell.[130] If zinc-containing cold aids are used, do not exceed the daily UL.

Table 5.6: Summary Chart Minerals

Key:

RDA = Recommended Dietary Allowances   NE = Niacin Equivalents

AI = Acceptable Intakes   P = Pregnancy; L = Lactation

RAE = Retinol Activity Equivalents

Micro-nutrient	RDA/AI (daily)	Primary Functions	Consider-ations	Deficiencies, Excesses	Richest Sources
Calcium	RDA Units—g 0–6 m—200 (AI) 7–12 m—260 (AI) 1–3 y—700 4–8 y—1,000 9–18 y—1,300 19–50 y (F)—1,000 >50 y (F)—1,200 19–70 (M)—1,000 >70 y (M)—1,200 P+L—1,000	Structural component of bones and teeth Muscle contraction Nerve cell transmission Blood clotting Blood pressure regulation Regulation of metabolism	Plant-exclusive eaters can ensure adequate intakes by regularly consuming calcium-rich plant foods and calcium-fortified foods. Calcium fortified non-dairy milks make meeting the RDA much easier, especially for children and teens.	*Deficiency:* osteopenia, osteoporosis, bone fractures *Excess:* calcification of blood vessels and soft tissue; constipation, reduced iron and zinc absorption. Do not exceed UL of 2,500 mg for children ages 1–8 years and adults 19–50 years; 3,000 mg for those 9–18 years and 2,000 mg for those 51+ years.	*Plant Sources:* low-oxalate greens, calcium-set tofu, fortified non-dairy milks, legumes, almonds, chia seeds, tahini, blackstrap molasses *Animal Sources:* milk and milk products (e.g., milk, yogurt, cheese), fish with bones (e.g., sardines)

Chloride	AI Units—mg 0–6 m—0.18 7–12 m—0.57 1–3 y—1.5 4–8 y—1.9 9–50 y—2.3 51–70 y—2.0 >70 y—1.8 P+L—2.3	Regulation of body fluids Electrolyte balance Acid-base balance Production of hydrochloric acid Nerve transmission	Excesses, generally associated with high intakes of salty, processed, and fast foods.	Deficiency: rare; muscle and liver damage, nonalcoholic fatty liver disease Excess: fishy body odor, vomiting, sweating, salivation, low blood pressure, liver damage.	Plant Sources: table salt, soy sauce, condiments, seaweed, tomatoes, lettuce, celery, olives, processed foods, rye. Animal Sources: processed meat, small amounts in milk and meat.
Chromium	AI Units—mcg 0–6 m—0.2 7–12 m—5.5 1–3 y—11 4–8 y—15 9–13 y (F)—21 9–13 y (M)—25 14–18 y (F)—24 19–50 (F)—25 14–50 y (M)—35 >50 y (F)—20 >50 y (M)—30 P—30 L—45	Carbohydrate metabolism and storage Insulin action (facilitates binding of insulin to receptors)	Plant-based diets can provide sufficient amounts. Chromium is reduced with food processing. Diets high in simple sugars (<35% of calories) can increase urinary excretion of chromium. Chromium levels are reduced with aging. Many interactions with prescription medications.	Deficiency: extremely rare (usually IV feeding without chromium); glucose intolerance, insulin resistance, diabetes Excess: no UL established as unlikely to cause adverse effects.	Plant Sources: broccoli*, grape juice, whole grains, potatoes, garlic, spices, orange juice, apples, bananas, green beans. Animal Sources: beef, seafood, dairy *Broccoli is an exceptional source with about 22 mcg per cup. Most foods have 2 mcg or less per serving
Copper	RDA Units—mcg 0–6 m—200 (AI) 7–12 m—220 (AI) 1–3 y—340 4–8 y—440 9–13 y—700 14–18 y—890 19+ y—900 P—1000 L—1,300	Energy production Iron metabolism Formation of connective tissue, bones, and red blood cells Produces color in skin, eyes, and hair Defends against oxidative damage Brain development Nervous and immune system function Gene activation	Sufficient in most dietary patterns; higher in plant-based diets; lower absorption. Copper supplements best avoided as copper can act as a pro-oxidant. High doses of zinc supplements can interfere with copper absorption so the UL for zinc is 40 mg/d for adults.	Deficiency: rare; extreme fatigue, light patches of skin, high cholesterol, connective tissue disorders, weak and brittle bones, loss of balance and coordination; elevated risk of infection. Excess: liver damage, cramps, nausea, diarrhea, vomiting. Do not exceed the UL of 10,000 mcg/day for adults (lower UL for children and teens).	Plant Sources: nuts, seeds, very dark chocolate, bran cereals, whole grains, potatoes, mushrooms, tofu, legumes, coconut, fruits, and vegetables Animal Sources: shellfish, organ meats, turkey, dairy products

Table 5.6: Summary Chart Minerals *(continued)*

Micro-nutrient	RDA/AI (daily)	Primary Functions	Consider-ations	Deficiencies, Excesses	Richest Sources
Fluoride	**AI** **Units—mg** 0–6 m—0.01 7–12 m—0.5 1–3 y—0.7 4–8 y—1 9–13 y—2 14–18 y—3 19+ y (F)—3 19+ y (M)—4 P+L—3	Formation of bones and teeth Prevention of tooth decay	Evidence for fluoride being essential is inconclusive.	*Deficiency:* increased risk of dental caries. *Excess:* dental fluorosis, diarrhea, sweating, weakness, adverse effects of bone, muscle, kidney, and nervous tissue. Toxic in excess. UL is 10 mg/day for adults (lower UL for children).	*Plant Sources:* tea (in leaves), grapes, grape juice, potatoes *Animal Sources:* fish and seafood, dairy products, eggs *Other sources:* fluoridated or naturally occurring water, tea, coffee, and other foods prepared with water containing fluoride.
Iodine	**RDA** **Units—mcg** 0–6 m—110 (AI) 7–12 m—130 (AI) 1–8 y—90 9–13 y—120 14+ y—150 P—220 L—290	Component of thyroid hormones Energy metabolism Immune function	Plant-based eaters can ensure adequate intakes with judicious use of iodized salt and/or seaweed, or supplements. Sufficient intakes are critical in pregnancy and lactation. Goitrogen-containing plant foods can trigger thyroid problems in those who consume insufficient iodine.	*Deficiency:* depressed thyroid hormone production, goiter; stunted growth, lower IQ, mental retardation, and delayed sexual development in infants and children. *Excess:* enlarged thyroid, inflammation of thyroid gland, increased risk of thyroid cancer. UL set at 1,100 mcg/day for adults (lower UL for children and teens).	*Plant Sources:* seaweed, grain products, some fruits and vegetables *Animal Sources:* fish, seafood, dairy products, eggs *Other sources:* iodized salt

Iron	**RDA Units—mg** 0–6 m—0.27 (AI) 7–12 m—11 1–3 y—7 4–8 y—10 9–13 y—8 14–18 y (F)—15 14–18 y (M)—11 19–50 (F)—18 19+ y (M)—8 >50 y (F)—8 P—27 L—9	Component of red blood cells Transports oxygen throughout the body Production of cellular energy Immune system function Physical growth Neurological development Synthesis of some hormones	Intakes are plentiful in plant-based eaters, but absorption is lower from plant compared to animal foods. Heme iron (from blood) can increase free-radical reactions. Vitamin C-rich foods enhance absorption; phytates inhibit absorption. Infants require iron from solid foods by 6 months of age.	*Deficiency:* anemia, GI upset, weakness, fatigue, irritability, lack of concentration, reduced immune response, low tolerance to cold temperatures. Risk higher in low birth weight or premature babies. *Excess:* stomach upset, constipation, nausea, stomach pain and vomiting, reduced zinc absorption. High dose supplements can cause serious poisoning in children. UL is 45 mg/day for teens and adults and 40 mg/day for infants and children.	*Plant Sources:* beans, tofu, nuts, seeds, fortified grain products, whole grains, some vegetables, dark chocolate, blackstrap molasses *Animal Sources:* meat, poultry, seafood
Magnesium	**RDA Units—mg** 0–6 m—30 (AI) 7–12 m—75 (AI) 1–3 y—80 4–8 y—130 9–13 y—240 14–18 y (F)—360 14–18 y (M)—410 19–30 (F)—310 19–30 (M)—400 31+ (F)—320 31+ (M)—420 P 19–30 y– 350 P 31–50 y– 360	Cofactor in over 300 enzyme systems Protein synthesis Muscle and nerve function Energy production Blood glucose control Structure of bones and teeth Active transport of calcium and potassium across cell membranes—affects nerve impulses, muscle contraction and heart rhythm	Intakes generally higher in plant-based eaters; intakes in the general population often below the RDA. High phytate diets can reduce absorption. Older adults are at increased risk of deficiency as intakes are lower and renal excretion increases.	*Deficiency:* fatigue, weakness, loss of appetite, nausea, vomiting. Severe deficiency can lead to numbness, tingling, muscle cramps, seizures, and arrythmias. *Excess:* no excess from food; too much from supplements can cause diarrhea, nausea, abdominal cramping, and heart failure. Do not exceed UL of 350 mg per day for those 9 years or more (lower UL for younger children)—the UL applies only to supplements.	*Plant Sources:* green leafy vegetables, nuts, seeds, legumes, soy products, whole grains, potatoes, avocados, other vegetables and fruits, some fortified foods *Animal Sources:* fish, meat, dairy *Other sources:* water (although amount varies significantly)

Table 5.6: Summary Chart Minerals *(continued)*

Micro-nutrient	RDA/AI (daily)	Primary Functions	Consider-ations	Deficiencies, Excesses	Richest Sources
Manganese	**AI** Units—mg 0–6 m—0.003 7–12 m—0.6 1–3 y—1.2 4–8 y—1.5 9–18 y (F)—1.6 9–13 y (M)—1.9 14–18 y (M)—2.2 19+ y (F)—1.8 19+ y (M)—2.3 P—2.0 L—2.6	Cofactor for many enzymes Energy production Synthesis of DNA, RNA and protein Cell signaling Bone and cartilage formation Reproduction Blood clotting Wound healing	Intakes meet or exceed AI in plant-based eaters.	*Deficiency:* rare, weak bones, poor growth in children; skin rashes, loss of hair color in men; mood changes *Excess:* none from food; water can have high levels; inhalation of magnesium dust in welding and mining. Toxicity symptoms include tremors, muscle spasms, hearing loss, mood changes, irritability, headaches. Do not exceed the UL of 11 mg for adults (lower UL for children and teens)	*Plant Sources:* whole grains, nuts, seeds, brown rice, legumes, leafy greens, potatoes, some fruits and vegetables, berries, coffee, tea, spices (especially black pepper). *Animal Sources:* seafood (especially mussels, oysters, clams)
Molybdenum	**RDA** Units—mcg 0-6 m – 2 (AI) 7-12 m – 3 (AI) 1-3 y – 17 4-8 y – 22 9-13 y – 34 14-18 y – 43 19+ y – 45 P+L– 50	Cofactor needed for 4 enzymes Metabolism of sulfur-containing amino acids Breakdown of some drugs and toxic compounds	Intakes meet or exceed RDA in plant-based eaters	*Deficiency:* very rare (only in those with genetic disorder); seizures and brain damage, death usually within days of birth. *Excess:* none from food; high levels from environmental exposure can lead to painful joints, gout-like symptoms. UL is set at 2,000 mcg for adults (lower UL for children, teens).	*Plant Sources:* legumes, whole grains, nuts, seeds, rice, potatoes, bananas, leafy greens *Animal Sources:* dairy products, beef, poultry, eggs

Phosphorus	**RDA** **Units—mg** 0–6 m—100 (AI) 7–12 m—275 (AI) 1–3 y—460 4–8 y—500 9–18 y—1,250 19+ y—700 P + L—700	Structural component of bones, teeth, DNA, RNA and all cell membranes Energy metabolism Acid-base balance Regulation of gene transcription Enzyme activation	Intakes generally meet or exceed the RDA in all dietary patterns. Plant-based eaters are protected against excess from food as phosphorus is less well absorbed from plant foods (phosphorus is stored as phytates— released with soaking, sprouting, yeasting, fermenting, leavening).	*Deficiency:* poor appetite, anemia, muscle weakness, bone pain, rickets, osteomalacia, loss of muscle control, confusion. Most likely in premature infants, those with genetic disorders, and with severe malnutrition. *Excess:* possibly increased risk of chronic disease, hormonal changes, calcification of soft tissues. Excretion is reduced in chronic kidney disease, so levels can get too high.	*Plant Sources:* legumes, nuts, seeds, potatoes, vegetables, grains, fruits *Animal Sources:* dairy products, meat, poultry, fish, eggs
Potassium	**AI** **Units—mg** 0–6 m—400 7–12 m—860 1–3 y—2,000 4–8 y—2,300 9–18 y (F)—2,300 9–13 y (M)—2,500 14–18 y (M)—3,000 19+ y (F)—2,600 19+ y (M)—3,400 P—2,900 L—2,800	Fluid balance— main regulator of fluids inside cells Transmission of nerve impulses Muscle contraction Acid-base balance Maintenance of electrical gradients	Plant-based eaters easily meet or exceed the AI; omnivores more commonly fall short. Magnesium depletion can increase urinary potassium losses.	*Deficiency:* increased blood pressure, elevated kidney stone risk, bone turnover, urinary calcium excretion. Most common with laxative abuse, inflammatory bowel diseases, diuretics, and certain medications. *Excess:* none from food except in those with kidney disease. High intakes from supplements association with adverse gastrointestinal side effects. No UL has been set.	*Plant Sources:* fruits, vegetables, legumes *Animal Sources:* dairy products, meat, poultry, eggs, fish

Table 5.6: Summary Chart Minerals *(continued)*

Micro-nutrient	RDA/AI (daily)	Primary Functions	Consider-ations	Deficiencies, Excesses	Richest Sources
Selenium	RDA Units—mcg 0–6 m—15 (AI) 7–12 m—20 (AI) 1–3 y—20 4–8 y—30 9–13 y—40 14+ y—55 P—60 L—70	Constituent of antioxidant enzymes called selenoproteins Reproduction Thyroid hormone metabolism DNA synthesis Protection from infection	Plant-based eaters generally have adequate intakes—similar to omnivores. Amounts in plants vary widely depending on soil content. Brazil nuts contain 70–90 mcg per nut. Limit to not more than 3–4 nuts a day for adults, and 1–3 per day for children (lower end of range for younger children).	*Deficiency:* male infertility, increased risk of certain diseases; could exacerbate iodine deficiency. *Excess:* garlic breath, metallic taste in mouth, hair or nail loss or brittleness, lesions of skin and nervous system, nausea, diarrhea, skin rashes, fatigue, irritability. Toxic in excess. UL is 90 mcg for 1–3 years, 150 mcg for 4–8 years, 280 mcg for 9–13 years, 400 mcg for 14+ years.	*Plant Sources:* Brazil nuts, whole grains, nuts, seeds, legumes, some vegetables and fruits *Animal Sources:* fish, seafood, organ meats, dairy, meat
Sodium	AI Units—mg 0–6 m—110 7–12 m—370 1–3 y—800 4–8 y—1,000 9–13 y—1,200 14+ y—1,500 P + L—1,500	Fluid balance—main regulator of fluids outside cells Transmission of nerve impulses Muscle contraction Acid-base balance Maintenance of electrical gradients Nutrient absorption and transport Maintenance of blood pressure and blood volume	Plant-based eaters generally have lower intakes than omnivores, although intakes may still exceed the Chronic Disease Risk Reduction (CDRR) level of 2,300 mg per day (CDRR—1,200 1–3 y; 1,500 4–8 y; 1,800 9–13 y). Intakes vary depending on the amount of processed foods eaten. Generous potassium intake can help counteract the blood pressure raising effects of sodium.	*Deficiency:* hyponatremia—headache, nausea, vomiting, muscle cramps, fatigue, fainting, dizziness, disorientation, falls, bone loss and fractures. Generally induced by extreme exercise and excessive water intakes, fluid retention, prolonged vomiting or diarrhea or medications. *Excess:* increased blood volume and blood pressure, depressed endothelial function, increased cardiovascular risk, gastric cancer and osteoporosis (due to increased calcium losses in urine).	*Plant Sources:* condiments, soy or tamari sauce, liquid aminos, pickles, sea vegetables, fermented vegetables, olives, ready-to-eat cereals, breads, crackers, prepared foods, salty snacks, tomato juice, tomato sauce *Animal Sources:* processed meat, cheese, cottage cheese, fast foods, prepared foods *Other sources: salt, sodium-based additives (MSG, sodium bicarbonate, sodium nitrate, sodium benzoate)*

Zinc	**RDA**	Cellular	While the RDA	*Deficiency:* growth	*Plant Sources:*
	Units—mcg	metabolism	is usually met,	retardation in infants	Legumes, nuts,
	0–6 m—2 (AI)	Required for	intakes can be	and children, delayed	seeds, whole
	7–12 m—3 (AI)	function of about	low in some	sexual development in	grains, fortified
	1–3 y—3	100 enzymes	individuals. Be	adolescents, impaired	foods (e.g.
	4–8 y—5	Production of	sure to include	immune function, hair	breakfast cereals,
	9–13 y—8	protein and DNA	plenty of zinc	loss, diarrhea, loss	some meat
	14–18 y (F)—9	Immune system	sources daily.	of appetite and taste,	analogs), peas
	19+ (F)–8	function	Phytates	weight loss, poor wound	*Animal Sources:*
	14+ y (M)—11	Cell division	(storage form of	healing, eye and skin	oysters (highest
	P—11	Wound healing	phosphorus in	lesions, impotence	content of all
	L—12	Growth and	foods) inhibits zinc	in men.	foods), meat,
		development	absorption; those	*Excess:* nausea,	poultry, seafood,
		of fetus during	with high intakes	vomiting, loss of	fish, dairy
		pregnancy,	of phytates may	appetite, abdominal	
		infants, children,	need 50% higher	cramps, diarrhea,	
		and adolescents	intakes of zinc.	headaches, low copper	
			Absorption is	status, reduced immune	
			higher from animal	function, urinary	
			compared to plant	disfunction. Do not	
			foods.	exceed the UL of 40	
				mg for adults (lower	
				UL for children and	
				adolescents).	

Sources: [131, 132, 133, 58, 59, 60, 134]

MINERALS... A FINAL WORD

In summary, when we move towards a whole food, plant-based diet, our intakes of potassium, magnesium, and copper generally rise compared to those eating omnivorous diets. Intakes of most other minerals are typically well within recommended ranges. The bottom line is, with a little care and attention, it is not difficult to meet recommended intakes for minerals in varied plant-based diets.

In our next chapter, we discuss the finer details of designing a healthful plant-based diet, and provide the practical tools you need to succeed in this task.

Chapter 6

What Makes
a Healthy Diet?

"Eat your vegetables, have a positive outlook,
be kind to people, and smile."

—*Dan Buettner*

What makes a healthy diet? While the question has sparked lively debate over many decades, we actually know the answer. We know that dietary patterns that emphasize whole plant foods such as vegetables, fruits, legumes, whole grains, nuts, and seeds are strongly associated with increased health and longevity. We know that Western-style dietary patterns featuring highly processed foods, fast foods, fatty animal products, and sugar-laden beverages are strongly associated with reduced health and longevity.[1] Not surprisingly, people who shift from a Western-style diet to a less processed plant-predominant diet experience remarkable improvements in health.[2] And people who make healthier diet and lifestyle choices not only live longer but they live better. They extend the number of years that they are able to do the things they need and want to do. They increase their odds of being physically active and socially engaged into their eighties, nineties, and beyond. As the famous saying goes, "In the end, it's not the years in your life that count. It's the life in your years." Hear, hear!

There are two primary prerequisites for a healthy diet:

1. **The diet must be nutritionally adequate.** The diet must provide the necessary amounts of macronutrients and micronutrients humans require to both survive and thrive.
2. **The diet must minimize risk of chronic disease.** The diet must be designed to minimize the risk of death and disability induced by our leading killers such as heart disease, cancer, and type 2 diabetes.

The first prerequisite for a healthy diet concerns nutritional adequacy or meeting our needs for both macronutrients and micronutrients. These nutrients were covered in some depth in the previous two chapters. There is no question that a wide variety of dietary patterns can provide the macronutrients humans require. As we saw in the previous chapter, micronutrients can vary substantially with different dietary patterns. It is generally best to focus on the overall dietary pattern rather than on one or more single nutrients. Regardless of the dietary pattern chosen, if sufficient energy (calories) is provided from a variety of healthy whole foods, essential nutrients, with a few exceptions (e.g., vitamin B12 in plant-based diets), are taken care of.

Malnutrition is a consequence of nutritional inadequacy. Most of us associate malnutrition with starving children in developing countries. What many people don't realize is that there are three broad categories of malnutrition: undernutrition, micronutrient-related malnutrition, and overconsumption. Undernutrition (wasting, stunting, and underweight) are the result of insufficient calories, macronutrients, and micronutrients. Micronutrient-related malnutrition involves a lack of vitamins and minerals. The micronutrients most commonly lacking worldwide are vitamins A and D, folate, iodine, iron, and zinc.[3] In plant-based families, vitamin A and folate are generally sufficient, but iodine, iron, zinc, and vitamin B12 may fall short if reliable sources are not provided. While few people associate overconsumption with malnutrition, it is the most prevalent form of malnutrition worldwide.[4] Overconsumption leads to overweight, obesity, and diet-related chronic disease. Excess fat accumulation due to imbalances in energy (calorie) consumption negatively affects multiple body systems and increases risk of disease and death. Micronutrient deficiencies are common with overconsumption, as the chosen foods are typically high in fat and sugar, and low in vitamins and minerals.[5]

Plant-based diets can be designed to ensure adequate nutrition at every stage of the lifecycle. The balance of this chapter and Chapters 7 and 8 will provide you with the practical tools you need to do just that.

The second prerequisite of a healthy diet is that it minimizes the lifetime risk of chronic disease. In this space, plant-based diets shine. Research suggesting disease-risk reduction in those eating plant-centered diets is strong and consistent.[2,6,7] What gives these diets an advantage? Whole food, plant-based diets concentrate the dietary components that have been shown to be most effective in preventing disease—fiber, phytochemicals, plant enzymes (convert certain phytochemicals into active forms), antioxidants, plant sterols and stanols, and pre-biotics (food for our gut microbiome). They also minimize the dietary components that are most strongly associated with increasing disease risk—saturated fat, trans fatty acids, refined carbohydrates, pro-oxidants (components that increase oxidative stress), pro-inflammatory compounds (e.g., Neu5Gc in meat and TMAO produced from carnitine in meat), environmental contaminants, products of high-temperature cooking, food additives, and salt. These components are concentrated in two categories of foods: highly processed foods and animal products. So, when we choose whole plant foods, we load up on the most powerful disease protectors, and put a lid on the most harmful disease promoters. When our children are exposed to healthy choices from their first bites of solid food, their palates are trained to appreciate the flavors of whole foods, and the initiation of lifelong healthy habits take root.

TOOLS OF THE TRADE...
FOOD GUIDES THAT WORK FOR YOU

As parents or guardians of children, we are tasked with ensuring that our family table is a place where cultural traditions are honored, community is celebrated, and each family member is well nourished. Sometimes, balancing nutrition with joy and connection can be challenging for parents. A variety of tools have been developed over the decades to support families in putting together meals that supply the nutrients we need to thrive at every stage of the lifecycle. Perhaps, the most well recognized are food guides. Food guides attempt to offer nutrition plans that ensure adequate nutrition for people of all ages (excluding infants). This is no small feat. Guides are generally designed to help ensure sufficient protein, fats, carbohydrates, and fiber and adequate intakes of vitamins and minerals. National governments develop food guides based on the food culture of their country, so they look very different from one nation to the next. The United States Department of Agriculture (USDA) released its first food guide in 1916. As nutritional science evolved, revisions were made. Today, the guide in is the shape of a plate with five groups—vegetables, fruits, grains, protein foods, and dairy. Within the dairy group, calcium-fortified soy milk is an option for nondairy consumers. Canada's current food guide has only three groups—vegetables and fruits, grains, and protein foods (with an emphasis on plant-based choices such as legumes, nuts, seeds, and tofu over animal-based choices such as meat, poultry fish, eggs, and yogurt). This guide does not include a separate food group for dairy foods.

The Plant-Based Plate diagram provided here is designed to assist you in putting together menus that nourish every member of your family (from the age of one year and beyond) by offering a visual representation of the foods that might be included at each meal. Of course, the specific choices from each group will vary from meal to meal and day to day. While not every meal will necessarily include foods from every group, aim for a minimum of three to four food groups at each meal. Each food group provides a target number of servings to consume over the course of the day. The number of servings is set to help ensure the nutrients represented in each group are provided in adequate amounts. You will notice different serving sizes based on calorie (energy) intakes. For toddlers one to three years of age, total energy needs are about half that of adults, so serving sizes are half that of adult servings. For children ages four to eight, energy needs are about three-quarters that of adults, so serving sizes are about three-quarters that of adult servings. By nine to ten years of age, energy needs are similar to adults, so serving sizes are the same.

The guide also includes a section labelled "Add Ons." These are nutrients that could potentially be lacking even if all of the suggested servings from each group are consumed. You may wonder if the recommended number of servings from each group are more than you or your family members could consume in a single day. Rest assured that the servings sizes are small, and most people do meet the mark. If you fall short, it does not mean you will not meet nutrient needs, but you will want to ensure that you are including a wide variety of foods with a focus on nutrient-dense choices (foods with a lot of nutrients per calorie). In addition to the food guide image, details about serving sizes and specific choices are provided in the Plant-Based Plate chart that accompanies the guide. Finally, we dive into the details of each food group to help you feed your family for health and with joy.

Figure 6.1: The Plant-Based Plate

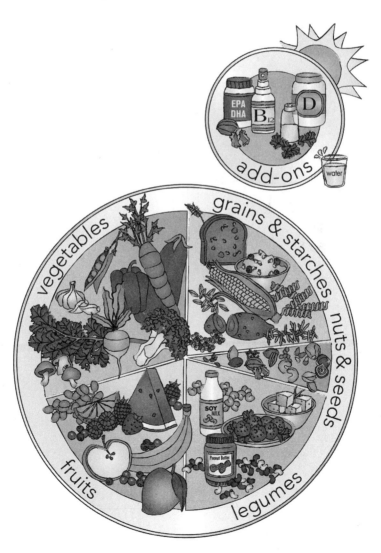

Table 6.1: The Plant-Based Plate Serving Sizes

Food Group Servings/ Day	Serving Size 1–3 years 1000–1400 kcal	Serving Size 4–8 years 1400–1600 kcal	Serving Size 9+ years 1800–2800 kcal	Notes
Vegetables 3+	¼ cup raw *or* cooked vegetables ½ cup raw leafy vegetables ¼ cup vegetable juice	⅓ cup raw *or* cooked vegetables ¾ cup raw leafy vegetables ⅓ cup vegetable juice	½ cup raw *or* cooked vegetables 1 cup raw leafy vegetables ½ cup vegetable juice	Choose a rainbow of colors. At least: 2 green, 1 each of orange-yellow, pink-red, purple-blue, white-beige.
Fruits 3+	¼ cup raw *or* cooked fruit 1 medium fruit 2 tbsp dried fruit ¼ cup fruit juice	⅓ cup raw *or* cooked fruit 1 medium fruit 3 tbsp dried fruit ⅓ cup fruit juice	½ cup raw *or* cooked fruit 1 medium fruit ¼ cup dried fruit ½ cup fruit juice	Choose a rainbow of colors. Include berries, citrus fruits, melons, and others.
Grains & Starches 3+	Grains: ¼ cup cooked grains ½ slice of bread ½ oz cold cereal Starches: ¼ cup cooked starchy vegetable ½ cup fortified oat milk	Grains: ⅓ cup cooked grains 1 slice of bread ¾ oz cold cereal Starches: ⅓ cup cooked starchy vegetable ¾ cup fortified oat milk	Grains: ½ cup cooked grains 1 slice of bread 1 oz cold cereal Starches: ½ cup cooked starchy vegetable 1 cup fortified oat milk	Make at least ½ your grains whole grains. Serving size same for sprouted and cooked grains. Minimize highly processed grains. Adjust number of servings to meet energy needs.
Legumes 3+	¼ cup cooked beans, split peas, or lentils, tofu, tempeh ½ cup sprouted lentils *or* peas 2 tbsp peanuts 1 tbsp PB ½ cup fortified soy or pea milk ½ veggie patty 1 oz meat alternative	⅓ cup cooked beans, split peas, or lentils, tofu, tempeh ¾ cup sprouted lentils *or* peas 3 tbsp peanuts 1½ tbsp PB ¾ cup fortified soy or pea milk 1 veggie patty 1½ oz meat alternative	½ cup cooked beans, split peas, or lentils, tofu, tempeh 1 cup sprouted lentils *or* peas ¼ cup peanuts 2 tbsp PB 1 cup fortified soy or pea milk 1 veggie patty 2 oz meat alternative	Select at least 1 whole legume choice, when possible—beans, lentils *or* peas Include one or more choices with each meal. PB= peanut butter
Nuts and Seeds 1+	2 tbsp nuts *or* seeds 1 tbsp nut *or* seed butter ½ cup fortified nut *or* seed milk	2 tbsp nuts *or* seeds 1½ tbsp nut *or* seed butter ¾ cup fortified nut or seed milk	3 tbsp nuts *or* seeds 2 tbsp nut *or* seed butter 1 cup fortified nut *or* seed milk	Include at least 1 omega-3 rich choice. Go for variety in both nuts and seeds.
Add Ons	*Recommendations*			
Vitamin B12	Ensure sufficient vitamin B12 through supplements, fortified foods, *or* a combination of the two.			
Vitamin D	Ensure sufficient vitamin D through safe sun, supplements, fortified foods, *or* a combination of these options.			
Iodine	Ensure sufficient iodine through a supplement, iodized salt, sea vegetables, *or* a combination of these options.			
Essential Fatty Acids	Ensure sufficient omega-3 rich fatty acids by including adequate ALA-rich foods. A DHA/EPA supplement may be warranted for those with increased needs or reduced ability to convert plant to long-chain omega-3s.			

TOP 10 HEALTHY EATING TIPS

1. **Eat a variety of foods from each food group.** The greater the variety of foods included from each group, the greater the diversity of nutrients, fiber, phytochemicals, and antioxidants you will consume. When you make healthy choices from each food group, you establish healthy eating patterns that offer a lifetime of protection.

2. **Make water your beverage of choice.** Beverages can easily be the downfall of any dietary pattern. They may contain unwanted sugars, sodium, saturated fat, caffeine, and/or alcohol (in adult beverages). Water is critical to overall health and is the most effective beverage for quenching thirst. To increase water intake, drink it hot or cold, drink it with your meals and between your meals, drink it during physical activity, and carry a reusable water bottle with you. To provide a flavor boost, add fruit pieces, lime, lemon, mint, cucumbers, cinnamon sticks and/or a frozen juice cube. Use soda water as a base to make it fizzy.

   > To provide a flavor boost, add fruit pieces, lime, lemon, mint, cucumbers, cinnamon sticks and/or a frozen juice cube.

3. **Skip the highly processed foods.** Highly processed foods are major contributors to the excess consumption of unhealthy fats, refined sugars and starches, salt, and potentially harmful food additives. Examples of highly processed foods are fast foods, deep-fried foods, sweet baked goods, sugar-laden ice creams and frozen treats, salty snacks, candy bars, candies, and sweet beverages. While you don't have to eliminate these foods altogether, consider reserving them as occasional foods in your family's diet. To curb intake of highly processed foods, start by slowly replacing some of these foods with healthier options. For example, instead of store-bought cookies and muffins, try making homemade baked goods with nutritious ingredients; swap out French fries for oven-baked "fries."

4. **Keep sodium intake moderate.** Over 70 percent of our sodium comes from processed food, about 15 percent is naturally present in whole food and only about 10 percent comes from salt added during cooking and at the table.[8] The balance comes mostly from water and dietary supplements. So, reducing processed foods will put a major dent in your sodium load.

Be aware of foods that are hyperconcentrated in sodium such as pickles and olives, as generous intakes can quickly lead to excess. You can easily adjust the amount used in cooking and at the table, if need be. Kids can overconsume sodium as well, and as diet habits are formed in childhood, reducing intake can help promote long-term health.

5. **Read food labels.** Food labels can supply information that will help you to make more healthful choices. The most valuable information is provided in the nutrition facts and ingredient list. The Nutrition Facts provide information about serving size, calories, and some nutrients (as a percent of the Daily Value). The ingredient list tells you about the ingredients in order of their weight in the product. It is common practice to try to fool customers by including multiple forms of less desirable ingredients such as sugar, so they all end up lower on the ingredient list. For example, instead of listing 16 grams of cane sugar per serving, a manufacturer might list 4 grams each of cane sugar, dextrose, maltose, and corn syrup. You can use the food label to help you compare products and choose those with less sugar, less salt, less fat, and more fiber. Additionally, nutrition claims ("high in fiber," "low in sugar," or "high in protein") are often depicted on a label. Foods must meet specific criteria to make these claims, and generally the healthiest foods (think broccoli!) don't require a label to convince you of their nutritional benefit.

6. **Be savvy about food marketing.** Food marketing is advertising that attempts to sell you a product. Most marketing is for products that are highly processed like presweetened cereals or toaster pastries, rather than for broccoli or blueberries. A significant amount of this advertising is directed towards children. Food marketing is designed to convince you or your children that a product is superior to its competitor's (for example, in taste, convenience, or nutrition) or that it will provide you with some desirable outcome—higher energy, more strength, better looks, or a more robust social life. Being savvy about marketing will help you and your children to avoid being deceived by a sales pitch.

7. **Prepare meals at home.** Cooking your own food means that you control what goes into your meals, including the amount of fat, sugar, and salt. You will be reducing highly processed foods and saving money for healthier

foods such as fresh vegetables and fruits. It's perfectly alright to purchase some ready-to-eat greens, pre-cut or frozen vegetables, pasta sauces, salsa, pre-seasoned tofu, or ready-to-eat veggie burgers to reduce meal prep time.

8. **Make your foods appealing and enjoyable.** Making foods appealing and enjoyable leads to more positive eating experiences for your family. Take the time to present your food attractively by using colorful vegetables and fruits, herbs, and sauces. Kids love fun food, like bear-shaped pancakes or fruit plated in a flower shape. Be creative, adventurous, and open to experiencing new flavors. Weave in traditions from your family's culture. Set an attractive table, light some candles, put on some soft music, and enjoy the company.

9. **Eat with others.** When you eat with others—family, friends, colleagues, or neighbors, you will connect in a valuable way. Eating together allows you to share your cultural traditions, to explore new foods, and to have quality time with others. Enjoy your meal at a leisurely pace, and get rid of distractions such as TV and cell phones.

10. **Eat mindfully.** Being mindful about your food choices means being more conscious about where your food comes from, how it is selected, and how it arrives on your table. It means experiencing your food's appearance, taste, and texture, and appreciating the effort that went into procuring and preparing the food. It means being aware of your eating behaviors and trying to take steps to improve them, such as removing distractions, slowing down to enjoy your food, spacing meals and snacks, and creating an inviting environment.

MAKING THE MOST OF EACH FOOD GROUP

Vegetables

Vegetables, particularly non-starchy vegetables, are our most nutrient-dense foods. In other words, they contain more nutrients per calorie than any other food. Vegetables are key sources of vitamins (vitamin A, vitamin C, vitamin K, and folate), minerals (calcium, iron, potassium, and magnesium), antioxidants, phytochemicals, and fiber. They are strongly and consistently associated with longevity and disease risk reduction.[9,10] Yet, only 9 percent of American adults, and 2 percent of high school students meet recommended intakes.[11,12]

In our Plant-Based Plate, the vegetable group includes only non-starchy vegetables, while starchy vegetables are part of the grains and starches group. Some
vegetables thought to be starchy, such as beets, carrots, kohlrabi, rutabaga, and
turnips, are actually classified as non-starchy.

The Pick of the Crop

- **Dark leafy greens.** These are the most nutrient-dense of all food, which
  means that they have the most nutrients per calorie. Include them not only
  in salads, but in soups, stews, main, and side dishes. Select a variety of dark
  greens as they each have their own unique nutrition profile.
- **Cruciferous vegetables.** Arugula, bok choy, broccoli, Brussels sprouts, cabbage, cauliflower, kale, radish, and turnips are all a part of the cruciferous
  vegetable family. These vegetables contain phytochemicals (e.g., glucosinolates) known for their powerful anti-cancer effects.[13]
- **Allium vegetables.** This family includes chives, garlic, leeks, onions, and scallions. These foods are rich in a type of fiber that helps to promote a healthy
  gut microbiome. They have anti-inflammatory, antioxidant, antimicrobial,
  and prebiotic activities.[14]
- **Sprouts.** When we grow sprouts (e.g., broccoli, pea, radish, sunflower), an
  army of phytochemicals is produced to protect the vulnerable little plants.
  These phytochemicals are typically many times more concentrated than they
  are in the mature plant.[15, 16] Sprouts are delicious in sandwiches, salads, and
  in breakfast or dinner bowls.
- **All other brightly colored vegetables.** Variety and color help to maximize
  the range of protective compounds in your produce. In the green category,
  choose asparagus, celery, Brussels sprouts, cabbage, snow peas, pea shoots,
  sunflower sprouts, or zucchini; in the yellow-orange category, select carrots,
  golden beets, golden cauliflower, yellow or orange tomatoes, and peppers;
  in the pink-red category, pick tomatoes, red onions, beets, red pepper, and
  watermelon radishes; in the purple-blue category go for purple carrots, cabbage, cauliflower, eggplant, or peppers; and in the white-beige category, try
  cauliflower, daikon, garlic, jicama, kohlrabi, salad turnips, and sweet onions.
- **Fresh, local, and organic.** Nothing beats homegrown vegetables, so consider

starting a garden, growing some herbs, and/or sprouting. Kids love to see things grow, so involve them in the process. Frequent farmer's markets and produce stands. When it is accessible and affordable, opt for organic to minimize pesticide exposure.

Boosting Veggies

- **Stock up and prepare.** Keep a good variety of veggies on hand, but not more than what you will eat in a week. Wash, prep and store some veggies in containers in the refrigerator for instant use.
- **Make it easy.** Buy some produce that is prepared for you, such as grated carrots, triple-washed greens, frozen vegetables, or tomato products.
- **Make a huge bowl of salad to last a few days.** Use the salad as a base for your lunch, or as an addition to dinner. Include a variety of greens and a rainbow of vegetables. To turn your salad into a full meal, top with grains or cooked starchy vegetables, beans, nuts, and seeds. Reserve items that will go bitter or discolor and add just before serving.
- **Slip veggies in.** Dice veggies into soups and scrambles, chop veggies into stews and casseroles, grate veggies into loaves and patties, and blend veggies into soups, sauces, dips, and dressings.
- **Get creative.** Add veggies to savory oatmeal, use collard leaves to make a wrap, or add frozen peas, fresh carrots, and cucumber to your smoothies.

Common Questions

Are frozen, canned, and jarred vegetables good choices?

Fresh is generally best for maximum nutrition. However, vegetables are usually frozen soon after they are picked, so their nutrients are well preserved, and they are super convenient. Plain is best, rather than those in creamy or buttery sauces. Canned vegetables lose some of their water-soluble nutrients during processing. They are often high in added sodium, may have added sugar, and are common sources of BPA (found in linings of cans), so are less desirable choices. When used, look for low or no added sodium options, and cans with BPA-free lining. Some canned vegetables, such as diced tomatoes, can make meal preparation easier, so do have an important place in the pantry.

What are the best ways to cook vegetables?

Steaming results in the greatest nutrient retention. Sautéing, microwaving, and blanching also minimize nutrient losses. Boiling causes greater losses of vitamins and minerals through heat and discarded water (water can be saved for soups!). However, boiling reduces oxalates, so can be useful for those who need to limit their intake. Baking or roasting are also good choices, though they do diminish vitamin (but not mineral) content. The least-desirable cooking methods are those that use very high temperatures and concentrated oils, such as deep-frying.

How can I make tough greens like kale more enjoyable in salads?

The easiest way to make raw, tough greens more palatable in salads is to slice the greens matchstick thin and distribute through the salad with more tender greens. You can also massage greens to help tenderize the leaves (to add flavor, you can massage with a little olive oil and lemon). Another option is to lightly steam, and dice before using. This works especially well in grain or legume-based salads.

Fruits

The evidence that fresh fruits are protective to health is rapidly accumulating. Fruit is an important source of fiber, phytochemicals, vitamins A and C, and potassium. Studies suggest that fruit intake improves gastrointestinal health, promotes healthy weight, reduces risk of heart disease, type 2 diabetes, and cancers, especially colorectal and lung cancers. It also appears to offer protection against asthma and other respiratory diseases, bone loss, and even depression.[17, 18] Only about 12 percent of the Western population meets recommended intakes for fruit.[11]

Pick of the Crop

- **Berries.** With more fiber, a unique complement of phytochemicals, and less sugar than most other fruits, berries are an exceptional choice.
- **Citrus fruits.** High in fiber, phytochemicals, vitamin C and other antioxidants, folate, thiamin, potassium, and magnesium, citrus fruits such as grapefruits, lemons, limes, oranges, pomelos, and tangerines are excellent choices. Some evidence suggests that citrus fruits can help reduce the risk of kidney stones.[19]

- **Melons.** As very high-water fruits, melons provide a surprising array of nutrients. For example, watermelon is an excellent source of lycopene (a powerful antioxidant associated with prostate cancer prevention),[20] pro-vitamin A carotenoids, vitamin C, and potassium.
- **Tree fruits, tropical fruits, vine fruits, and all others.** There are no unhealthy fresh fruit choices; each variety provides a distinct nutrition profile. Purchase fruits that are local, in season, fresh, and organic, when accessible and feasible. Frozen fruits are also good choices.

Boosting Fruits

- **Enjoy fruit with your morning meal.** Add to hot or cold cereal, chia pudding, yogurt, smoothies and smoothie bowls, pancakes, French toast, and waffles. If you are having a savory breakfast such as scrambled tofu, include a fresh fruit or fruit bowl along with it.
- **Add fruit to salads.** Enjoy some berries, sliced mango, apples or pears, or sliced oranges or grapefruit on your salad.
- **Make fruit your go-to snack or dessert.** Prepare a variety of fruits and arrange attractively on a plate. It is amazing how rapidly fruit disappears when it is cut up versus when it is sitting unprepared in a bowl. Serve fruit with a dip like nut butter and top with a sprinkle of cinnamon. Use fruit as a base for delectable treats like fruit salad, fruit-based ice cream, fruit crisp, or baked fruit.
- **Use fruit as your sweetener of choice in treats.** Use dried fruits such as dates, prunes, raisins, or pears to replace other sweeteners in muffins, cookies, and other homemade goodies.
- **Stew fruit in season and freeze for amazing breakfast and dessert toppings.** Fruit can be stewed with just enough water to prevent sticking on a very low temperature—no sugar required. Wonderful choices are Italian prune plums, blueberries, apricots, peaches, and nectarines.
- **Keep some precut fruit in the refrigerator for easy use.** This works only for choices that do not brown, like melons, pineapple, mango, papaya, and strawberries.
- **Carefully select canned fruits.** If choosing canned or jarred fruits, go for those packed in water or juice rather than light or heavy syrup. Canning does cause nutrient losses, so opt for fresh or frozen most often.

Common Questions

How much fruit is too much?

Although fruit is our most significant source of naturally occurring simple sugars, research does not suggest an upper limit for fruit intake. If you love fruit, let your gut be your guide. Arguments made against high fruit intake, particularly for those with blood sugar issues, such as diabetes, are not well supported by the literature.[21, 22]

Is the fructose in fruit harmful?

The fructose in fresh fruits is present in relatively small amounts and is easily managed by the body. On the other hand, the body's ability to handle fructose can be quickly overwhelmed when fructose is added to beverages and other highly processed foods. So, while it is best to minimize fructose in beverages and highly processed foods, fructose from fruit is not a problem![23, 24]

Are dried fruits healthy foods?

Dried fruits are healthy foods. They are loaded with fiber, antioxidants, phytochemicals, and micronutrients. Dried fruits make an exceptional replacement for concentrated sugars. There are, however, a few caveats. First, because dried fruits are much smaller than their fresh counterparts, it is easy to eat a lot of them in a short time and overconsume calories. Also, some dried fruits have sugar added, so it is preferable to stick to those that do not. Many light-colored dried fruits are treated with sulfites to preserve color, and some individuals are sensitive to these additives. For many years, consumers were cautioned that dried fruits contribute to dental caries by sticking to teeth. More recent evidence suggests that dried fruits inhibit bacteria that contribute to caries and don't stick to teeth more than other foods.[25, 26]

Are fruit juices recommended as part of the daily diet?

No, fruit juices are not recommended as part of the daily diet, particularly as a primary beverage for children. Fruit juices are fruit minus the fiber and many protective phytochemicals that are associated with the fiber. It is better to eat the whole fruit and drink water. Whole fruit is high in fiber and helps to slow the absorption of sugar that occurs naturally in fruit. Fruit juice produces a greater spike in blood sugar and is less filling than whole fruit.[27] One study in children reported that the intake of fruit juice was associated with increased body fat, while whole fruits were associated with reduced body fat.[28] This is not to say that unsweetened fruit juice cannot be part of a healthy diet, but it is best consumed only on occasion and in moderation. It may be preferable to include a small glass of orange juice at breakfast than to have no fruit at all. The orange juice adds vitamin C, which enhances iron absorption, and increases the potassium content of the meal. One hundred percent unsweetened fruit juices are preferable to beverages with added sugars. Fresh pressed or fresh squeezed are best, often providing some fruit pulp. Fruit "drinks" contain only a small percent of fruit juice—they are largely sugar (or artificial sweeteners) with food colors and flavors.

Grains and Starches

Grains and starches are concentrated carbohydrate sources and important energy-giving foods. Grains include barley, corn, farro, Kamut, millet, oats, rice, rye, sorghum, spelt, teff, and wheat. Pseudograins, although not botanically grains, are also included in this group because they are used like grains. Examples of pseudograins include amaranth, buckwheat, quinoa, and wild rice. Starches refer primarily to starchy vegetables such as breadfruit, cassava, corn, parsnips, peas, potatoes, pumpkin, taro, sweet potatoes, and winter squash.

Grains provide about half the world's protein and fiber. Whole grains are rich in B vitamins (especially thiamin and niacin) and vitamin E. They're good sources of copper, iron, manganese, magnesium, phosphorus, selenium, and zinc, plus a variety of phytochemicals and antioxidants. Whole grains are consistently associated with reduced risk of many chronic diseases.[29] Refined grains are grains that have had their bran and germ removed. Examples of refined grains are white rice and white flour products. Most of the grains consumers eat are refined. These products are less desirable, as most of the fiber, vitamins, and minerals have been significantly reduced during processing. Enriched grains have some nutrients, such as thiamin, riboflavin, niacin, folic acid, and iron added back. Most of the grains in the diet should be whole rather than refined grains, although it is perfectly okay to include some refined grains, especially for young kids who need to boost energy intakes.

Starchy vegetables are good sources of fiber (especially if you eat the skin), vitamin A (as carotenoids in the more colorful options such as sweet potatoes and squash), vitamin C, and potassium. Starchy vegetables have a bad rap because the most popular offerings are highly processed forms such as french fries or potato chips. When simply prepared by steaming, boiling, or baking, starchy vegetables are wonderfully healthful foods that are low in fat, high in fiber, and rich in antioxidants.

Pick of the Crop

- **Colorful grains and starchy vegetables.** Colorful grains and starchy vegetables such as black barley, red or black quinoa or rice, orange or purple sweet potatoes, and winter squash provide a wide array of antioxidants and phytochemicals.
- **Nutrient-dense whole grains.** Among the most nutritionally impressive grains are amaranth, buckwheat, oats, quinoa, teff, and wheat (including kamut and spelt).
- **Unprocessed or minimally processed whole grains.** As mentioned previously, whole grains provide fiber and many beneficial nutrients. They are more slowly absorbed than refined grains making them more satiating.
- **Peas and corn.** These are very high fiber options. Peas are particularly rich in protein, while corn is a rich source of zeaxanthin and lutein—carotenoids associated with eye health.

Boosting Whole Grains and Starchy Vegetables

- **Include a starchy vegetable or whole grain with each meal.** This adds fiber, nutrients, and calories, making meals more satisfying.
- **Get familiar with intact grains.** Cook up a batch and use it as a breakfast cereal, as a topping for salads, or as a hearty addition to soups and stews. Information on cooking intact grains is provided in Chapter 15.
- **Add starchy vegetables to soups and salads.** Top salads with cubed and steamed squash or sweet potatoes. Add potatoes, parsnips, or squash to soup.
- **Serve stuffed baked potatoes for dinner.** Stuffed sweet potatoes offer a nutritional advantage, but regular baked potatoes are nutritious as well, especially when accompanied by a bean-based filling.
- **Enjoy grains with a vegetable curry or stir-fry.** Grains that pair particularly well with these dishes are rice (black, red, or brown) and quinoa.

Common Questions

Do I need to buy organic oats and wheat products to avoid glyphosates?

Glyphosate is an herbicide (weed killer) in Roundup that is considered a probable carcinogen.[30] Roundup is commonly sprayed on grains, such as wheat, barley, and oats to speed drying so the crop can be harvested more quickly. According to the Environmental Protection Agency (EPA), one to two-year-old children are likely to have the highest exposure, with intakes often significantly exceeding current standards. The Environmental Working Group (EWG) tested twenty-nine oat-based products and reported some of the highest levels in rolled oats, commercial granola, and ready-to-eat breakfast cereals. The only products that had no detectable glyphosate were organic, although some organic products did contain small amounts due to cross contamination from other fields.[31] So, yes, do opt for organic oat and wheat products when they are accessible to you.

Should everyone avoid gluten?

No. Most people can tolerate gluten, and many very healthy populations around the world eat gluten-containing grains (wheat, barley, rye, and triticale (wheat/rye hybrid)) as dietary staples. Of course, those with celiac disease (about 1 percent of the population) need to be very vigilant about avoiding gluten, while those on the gluten-sensitivity spectrum (an estimated 6 to 10 percent of the population) need to completely avoid or reduce gluten in their diets.

What breads are healthiest?

Usually the denser the bread, the more slowly the nutrients are absorbed and the more healthful it is. Very heavy breads, such as German pumpernickel, (those that you can practically stand on!) are outstanding choices. While you might expect children would prefer light, fluffy breads, their preferences have a lot to do with their exposures. If a child grows up eating dense black bread, they are likely to love it their whole lives. Other great breads are sprouted grain breads and breads that are 100 percent whole grain. Whole grain breads that contain seeds such as flax, chia, or sunflower are also excellent choices. If you do include white bread on occasion, sourdough is a great choice.

Legumes

Legumes (beans, lentils, chickpeas, split peas, peanuts) are the protein pow-
erhouses of the plant kingdom and are our principal sources of iron and zinc.
They are also our most concentrated sources of fiber, and they deliver a wonderful complement of phytochemicals. In plant-based diets, legumes serve as
meat replacements. They provide many of the benefits of meat but without the
saturated fat and cholesterol. Meat contains none of the protective fiber or phytochemicals we get from legumes. Studies show that replacing animal protein
with plant protein reduces death and disease.[32, 33]

Pick of the Crop

- **Cooked beans, lentils, chickpeas, and split peas.** These legumes are exceptional choices, brimming with fiber, plant protein, vitamins, minerals, and
  phytochemicals. They also give you the biggest bang for your buck!
- **Sprouted mung beans, peas, and lentils.** For a burst of phytochemicals,
  sprout legumes. Sprouted mung beans, peas, and lentils are safe to consume
  raw, though larger beans must be cooked after sprouting.
- **Soy products.** Tofu and tempeh have a rich history of use in long-lived
  populations. Tempeh, a fermented product, is relatively high in fiber. Tofu
  is extremely versatile and provides readily available plant protein. More processed soy foods such as veggie meats provide abundant available protein,
  and can add variety and enjoyment to the diet. Go for organic, if possible.
- **Bean pasta.** Rapidly rising stars, bean pastas are available in many forms.
  They boast about half the carbohydrate, double the fiber, and triple the
  protein of regular pasta. While a regular pasta and marinara dinner may be
  lacking in protein, iron, and zinc, replacing wheat pasta with adzuki bean,
  chickpea, lentil, or black bean pasta provides a seamless supply of nutrients.
- **Peanuts, peanut butter.** While commonly considered "nuts" in a culinary
  sense, peanuts are technically legumes. From a nutritional perspective, they
  are more like nuts than legumes, although they are about one third higher
  in protein (¼ cup peanuts provides about 9 grams of protein compared to an
  average of about 6 grams in most nuts). They are rich sources of manganese
  and magnesium.

Boosting Legumes

- **Add beans to breakfast.** Many people around the world enjoy beans or lentils with their morning meals. If this strikes you as unusual, think of beans on toast, breakfast burritos, or scrambled tofu. Add lentils to your breakfast grains (you can cook them together) or beans to your savory steel cut oats.
- **Add legumes to salads.** Add chickpeas, black beans, grilled tempeh, smoked or baked tofu, or peas to a full meal salad. Make a bean-based side salad.
- **Enjoy bean, lentil, or pea soup.** Bean soups are classic comfort foods—think pea soup, lentil soup, or bean and barley soup.
- **Make legumes the main event.** Get creative when it comes to lunches and dinners. For centuries, numerous cultures have relied on legumes as dietary staples. Mexican, Indian, South American, Asian, and African cuisines include many beautifully flavored legume dishes.
- **Go for bean-based spreads, dips, and dressings.** Make hummus with chickpeas, or similar bean-based dips with black or white beans. Use lentils as a base for a spread and white beans or chickpeas in a salad dressing.

Common Questions

How can we reduce the gas production experienced when eating beans and lentils?

Beans and lentils cause gas because they contain a very healthy type of carbohydrate (oligosaccharides) that isn't broken down and digested in the small intestine. It makes its way into the large intestine and provides a feast for our beneficial bacteria. Gas is a by-product. The following suggestions will help to keep gas production tolerable:

- *Reduce the oligosaccharides in beans.*
  - ✓ Use the hot soak method for cooking dried beans. (see Chapter 15) This involves bringing beans to a boil and then letting them soak for twenty-four hours. Discard soaking water and use fresh water to cook. The hot soak method reduces oligosaccharides more than the traditional soak (no pre-boiling).
  - ✓ Buy only as many dried beans as you can use within a few months and avoid eating beans that are older than one year, as they become less digestible.

✓ Sprout legumes before cooking them. Sprouting converts oligo-saccharides into more-digestible sugars.

✓ Some canned beans have fewer oligosaccharides as they are very well cooked, though they are more costly. Rinse well.

- *Start with small portions, then gradually increase your intake.* In this way, healthy gut flora will flourish and become accustomed to the dietary shift, and with unhealthy flora being crowded out.

- *Cook beans thoroughly.* When beans are undercooked, they're more difficult to digest and more gas producing.

- *Select small legumes, as they are easier to digest.* The least problematic are skinless, split legumes, such as mung dal (split mung beans), red lentils, and split peas. In general, these will produce less gas than large beans, such as lima or kidney beans.

- *Pick options with fewer oligosaccharides.* Choose tofu and bean products that are fermented, such as tempeh.

- *Use seasonings that counteract the production of intestinal gas.* Black pepper, cinnamon, cloves, garlic, ginger, turmeric, and the Japanese seaweed kombu are all prized for their ability to diminish gas production.

- *Improve your gut flora.* Use probiotic-rich fermented foods, such as fermented vegetables, nut cheeses, yogurts, and other dishes.

- *Consider a digestive enzyme supplement.* Find one that is targeted towards bean digestion.

Are canned beans healthy?

Yes, canned beans are healthy choices. However, they can be high in sodium, so if this is a concern, select no or low sodium options, or rinse beans well. Many companies also offer BPA-free can linings, so if accessible, chose these. A good alternative to canned beans is cooking your own beans in large batches and freezing them in 1½- or 2-cup (375- or 500-ml) portions in freezer bags or jars. If you have an Instant Pot or similar pressure cooker, cooking beans is a breeze.

Aren't the lectins in beans dangerous for people?

While beans do contain lectins, they are easily destroyed by standard cooking practices, so are perfectly safe. For bean cooking instructions, see

Chapter 15. The lectins in raw (or very undercooked) beans such as kidney beans can cause a food poisoning-like reaction, but this is a rare occurrence as most large beans are unpalatable if undercooked. It is interesting to note that there are many different types of lectins in food. Some lectins have been shown to reduce cancer risk.[34]

Nuts and Seeds

Nuts and seeds are the most nutritious sources of healthful fats and essential fatty acids in plant-based diets. They are brimming with trace minerals, antioxidants (particularly vitamin E), and phytochemicals. Generally, the fat in nuts is mostly monounsaturated (with the exception of walnuts), while the fat in seeds and walnuts is mostly polyunsaturated. Omega-6 fatty acids predominate in poppy, pumpkin, sesame, and sunflower seeds, while omega-3 fatty acids predominate in chia seeds and flaxseeds. Hempseeds and walnuts contain a healthy balance of the two essential fatty acids. While nut and seed oils can be rich sources of essential fatty acids and can add flavor to foods, these sources lack the fiber, trace minerals, and phytochemicals provided by the whole foods.

Nuts and seeds are associated with longevity and disease risk reduction, particularly for cardiovascular disease and diabetes.[35, 36]

Pick of the Crop

- **Omega-3 rich choices.** Chia, flax, or hemp seeds, and walnuts are excellent omega-3-rich choices. The absorption of omega-3 fatty acids is improved by grinding flaxseeds (this is not necessary for chia or hempseeds).
- **Pumpkin, hemp, and other seeds.** Seeds are higher in protein and fiber and more concentrated in essential fatty acids (both omega-6 and omega-3 fatty acids) than nuts (except for walnuts). Hemp and pumpkin seeds are higher in protein than other seeds. Sunflower seeds are brimming with vitamin E, while chia seeds provide abundant calcium.
- **Almonds, Brazil nuts, cashews, and other nuts.** Go for variety. Each type of nut seems to have a claim to fame in the nutrition department. For example, almonds are richest in vitamin E, calcium, riboflavin and niacin; Brazil nuts top the charts for selenium and magnesium; cashews contain the most iron and zinc; hazelnuts are number one for folate; pistachios are

best for B6, walnuts stand out for omega-3s, and pecans are phytochemical champions.

- **Raw, soaked and dehydrated, or roasted.** Choose nuts and seeds that are raw, soaked, or lightly roasted. Soaking and dehydrating can increase the content and availability of nutrients, phytochemicals, and antioxidants. Roasting brings out flavor in nuts and seeds, but can cause the formation of products of oxidation. If you are roasting your own, keep temperatures low. Do not allow nuts and seeds to get dark brown. If purchasing roasted nuts or seeds, select unsalted, dry roasted, if possible.

Boosting Nuts and Seeds

- **Add omega-3s to your breakfast bowl.** Add ground flaxseeds, chia seeds, hemp seeds or walnuts to hot or cold cereal. Make a mix of seeds and walnuts, and store in a mason jar in the refrigerator so you can conveniently enjoy their combined benefits.
- **Add 1 to 2 tablespoons nuts or seeds to salads.** Almonds, pumpkin seeds, and sunflower seeds are excellent choices.
- **Use seeds, nuts, or their butters as a salad-dressing base, in sauces, and in spreads.** Nuts and seeds can dramatically increase the nutritional value of dressings (e.g., lemon tahini dressing), sauces (e.g., miso ginger tahini sauce), and spreads (e.g., snickerdoodle hummus). See recipes in Chapter 15.
- **Select nut-based cheeses, creams, and milks.** Whether homemade or store-bought, nut-based dairy replacements are becoming more widely available and are scrumptious.
- **Spread on nut and seed butters.** Nut and seed butters are great in wraps, or on sandwiches, bread, toast, pancakes, waffles, or crackers. They provide far more nutrition than butter or margarine.
- **Use nuts or seeds in main dishes.** Add walnuts or sunflower seeds to patties or loaves, add pine nuts or hazelnuts to pilafs, or throw a few peanuts or cashews into a stir-fry.
- **Include nuts or seeds with snacks, desserts, baked goods, and smoothies.** Pack along a few nuts or trail mix. Spread nut or seed butters on celery or apples. Use nuts or seeds to top fruit salad, fruit-based ice cream, or baked

fruit. Add nuts and seeds to energy balls, cookies, granola, muffins, and other homemade delights.

Common Questions

Aren't nuts and seeds high in fat and calories?

Yes, about 75 to 85 percent of the calories in nuts and 55 to 75 percent of the calories in seeds are from fat. However, they are among the most healthful sources of fat in the food supply. They do provide 500 to 800 calories per cup, so consume accordingly.

Is coconut a nut and is it a healthy choice?

Coconuts are not technically "nuts" but rather fruits. Unlike true nuts, which feature monounsaturated fats, and seeds, which have mostly poly-unsaturated fats, coconut contains mostly saturated fat. Because of its high saturated fat content, it is best to eat coconut in moderation, and in its whole form (as opposed to coconut oil). Fresh or dried coconut provides a good mix of vitamins and minerals, phytochemicals, and dietary fibers. Enjoy coconut in breakfast bowls, in main dishes, and in desserts and baked goods.

FINAL THOUGHTS

Eating a diet that is predominantly or exclusively whole plant foods can open up a world of culinary adventure. Be bold in your explorations and take your children on the journey with you. Remember that variety and color are key to maximizing the advantages of plant-based diets.

In our next chapter, we explore maternal nutrition, and provide the essential information plant-based pregnant and lactating mothers require to ensure health for themselves and their little ones.

Chapter 7

Pregnancy and Lactation

"What good mothers and fathers instinctively
feel like doing for their babies is
usually best after all."

—*Benjamin Spock*

Whether you are planning for your first or your fifth child, a healthy pregnancy outcome is a top priority. All aspects of your health deserve special consideration—exercise, sleep, stress management, the use of potentially harmful substances, and of course, diet. Regardless of where you might be on the plant-based spectrum, you may be wondering if this way of eating will support and sustain optimal growth and development in the tiny being who will be sharing your food. Take a deep breath. You've got this. With a little care, you can rest assured that your diet will provide everything you need to adequately nourish both yourself and your baby.

PRECONCEPTION NUTRITION...
STARTING OUT ON THE RIGHT FOOT

Step number one on your journey to parenthood is to up your nutrition game prior to pregnancy. You want to enter pregnancy healthy and well nourished...and the sooner, the better. While it is often assumed that nine months is all it takes to ensure the health of your baby, the journey actually takes a little longer. Your choices as you approach the time of conception matter. They matter because the first few weeks of pregnancy (often before you even know you are pregnant) can profoundly impact your baby's development.

In terms of lifestyle choices, if you smoke, stop well before conception. Smoking increases risk of low-birth weight, preterm deliveries, and infant death.[1] If you take prescription drugs, talk to your doctor, as some are associated with birth defects. Avoid recreational drugs and exposure to hazardous chemicals. Get daily exercise, adequate rest, and practice relaxation techniques to help reduce stress. Make a doctor's appointment, so you can ensure that all systems are go. Many health conditions such as diabetes, high blood pressure, thyroid disease, and asthma can affect pregnancy outcomes.[1,2]

As for diet, you will want to make some changes if you are overweight or underweight. Achieving a healthy body weight prior to pregnancy helps to minimize pregnancy complications for you and your baby.[3,4] If you are overweight, incorporate regular exercise and adopt a well-balanced, high-fiber diet. Weight loss diets are generally inappropriate once you become pregnant. If you are underweight, build muscle through exercise and increase your energy intake. For many underweight individuals, this means regular, more calorically dense meals and snacks—more nuts, seeds, avocados, whole grains, starchy vegetables, and legumes in the diet. If you suffer from an eating disorder, seek treatment prior to conception, as eating disorders can seriously compromise nutritional status.[5]

Next, identify any potential shortfalls in your eating pattern, and incorporate strategies that cover these shortfalls. The top three considerations are: ensuring adequate nutrients, eating a variety of healthy foods, and minimizing harmful dietary constituents.

Ensuring Adequate Nutrients

During preconception, aim for a healthy, balanced diet that provides all essential nutrients. One nutrient that is critical during preconception is folate. Inadequate folate is associated with neural tube defects—serious abnormalities of the spinal cord and brain. Neural tube defects occur in the first few weeks after conception, often before a woman knows she is pregnant. For this reason, health authorities recommend that women who are planning on or capable of becoming pregnant take a daily supplement of 400 to 800 mcg folic acid (synthetic form of folate).[6] The upper limit (UL) for folic acid is 1000 mcg, so the line between adequate and excessive intakes is small (see pages 177–178). There is no UL for folate (the natural form of the vitamin) and some supplements offer this form, so this is a safe and reasonable option. The bottom line is that when you are trying to conceive you must meet the RDA for folate (600 mcg)—whether it comes in the form of folate, folic acid or both. Many people fall short of the RDA. The richest folate sources are plant foods such as greens, beans, lentils, avocados, asparagus, beets, oranges, and sunflower seeds, so whole food, plant-based eaters are at an advantage. Taking a prenatal supplement during the preconception period also helps boost iron, iodine, zinc, vitamin B12, and vitamin D status (read labels to verify nutrients included). Entering pregnancy well-nourished can help to offset adverse effects of nausea and food aversions that often accompany early pregnancy.

Eating a Variety of Healthy Foods

Another simple way of boosting nutrition during preconception is to follow the Plant-Based Plate (see page 149). Make changes to your diet where you see gaps in your eating patterns. For example, if your diet is lacking in leafy greens, throw some into your soup or smoothie, add a salad to your lunch or dinner, or switch from potato chips to kale chips as a snack. If you tend to forgo fruit, try adding a piece of fruit at each meal—perhaps some berries on your oatmeal at breakfast, an apple or orange at lunch, and a fruit salad with a little soy yogurt or cashew pear cream (see page 390) as a dinner dessert. If legumes are low, consider adding a bean, pea, or lentil soup to lunch, and throwing some chickpeas, kidney beans, edamame, or tofu into your dinner bowl. If you fall short on omega-3 fatty acids, sprinkle a tablespoon of chia or flaxseeds on your breakfast bowl, use hempseeds in your salad dressings, and sprinkle a few walnuts on your fruit bowl. Consider this simple fine-tuning an investment in your future family.

Minimizing Harmful Dietary Constituents

There are many potentially harmful compounds that are present in the food supply. Alcohol is particularly problematic, as there is no safe level of intake during pregnancy, so it is best eliminated prior to pregnancy.[1, 3, 4] It is also advisable to reduce exposure to pesticides and other endocrine disruptors, choosing organic produce when possible, and minimizing exposure to BPA and phthalates used in household personal care products and foods (such as canned foods and dairy products).[7, 8, 9] Environmental contaminants such as persistent organic pollutants have been associated with adverse pregnancy outcomes, so taking steps to minimize intakes may be protective.[10, 11] These chemicals tend to move up the food chain, and are generally more concentrated in animal products such as fish and dairy. Eating a plant-based diet, which is lower on the food chain is a valuable way of reducing exposure.

Preconception Nutrition Tips

1. Take a good quality prenatal supplement.
2. Aim to achieve the recommended servings in each food group.
3. Minimize harmful dietary components. Avoid alcohol completely.

PLANT-BASED PREGNANCY

During pregnancy, every nutrient the baby requires for growth and development comes from her mother. If the mother's diet is lacking, the mother and baby compete for nutrients.[12] As the mother's nutrient stores are depleted, the risk of complications rises, and the potential for long-term adverse health consequences for both mother and child grows. Fortunately, making the appropriate adjustments in food intake during pregnancy and lactation is easier than you might imagine, regardless of whether your dietary pattern is plant-based or mixed.

How Safe Are Plant-Based Diets During Pregnancy?

The safety of plant-based diets depends on your food choices, as it is for those eating mixed diets. When the diet is well planned, pregnant and lactating plant-predominant and plant-exclusive eaters meet all their nutrient requirements and can have very healthy babies.[13, 14]

Average birthweights of babies born to vegan mothers are not significantly different from those born to omnivorous mothers. Vegan pregnant women have fewer caesarean deliveries, less postpartum depression, and lower rates of neonatal and maternal mortality.[15] In addition, plant-based and plant-exclusive diets have been shown to protect against preeclampsia, pre-pregnancy obesity, and exposure to genotoxic chemicals (chemicals that can damage genetic material).[14, 15] The largest study to date of pregnant vegans examined the records of 775 women at a community called "The Farm" in Summertown Tennessee back in 1987.[16] The most novel finding that came out of this study was that only one vegan woman developed preeclampsia. That is a rate of 0.1 percent, compared to 5 to 10 percent of women in the general population. The authors concluded that it is possible to sustain a healthy pregnancy on a vegan diet and that such a diet could prevent most, if not all, of the signs and symptoms of preeclampsia.

Occasionally, less favorable reports of women consuming plant-predominant or plant-exclusive diets appear in the literature. Generally, these cases are associated with highly restrictive diets and refusal to supplement essential nutrients such as vitamins B12. The good news is that these failures are the exception, and appropriately planned, plant-based diets are both safe and adequate.

Energy Needs and Weight Gain

When you are pregnant, it is true that you are eating for two, but your caloric requirements reflect the size of the second person. During the first trimester, you do not need any additional calories—your non-pregnant calorie intake is perfect. During the second trimester, you need an extra 340 calories a day, and in the third trimester, as the baby's growth accelerates, an additional 450 calories a day are recommended.[17] Of course, the exact amount will vary depending on your size, metabolism, and activity level. You can obtain 340 calories by eating a slice of whole grain bread with almond butter and banana slices, plus a cup of soy milk.

Adding another slice of whole grain bread to this meal (to make an almond butter and banana sandwich) will get you to 450 calories. No weight gain is expected during the first trimester. During the second and third trimesters, weight gain goals are about 1 pound per week for those of normal weight, 1.1 to 1.3 pounds per week for those who are underweight, 0.6 pounds per week for those who are overweight, and 0.5 pounds per week for those who are obese.[17] The total weight gain goal for a normal weight individual is about 25 to 35 pounds, however, it is more for those who are underweight, and less for those who are overweight. If you are having more than one baby, your weight gain goals will be higher. Table 7.1 provides the recommended weight gain according to pre-pregnancy weight status and whether a single baby or twins are expected.

Women who gain the appropriate weight during pregnancy have fewer adverse pregnancy outcomes. Gaining too little weight can increase risk of low birth weight and preterm birth.[18] Gaining too much weight can increase risk of preeclampsia, hypertension, caesarean sections, and large for gestational age babies.[19]

Table 7.1: Weight Gain Recommendations

PRE-PREGNANCY WEIGHT STATUS	WEIGHT GAIN RECOMMENDED ONE BABY (pounds)	WEIGHT GAIN RECOMMENDED TWINS (pounds)
Underweight (BMI<18.5)	28–40	50–62
Normal Weight (BMI 18.5–24.9)	25–35	37–54
Overweight (BMI 25–29.9)	15–25	31–50
Obese (BMI ≥30)	11–20	25–42

Source:[17]

Notable Nutrients

During pregnancy, the demands for essential nutrients rise, as the mother's body must support and sustain new life. The recommended intakes for both macro- and micronutrients are increased, as many are during lactation as well. Table 7.5 provides the recommended dietary allowances for micronutrients for nonpregnant, pregnant, and lactating females ages nineteen to fifty years.

The macronutrients that deserve special consideration during pregnancy are protein and essential fatty acids (particularly omega-3 fatty acids). The micronutrients that require attention are folate, vitamin B12, choline, vitamin D, calcium, iodine, iron, and zinc. In the section that follows, we will consider the dietary adjustments recommended to ensure these notable nutrients are adequately provided. Recommendations for lab tests and dietary supplements will also be reviewed.

Protein

Extra protein is needed so your baby can build her skeleton, skin, muscles, and all other body tissues. Your body needs a little extra protein, too, as your blood volume and uterus expand. While your energy needs rise during the second and third trimesters by about 15 to 20 percent, protein needs increase by about 50 percent. This means that during pregnancy women need to consume more protein-rich foods. Adults need about 0.8 grams (g) of protein per kilogram (kg) body weight (1 kg = 2.2 lbs.). During pregnancy, the RDA increases to 1.1 g/kg, or an additional 25 grams of protein per day (on average). For twins, that amount doubles to 50 grams additional protein per day. Those eating plant-based may need to add an extra 10 percent to compensate for reduced digestibility of protein from high-fiber plant foods. That would mean about 1.2 grams of protein per kilogram body weight or an additional 28 grams of protein daily.

How do we achieve these high protein intakes on plant-based diets? Here are some simple tips:

- Include at least one protein-rich choice at each meal and each snack.
- Select protein-rich non-dairy milks such as soy or pea milk rather than low protein options such as almond milk.
- Eat lentils and beans at least twice a day. Add to soups, salads, breakfast, and dinner bowls. Use to make dips and spreads. Select beans or lentil-based pastas.
- Add in soy options—tofu, tempeh, edamame, and veggie meats.
- Add seeds (e.g., hemp and pumpkin), nuts (e.g., almonds), and peanuts to breakfast bowls, salads, and main dishes.
- Spread nut or seed butter on your toast instead of butter, margarine, or jam.

- Add whole food protein-rich foods to smoothies (e.g. soy milk, tofu, frozen peas, hempseeds, nut or seed butters).

Lab Tests: Blood test are not routinely done to assess protein status in pregnancy. However, total serum protein and albumin tests may be ordered. Healthy values decrease by about 30 percent compared to non-pregnant values due to increases in blood volume.[17]

Supplements: It is preferable to increase protein intake using high-protein foods such as tofu, lentils, beans, and hempseeds rather than with protein supplements. Many protein powders contain sugars, colors, artificial flavors, thickeners, herbs, caffeine, artificial sweeteners, and added vitamins and minerals (with a prenatal multi, the added vitamins and minerals in protein powders could bump you beyond the upper limits). In addition, protein powders, including organic products, may contain heavy metals and bisphenol A (BPA). If after consulting your health care provider, you are advised to add a supplement, do some digging before purchasing. Go to the Clean Label Project to check levels of environmental contaminants in the product you are considering.

Omega-3 Fatty Acids

Babies need long-chain omega-3 fatty acids (DHA and EPA) to support the growth and development of the brain, nervous system, retina, and cell membranes. Higher intakes of long-chain omega-3 fatty acids are associated with improved health outcomes, including better birth weights and fewer preterm births.[20] Plant foods contain minimal DHA and EPA, so plant-exclusive eaters must rely either on conversion of ALA (the plant omega-3) to DHA and EPA, or take DHA and EPA directly as a microalgae supplement. The RDA for ALA is 1.4 mg during pregnancy, although experts suggest this level be doubled to 2.8 mg for those who are not consuming EPA and DHA directly.[21, 22] This amount of ALA can be obtained by consuming about 1 tablespoon of chia seeds, 1½ tablespoons of ground flaxseed, 3 tablespoons of hempseeds, or ¼ cup walnuts. While conversion appears to be significantly enhanced in women of child-bearing age, levels of DHA and EPA are reduced compared to omnivores. No dietary reference intakes have been set for DHA and EPA, however health organizations recommend a minimum of 200 to 300 mg DHA and EPA per day during pregnancy, with at least 200 mg

DHA.[23, 24] Based on the current evidence, it seems prudent to aim for similar levels of intake from microalgae-based supplements for plant-based pregnant women who do not consume fish.[25, 26]

For plant-predominant eaters who include eggs, about 25 to 150 mg DHA are provided per egg (with higher amounts found in omega-3-rich eggs—from chickens fed fish meal or flaxseeds). Those who include fish can achieve significantly higher intakes, particularly if eating omega-3 rich choices such as salmon, sardines, and herring. One 3-ounce serving provides about 500–1500 mg DHA/EPA. However, fish is the primary source of several dietary contaminants, including mercury, so microalgae may be a safer choice. The U.S. Food and Drug Administration (FDA) and the Environmental Protection Agency (EPA) provide fish advisories to help protect against excessive intakes.[27]

Lab Tests: Omega-3 fatty acid status is not routinely assessed, as tests are not widely available, normal ranges have not been established, and validity of tests is uncertain. Serum and plasma fatty acids levels are more reflective of the last meal consumed than long-term status.

Supplements: Based on the current evidence, it is advisable to take a 200 to 300 mg DHA/EPA supplement for those who do not consume fish regularly in the diet during pregnancy.

Folate

As you recall from our preconception discussion, folate is a critical nutrient, particularly during early pregnancy. As a result, the RDA increases from 400 mcg to 600 mcg DFE (dietary folate equivalents) for pregnant women (600 mcg DFE = 600 mcg food folate OR 360 mcg folic acid from fortified foods OR 300 mcg folic acid from supplements). This level of intake is easier to achieve on whole food plant-based diets than on diets higher in animal products, but it can still be challenging for some women to meet these needs. Prenatal vitamin supplements include folate or folic acid to help bridge any potential gap.

Lab Tests: Blood tests to measure folate status are not routinely performed during pregnancy, as the risks of inadequate intakes are so high that all pregnant women are advised to supplement.

Supplements: Taking a prenatal supplement almost always ensures sufficient folate. While there is no upper limit (UL) for folate from food (as there is no

toxicity related to food folate), the UL for folic acid from supplements and fortified foods is 1,000 mcg. In the case of folic acid, more is not better. In fact, there
is some evidence that folic acid intakes at or above the UL are associated with
lower scores on tests of cognitive development in four- to five-year-old children
compared to mothers taking 400 to 999 mcg folic acid.[28] With 600 to 800 mcg
folic acid often included in a prenatal supplement, and 50 to 100 mcg in a serving
of fortified foods such as cereal or bread, the numbers can add up quickly. If you
are using protein powders, energy bars or other supplements, check the label to
ensure that you are keeping below the UL. A good option for keeping folic acid
under the UL of 1,000 mcg is to select a prenatal supplement that uses food folate
in its formulation rather than synthetic folic acid.

Vitamin B12

The nutrient of greatest concern in the diets of plant-based eaters, particularly
those who are plant-exclusive, is vitamin B12. The RDA for vitamin B12 during
pregnancy increases to 2.6 mcg (from 2.4 mcg). This nutrient is necessary for red
blood cell formation, DNA synthesis, and neurological function. During pregnancy,
intestinal absorption of vitamin B12 increases and the mother's dietary intake
supplies B12 to the fetus. However, if the mother does not get sufficient B12 from
foods or supplements, her B12 stores are not used to supply B12 to the fetus. In
other words, if there is a B12 tug-of-war between mother and infant, the mother
wins.[29] Inadequate intakes, particularly during the first trimester, have been associated with an increased risk of neural tube defects and neurological problems in
the baby and increased risk of preeclampsia, macrocytic anemia, and neurological
impairment in the mother.[29] Plant foods, including seaweed, fermented foods, and
organic produce, are not considered reliable sources. While some vitamin B12
can be obtained from vitamin B12 fortified foods, supplements are more reliable
sources and are advised for all pregnant women following plant-based diets.

Lab Tests: An assessment of vitamin B12 status is recommended for all those
consuming plant-based diets who have not been supplementing with at least 100
mcg B12 per day or 1,000 mcg twice a week. Lab tests routinely ordered to assess
B12 status include a complete blood count (CBC) and serum B12[30] However, serum
B12 is not a sensitive indicator of B12 status, and the increased blood volume
associated with pregnancy further compromises its utility. Serum methylmalonic

acid (MMA) and homocysteine are superior tests for detecting diminished B12 status.[31, 32] Hence, these tests are recommended for those who are at risk.

Supplements: Many prenatal supplements do not contain sufficient B12 to be relied upon as the sole source, and B12 absorption from multivitamins is not always reliable. The combination of a prenatal multi (with B12) plus at least two servings of B12-fortified foods providing 100 percent of the DV is another option. However, the safest option is to include a B12 supplement providing at least 1,000 mcg B12 twice a week, in addition to the prenatal supplement.[33]

Choline

Choline plays an important role in cell division, gene expression, and in the growth and development of the brain and nervous system. Adequate choline intake is associated with a reduced risk of neural tube defects, improved cognitive function, and better visual acuity in infants. Choline intakes of pregnant women in the United States fall short of the 450 mg Acceptable Intake (AI).[34] Plant-based eaters are not likely at an advantage here as animal products tend to be more concentrated sources. To meet the AI on a plant-based diet, eat a healthful, varied diet. The most concentrated plant sources are shiitake mushrooms, soyfoods (e.g., tofu and soy milk), legumes, quinoa, peanuts, almonds, and other nuts and seeds, vegetables (e.g., Brussels sprouts, broccoli, cauliflower, and peas), and fruits (e.g., oranges and bananas).

Lab Tests: Choline status is not routinely measured.

Supplements: Select a prenatal supplement that includes choline (many do not). Choline content ranges from about 50 to 300 mg depending on brand. Look for one that provides at least 100 mg per day, if possible. Studies suggest intakes as high as 900 mg per day are safe during pregnancy.[34]

Vitamin D

A lack of vitamin D during pregnancy has been associated with increased risk of preeclampsia, gestational diabetes, and low birthweight.[35, 36] Vitamin D plays a critical role in skeletal development and calcium balance in the growing fetus. Dietary vitamin D needs vary with exposure to sunshine. For those with limited exposure to warm sunshine (including those living in cooler climates for several months of the year), vitamin D-rich foods and/or supplements are key vitamin

D sources. Fatty fish, egg yolks, and fortified dairy products are main dietary sources of vitamin D for people eating mixed diets. Although there are some plant food sources such as mushrooms grown in sunlight and fortified non-dairy milks, vitamin D intakes in plant-exclusive eaters are typically lower than those of individuals who include vitamin D-rich animal products. Those with insufficient sun exposure and limited dietary sources, are well advised to supplement. While prenatal vitamins generally include vitamin D, amounts are not always sufficient to meet needs (check the label). The RDA for vitamin D remains at 600 IU (no change over non-pregnant RDA).

Lab Tests: Serum vitamin D is not routinely tested during pregnancy. However, for those who have limited sun exposure (or a lack of exposure to warm sunshine year-round), and who include few dietary sources of vitamin D, it is advisable to have vitamin D levels checked prior to conception.

Supplements: Most prenatal supplements contain 400–800 IU vitamin D, so this may be sufficient to maintain good vitamin D status, especially if food sources are also consumed. Some experts recommend 1,000 to 2,000 IU per day during pregnancy, especially if vitamin D status is in question.[37] Do not exceed the UL of 4000 IU per day.

Calcium

The calcium RDA remains unchanged during pregnancy, at 1,000 mg per day. Plant-predominant eaters who regularly include dairy products in their diet will typically meet the RDA. Those who are plant-exclusive and consume a variety of calcium-rich choices such as calcium-set tofu, beans, calcium-rich, low-oxalate greens, almonds, and chia seeds, can easily meet the RDA by adding 1 or 2 servings of calcium-fortified non-dairy beverages each day.

Lab Tests: Circulating blood levels of calcium are tightly regulated, so blood tests are not reliable indicators of status. Long-term shortages are evident in reduced bone density.

Supplements: Calcium supplements are recommended for those who do not meet the RDA. Calcium supplements may help to prevent preeclampsia, preterm birth, and complications due to high blood pressure.[38] Generally, a supplement containing 500–600 mg calcium is adequate. Do not exceed the UL of 2,500 mg calcium per day.

Iron

During pregnancy, red blood cell production dramatically increases, and iron absorption is enhanced to ensure sufficient iron for an expanding blood volume in the mother and a rapidly growing fetus. Iron deficiency during pregnancy is associated with preterm births, low birth weight, and cognitive impairments in the infant, so getting enough iron is considered a priority in pregnancy.[39] The RDA jumps 50 percent, from 18 mg to 27 mg per day! The Institute of Medicine suggests a further increase for vegetarians (1.8 times above those of meat-eaters or almost 49 mg per day), although this level of increase represents a worst-case scenario—a diet very rich in inhibitors of iron absorption (e.g., phytates and polyphenols), and low in enhancers of iron absorption (e.g., vitamin C and organic acids). Our goal would be to achieve a best-case scenario, with more moderate intakes of iron inhibitors and more generous intakes of enhancers, so that a smaller increase in the RDA would suffice. This means limiting intake of concentrated bran cereals, soaking, sprouting, fermenting, or yeasting grains and beans, keeping tea intake separate from meals, and including plenty of vitamin C-rich foods such as citrus fruits, strawberries, and red peppers with meals. Also, be sure to select iron-rich choices at each meal, such as lentils, beans, nuts, and seeds.

Lab Tests: The CDC recommends that all pregnant women be screened for iron deficiency anemia at their first prenatal visit.[39] A complete blood count (CBC), which includes hemoglobin, hematocrit, mean corpuscular volume and red blood cell distribution width, and serum ferritin (a measure of iron stores) are commonly used to assess iron status.[40]

Supplements: It is difficult to achieve the RDA for iron during pregnancy, so the CDC recommends that all pregnant women, at their first prenatal visit, begin taking an oral low dose (30 mg/day) supplement. Most prenatal supplements contain this amount of iron. If iron deficiency is diagnosed, a supplement of 60–120 mg/day is advised.[39]

Iodine

Most of us know that iodine is a necessary component of thyroid hormones, but fewer are aware that iodine is critical for the normal development of the brain and central nervous system of developing babies. While severe iodine deficiency resulting in intellectual disability is rare in developed countries, mild or moderate deficiencies resulting in lower than average intelligence may be relatively common. The RDA for iodine increases from 150 mcg in adults to 220 mcg during pregnancy.[41] The upper limit (UL) set by the Institute of Medicine (IOM) is 1,100 mcg, however, there is evidence that this UL may be too high during pregnancy. Excess iodine can negatively affect the fetal thyroid gland and cognition. The World Health Organization (WHO) recommends an UL of 500 mcg, and some experts suggest an UL of 250 mcg.[42] The main dietary sources of iodine are seaweed, seafood, and iodized salt (with much smaller amounts in whole plant foods, especially if grown in iodine-rich soil). Plant-based eaters could end up on either end of iodine intake spectrum, with low intakes in those who do not consume seaweed, seafood, or iodized salt, and high intakes for those eating kelp and other iodine-rich seaweed regularly. As seaweed is an extremely concentrated source of iodine, regular intakes could easily exceed recommended upper limits. For example, just one half a teaspoon of kelp powder provides over 1,100 mcg iodine. For this reason, seaweed is not recommended as a primary iodine source during pregnancy, although one or two servings a week is safe (note: avoid hijiki completely due to high arsenic content). That leaves us with iodized salt or supplements as our most reliable iodine sources. One-half teaspoon of iodized salt (containing about 150 mcg iodine), plus a variety of whole plant foods will provide sufficient iodine.

Lab Tests: Iodine status is typically measured using urinary iodine tests, as most of the iodine we consume is excreted in the urine. These tests are not routinely ordered during pregnancy and generally unnecessary if a reliable iodine source is supplied.

Supplements: The easiest way to ensure adequate iodine is to select a prenatal supplement that includes it—check the label as only about half the supplements available in the U.S. contain iodine and the amounts are quite variable. If a supplement provides 100 mcg, you could consume ¼ teaspoon of iodized salt and a variety of plant foods to reach the 220 mcg target. If it provides 150 mcg, you will be close to your target without adding iodized salt.

Zinc

Zinc is needed for cell duplication—a task that is greatly accelerated during pregnancy. It is also important for immune function, enzyme production, and for protein and DNA synthesis. Hence, needs for zinc increase from 8 to 11 mg during pregnancy. Due to reduced absorption, it is possible that plant-based eaters need up to 50 percent more zinc than meat eaters. The best plant sources are legumes, seeds (especially pumpkin seeds), nuts (especially pine nuts and cashews), and whole grains. By soaking, sprouting, fermenting, and leavening foods, zinc becomes more available for absorption.

Lab Tests: Zinc is not routinely measured, as lab tests are not reliable indicators of overall zinc status.

Supplements: Be sure your prenatal supplement contains zinc—ideally between 10 and 15 mg.

Practical Pointers for a Plant-based Pregnancy

Plant-based diets can provide excellent nutrition during pregnancy when they are well designed. Using the Plant-Based Plate will help you to ensure that nutrient needs are met. Table 7.2 provides a minimum suggested number of servings from each food group during pregnancy and lactation. Increase the number of servings to achieve your weight gain goals. A summary of recommended supplements is provided in Table 7.3.

Generous intakes of whole plant foods, such as vegetables, fruits, legumes, whole grains, nuts, and seeds help to maximize intakes of protective dietary factors such as antioxidants, phytochemicals, and fiber. Fiber is our source of prebiotics, or food for a healthy gut microbiome. A healthy gut microbiome can have long-term positive health implications for both mother and child.[43]

Table 7.2: The Plant-Based Plate for Pregnancy and Breastfeeding

FOOD GROUP	SUGGESTED SERVINGS—PREGNANCY (2ND–3RD TRIMESTER +340–450 CALORIES)	SUGGESTED SERVINGS—BREASTFEEDING (+500 CALORIES)
Vegetables	6	6
Fruits	4	4
Legumes	5	5
Grains	5–7	6–8
Nuts + Seeds	2	2

Table 7.3: Supplement Summary

SUPPLEMENT	PREGNANCY RECOMMENDATION	LACTATION RECOMMENDATION
Prenatal Multi-Vitamin	Daily	Daily
Vitamin B12	Single Nutrient Supplement 100 mcg/day *or* 1,000 mcg 2–3 x/wk	Single Nutrient Supplement 100 mcg/day *or* 1,000 mcg 2–3 x/wk
Vitamin D (If insufficient from sun, food, prenatal suppl)	Single Nutrient Supplement 600–1,000 IU/day	Single Nutrient Supplement 600–1,000 IU/day
Iodine	220 mcg (prenatal suppl + food)	290 mcg (prenatal suppl + food)
DHA/EPA	200–300 mg from a microalgae supplement; at least 200 mg DHA	200–300 mg from a microalgae supplement; at least 200 mg DHA

Potentially Unsafe Foods

There are several foods or food components that are potentially unsafe in pregnancy. Some must be completely avoided, while others can be consumed, but in limited amounts. Table 7.4 provides a list of these items for quick identification.

Table 7.4: Potentially Unsafe Foods

FOOD/ FOOD COMPONENT	NOTES	RECOMMENDED RESTRICTIONS
Alcohol	Can cause permanent birth defects such as fetal alcohol syndrome.	Avoid completely. No safe level of intake.
Artificial Sweeteners	Although many health authorities approve the use of artificial sweeteners during pregnancy, data regarding safety is limited, with some evidence suggesting increase in risk of preterm birth.	Minimize or avoid artificial sweeteners, including acesulfame K, aspartame, neotame, saccharin, and sucralose during pregnancy.

FOOD/ FOOD COMPONENT	NOTES	RECOMMENDED RESTRICTIONS
Caffeine	High caffeine intakes may adversely affect the health of both mother and infant. The ability to clear caffeine from the blood is reduced during pregnancy, and infants have minimal capacity to metabolize it. Coffee, caffeinated teas and energy drinks are all significant sources.	Limit caffeine intake to no more than 200 mg per day.
Raw Sprouts	Raw vegetable sprouts may contain bacteria that can cause illness in both the mother and the baby.	Avoid raw sprouts.
Unpasteurized Juices	Unpasteurized juices may contain bacteria that can cause illness in both the mother and the baby.	Avoid unpasteurized juices.
Raw and Unpasteurized Dairy Products	Raw and unpasteurized milk and cheese may contain bacteria called listeria, which is harmful to unborn babies.	Avoid raw and unpasteurized dairy products.
Fish/Shellfish	Large predatory fish such as bigeye tuna, king mackerel, marlin, orange roughy, shark and swordfish contain high levels of mercury. Raw and undercooked shellfish are at high risk of bacterial contamination.	Avoid bigeye tuna, king mackerel, marlin, orange roughy, shark and swordfish. Avoid raw and undercooked shellfish.
Prepared Foods	Ready-to-eat processed meats, pâtés, dressed and pre-packaged salads may contain listeria.	Avoid ready-to-eat processed meats, pâtés, dressed and pre-packaged salads.
Herbal Teas	Most commercial tea brands are safe to drink in moderation. Loose teas are not regulated, and best limited or avoided. Some herbal teas may increase risk of uterine contractions in early pregnancy, preterm births, and miscarriage; some have diuretic properties.	Avoid aloe, black and blue cohosh, buckthorn bark, chamomile, chicory root, coltsfoot, comfrey, dandelion, Dong Quai, ginseng, juniper, Labrador laxative teas, licorice root, lobelia, nettle leaf, penny-royal teas, sassafras, Senna leaf, and slippery elm bark teas.
Seaweeds	Hijiki seaweed contains high levels of arsenic. Kelp, dulse, arame and wakame contain high levels of iodine.	Avoid hijiki seaweed. Limit intake of other seaweed to 1–2 times a week. Nori is lower in iodine, so daily moderate intake is safe.

Sources: [44, 45, 27, 46, 47, 48, 49, 50]

Supplements to Avoid

Some supplements are unsafe to take during pregnancy. Although vitamin A is vital to the health of both mother and infant, too much preformed vitamin A (retinol from animal products and in supplements) can cause birth defects such as malformations of the eyes, skull, lungs, and heart (note: this does not apply to provitamin A carotenoids from plants).[51] Preformed vitamin A from animal products and supplements should not exceed the upper limit of 2,800 mcg.

Vitamin E is also best avoided as a single nutrient supplement during pregnancy due to a possible association with increased abdominal pain in the mother and premature rupture of the amniotic sac at term.[52] Herbal supplements are generally best avoided during pregnancy as several are associated with adverse side effects. Always check with your medical provider before taking supplements.

Morning Sickness

The first trimester can be the greatest challenge nutritionally, particularly for the 50 to 85 percent of pregnant women who suffer from nausea (and sometimes vomiting) that so often appears between the sixth and eighth week of pregnancy.[53] While commonly known as "morning sickness," the condition can occur at any time of day or night, or all day long. The good news is that "morning sickness" is an indication that hormonal changes necessary to support a healthy pregnancy are taking place. It does not generally pose a danger to mother or baby and typically resolves around the fourteenth to twentieth week of pregnancy.[54] However, a more severe form of the condition called hyperemesis gravidarum (affecting an estimated 0.3–1 percent of pregnant women), may require medical attention.[53] Fortunately, for most women, there are several things you can do to help alleviate symptoms of morning sickness:

1. **Eat small, frequent meals.** Large meals can make matters worse, while grazing helps to keep blood sugars from dipping down and triggering nausea.
2. **Stay well hydrated.** Dehydration can aggravate nausea. If you have a hard time drinking enough plain water, drink soda water flavored with fruits, cucumber and mint, or a splash of your favorite juice. Aim for 6 to 8 cups of noncaffeinated fluids each day.
3. **Be picky about your food.** Generally, avoid spicy, greasy, strong smelling

foods. Stick to bland foods like bananas, oatmeal, and toast, and include some protein with each meal. For example, almond butter on your banana, hempseeds on your oatmeal, and hummus on your toast. Eat what appeals to you and what agrees with you; avoid foods that aggravate your symptoms.

4. **Try natural anti-nausea aids.** Ginger is at the top of the list and is available in several forms—fresh root, beverages, powders, tablets, candies, and syrups. Raw ginger can be added to main dishes, dressings, water, or tea.

5. **Consider adding vitamin B6.** This vitamin may help alleviate some of the symptoms of morning sickness. Usual dosages are 10 to 50 mg twice a day.[53]

6. **Adjust timing of prenatal vitamins.** If they make you feel queasy, try taking them just before bed or with a meal.

7. **Try an alternative remedy.** Some women report relief using acupressure, acupuncture, hypnosis, or aromatherapy.

Infant Allergy

For many decades, the prevailing opinion was that pregnant and nursing moms should avoid potentially allergenic foods to help reduce the risk of severe allergic reaction in their infants. The weight of the evidence today suggests the opposite. It appears that allergen exposure during pregnancy and lactation induces tolerance to allergens and reduces the risk of allergies in your baby. While the current evidence is not yet conclusive, we certainly can say it is safe to include allergenic foods in your diet while pregnant.[55]

PLANT-BASED BREASTFEEDING

Your little miracle has arrived, and breastfeeding will continue to make you your baby's sole source of nutrition for another six months or thereabouts. Whether you plan to nurse for nine months or three years, your milk is exquisitely designed to provide a healthy balance of nutrients for your baby. Breastfeeding protects your baby's gut, reduces risk of infections, and appears to reduce risk for celiac disease, allergies, diabetes, and leukemia.[56] It provides some impressive advantages for you as well, reducing blood loss after delivery, and helping restore your uterus to its previous size more quickly. It also helps you return to your pre-pregnancy weight more quickly, lowers your risk of postpartum depression, prevents menstruation (helping to space pregnancies and conserve iron), reduces the risk of several diseases, including breast and ovarian cancer, type 2 diabetes, hypertension, and heart disease.[57, 58, 59] You will have no formula to purchase, nipples to sterilize, or bottles to warm, so it is both convenient and economical. And, of course, nursing your baby is a wonderful way to strengthen your maternal-infant bond.

NUTRITION KNOW-HOW FOR BREASTFEEDING MOMS

Your nutritional needs change only slightly from those of pregnancy, so most of the guidelines provided in the pregnancy section will work perfectly for you during breastfeeding as well. Table 7.5 provides the recommended nutrient intakes for women from nineteen to fifty years, as well as for pregnant and breastfeeding women. Let's explore the fine points of designing a diet to support a beautiful breastfeeding experience.

During pregnancy, your energy needs increase by an average of about 300 calories a day over the course of the pregnancy. When you are breastfeeding, you typically need an extra 500 calories a day. It is important that you are not on a weight loss diet, as this can compromise the quality of your diet, and nutrients available for your baby. However, because nursing uses up a lot of calories, you may notice a more rapid return to pre-pregnancy weight than is typical of those who are not nursing.

The RDAs for protein, calcium, thiamin, vitamin D, and vitamin K remain unchanged from that of pregnancy. The RDAs for copper, selenium, zinc, riboflavin, pantothenic acid, vitamin B6, vitamin B12, and choline increase slightly, while those of vitamin A, vitamin C, and iodine increase more significantly. For magnesium, potassium, and folate, the RDA decreases slightly below that of pregnancy, while for iron, it drops dramatically from 27 mg to 9 mg per day. This is because the lactating mother no longer has an increased blood volume, and menstruation generally does not resume with full time breastfeeding. It is commonly advised that breastfeeding mothers continue their prenatal supplements during breastfeeding (be sure the supplement includes iodine and vitamin D), although a switch to an iron-free formulation is quite acceptable. You may also continue your prenatal supplement for a few months and then switch to a regular adult multi-vitamin mineral supplement with iodine and vitamin D. If you are mostly or entirely plant-based, you will also need a vitamin B12 supplement (same level of intake recommendations for pregnant women). Compared to omnivores, plant exclusive eaters have significantly reduced levels of DHA/EPA in breast milk, so it seems reasonable to boost these levels by continuing with the 200–300 mg DHA/ EPA supplement suggested for pregnancy.

Table 7.5: Recommended Dietary Allowances for Pregnant and Lactating Women

NUTRIENT	NON-PREGNANT	PREGNANT	LACTATING
Minerals			
Calcium (mg/d)	1,000	1,000	1,000
Copper (mcg/d)	900	1,000	1,300
Iodine (mcg/d)	150	220	290
Iron (mg/d)	18	27	9
Magnesium (mg/d)	310–320	350–360	310–320
Potassium (mg/d)	2,600	2,900	2,800
Selenium (mcg/d)	55	60	70
Zinc (mg/d)	8	11	12
Vitamins			
Vitamin A (mcg RAE/d)	700	770	1,300
Thiamin (mg/d)	1.1	1.4	1.4
Riboflavin (mg/d)	1.1	1.4	1.6
Niacin (mg/d)	14	18	17
Pantothenic Acid (mg/d)	5	6	7
Vitamin B6 (mg/d)	1.3	1.9	2
Folate (mcg/d)	400	600	500
Vitamin B12 (mcg/d)	2.4	2.6	2.8

Table 7.5: Recommended Dietary Allowances *(continued)*

Choline (mg/d)	425	450	550
Vitamin C (mg/d)	75	85	120
Vitamin D (IU/d)	600	600	600
Vitamin E (mg/d)	15	15	19
Vitamin K (mcg/d)	90	90	90

Sources: [60, 61, 62, 41, 63]

As a breastfeeding mom, you will need extra fluids, so always have water handy, especially while nursing. Aim for about 8 to 12 cups of fluids a day—mostly water! Caffeine use should be limited, as in pregnancy. Alcohol use is best minimized, although it does not need to be strictly avoided as is necessary during pregnancy.

One of the unexpected benefits of choosing to eat plant-based is that the levels of environmental pollutants in your breast milk may be reduced compared to those eating mixed diets.[64, 65, 66] One American study found that the highest value for six contaminants in the breast milk of vegans was lower than the lowest value from the breast milk of women consuming mixed diets.[66] To further reduce potentially harmful environmental substances, choose organic foods when possible and practical.

Breastfeeding is a very new experience for both mother and baby, so it may not come as naturally as you might imagine. If you encounter difficulties, seek the assistance of a lactation consultant (look for someone who is an International Board-Certified Lactation Consultant). These are breastfeeding experts who help new moms with poor milk supply, positioning and latching issues, falling asleep at the breast, and just about every other breastfeeding challenge you might face.

In conclusion, there are so many reasons to experience a plant-based pregnancy and lactation. Ensuring nutritional adequacy is easy, with some planning. Our next chapter is just what you might have expected—nutrition during the growing years. We will navigate the nutrition challenges that accompany infancy, the preschool years, childhood, and adolescence.

Chapter 8

Childhood and Adolescence

"One thing I had learned from watching chimpanzees with
their infants is that having a child should be fun."

—Jane Goodall

T
he shift toward a plant-based diet is widely embraced as a wise choice for
disease risk reduction in adults. However, you might still expect to encounter a few raised eyebrows if you share your intention to raise children on a
plant-based diet. Infancy, childhood, and adolescence are characterized by constant
physical changes and unique physiological requirements. The notion that animal
products are necessary during these more nutritionally vulnerable periods is deeply
ingrained into our culture. However, this has more to do with culture than with
science. As you may recall from Chapter 1, the Academy of Nutrition and Dietetics
takes the position that appropriately planned vegan, and other types of vegetarian diets, satisfy the nutrient needs and promote normal growth at all stages of
the life cycle, including infancy, childhood, and adolescence. In this chapter, we
walk you through each of the stages of growth, provide you with tools you need

to navigate through the challenges, and offer a wealth of information that will set your mind at ease. We begin by reviewing the core concepts of nutrition for growing children, identify key aspects of each stage of development, and end by addressing many of the questions parents often have around nutrition for their families, including indications for laboratory testing and supplements.

CORE CONCEPTS FOR GROWING CHILDREN

Well-planned plant-based diets are safe and adequate for children of all ages.[1] The overall diet quality is what really matters. For families who are plant-predominant and include dairy products and eggs, studies suggest that there is little difference in growth and development compared to omnivorous children.[1,2] For those who are plant-exclusive, though fewer studies exist, adequate growth and development has been demonstrated in these children as well.[3,4]

As we dive into the particulars of nutrition for growing infants, toddlers, children, and adolescents, let's consider some of the core concepts that are paramount to raising healthy plant-based children of all ages.

1. **Promote optimal growth, development, and well-being.** Many dietary patterns can adequately support the growth and development of children. Well-planned plant-based diets are no exception. All diets for children should provide adequate calories and nutrients, including sufficient macro- and micronutrients.

2. **Prevent immediate childhood health concerns such as iron-deficiency anemia, dental caries, and over and under nutrition.** This means providing a variety of nutrient dense foods (in some instances, fortified) and supplements when indicated.

3. **Establish eating habits that support health throughout life and that prevent against chronic diseases** (such as cardiovascular disease, type 2 diabetes mellitus, obesity, hypertension, some forms of cancer, and osteoporosis). Eating patterns developed in childhood and adolescence profoundly impact our food choices in adulthood.[5,6,7,8] Plant-based dietary patterns can help to establish healthy habits. Research confirms that

children who grow up eating well-planned plant-based diets enjoy several important advantages.[1] For example, plant-based children:

- Are at lower risk for overweight or obesity (which reduces risk of chronic disease)
- Eat more vegetables and fruit
- Eat fewer sweets and salty snacks
- Have higher fiber intakes
- Eat less saturated fat

As a parent, you are at the top of the list of powerful role models in your child's life—you are their first teacher.

4. **Nurture children's natural ability to eat intuitively and with joy to provide a foundation for a healthy relationship with food.** Babies are born with an innate ability to eat intuitively. They generally want to eat when they are hungry and stop eating when they are full. As parents, we can encourage intuitive eating by honoring our child's appetite. We can help shape a healthy relationship with food by keeping experiences around food positive and pleasant. By exploring food together and avoiding food rewards and punishments, we can help our children become joyful, confident, healthy eaters.

INFANCY (BIRTH TO TWELVE MONTHS)

Adam and Martha were ecstatic (and exhausted!) parents of a newborn baby boy, Henry. Martha had great support from the lactation consultants before leaving the hospital but breastfeeding at home was not going well. With the support of lactation consultants and their pediatrician, Dr. Garcia, they decided to continue breast feeding but also to supplement with formula to ease some of their stress and anxiety. As plant-exclusive eaters, Adam and Martha were hoping for an option that was not cow's milk based. They had read that soy formula could be harmful to babies. Dr. Garcia addressed their concerns and reassured them that soy formula was safe and adequate for growing babies. Martha continued to breastfeed and offered supplemental soy formula until little Henry turned one. She also gave Henry a daily vitamin D supplement since he usually only had 8 or so ounces of formula a day.

Infancy is a period marked by rapid growth and development. During this critical time, babies are learning to sit, crawl, walk, talk, and explore the world around them. By six months of age, babies have doubled their birth weight and by one year of age they have tripled it. Proper nutrition is essential at this time and feeding offers an opportunity for caregivers to develop an emotional bond with their infant. The first year of life can be thought of in two stages when it comes to feeding: breast/formula feeding and introduction of solids.

The First Six Months… Best Milks for Baby

The decision about what milk to feed your baby is, for some parents, easy peasy, while for others, it is the source of sleepless nights. Although breastfeeding seems a natural choice and is recommended by health authorities, not all moms are able to, or choose to, breastfeed. According to the CDC's 2016 Breast-Feeding Report Care, just over half of American women were breastfeeding their babies at six months of age and almost a third were breastfeeding at twelve months of age.[9] While most moms start out breastfeeding, many stop within the first six weeks due to concerns about milk supply, fatigue, or the need to return to work.[10] Let's take a closer look at the options you have for feeding your baby during the first six months of life.

Breast Milk

Each mammal species produces a milk that is exquisitely designed to support the growth and development of their offspring. Humans are no exception. There is unanimous agreement in scientific circles that human breast milk is the best food for human infants. The evidence is simply overwhelming. Breast milk provides multiple advantages for your baby.[11, 12]

- ✓ Supplies an ideal balance of nutrients that adjusts over time (assuming adequate maternal intake):
  - Protein, including essential amino acids
  - Fats, including essential fatty acids
  - Carbohydrate
  - Vitamins and minerals
- ✓ Delivers protective antibodies, cytokines, antimicrobial agents, and oligosaccharides (which favorably shapes the gut microbiome).
- ✓ Guards against respiratory tract infections.

✓ Reduces risk of gastrointestinal infections.

✓ Decreases the risk of sudden infant death syndrome (SIDS).

✓ Diminishes incidence of asthma, celiac disease, allergies, atopic dermatitis, and eczema.

✓ Helps prevent childhood inflammatory bowel disease.

✓ Reduces risk of excess weight gain during adolescence and adulthood.

✓ Protects against both type 1 and type 2 diabetes.

✓ Decreases risk of leukemia, with greater protection conferred by breast-feeding at least six months.

The World Health Organization (WHO), the Institute of Medicine (IOM), and the American Academy of Pediatrics (AAP) all concur that breast milk should serve as the sole food during the first six months of life.[11] While older guidelines suggested the introduction of solid foods at four to six months, more recent research has established that health outcomes are improved with exclusive breastfeeding for a full six months. Babies who were given solids between four to six months had significantly greater incidence of respiratory tract infections, ear infections, and diarrheal disease.[11] It is recommended that breastfeeding continues for a full year and beyond. It is interesting to note that in most traditional societies, children wean between two and four years of age.[13] For women who cannot breastfeed or who produce insufficient milk, pasteurized donor milk from human milk banks is an option. It can be highly beneficial for high-risk infants, particularly those with very low birthweight. Unfortunately, donor milk from established milk banks is not always accessible or affordable and informal direct milk sharing without pasteurization exposes infants to a range of risks including bacterial and viral contamination.[14]

Infants who are exclusively breastfed should receive a vitamin D supplement of 400 IU daily beginning in the first few days of life and continuing until at least twelve months of age.[15] Many continue to require a vitamin D supplement throughout childhood and adolescence. In the United States, infant formula provides sufficient vitamin D if at least one quart (or one liter) is consumed per day. If a combination of breast milk and formula are used or formula drops below one quart per day, an infant supplement of 400 IU per day is recommended.[15] For plant-exclusive or close to plant-exclusive mothers, 1,000 mcg B12 at least twice a week (see Table 8.4) and 200–300 mg DHA/EPA per day, with at least 200 mg DHA is recommended. Breastfeeding mothers should also continue to take a prenatal supplement or an adult multi-vitamin.

Breast Milk Alternatives

Commercial infant formula is the only acceptable alternative to breast milk during the first year of life. All infant formulas in the United States must meet strict federal nutrition requirements prior to marketing their product. They have to include minimum amounts for twenty-nine nutrients and maximum amounts for nine nutrients.[16] The American Academy of Pediatrics (AAP) currently recommends that iron-fortified formula be used for all infants who are not breastfed, or who are only partially breastfed, from birth to one year of age.[17] If breast-feeding slows or stops prior to one year of age, an iron-fortified commercial infant formula should be used as the replacement. Apart from breast milk and commercial infant formula, no other substitutes can safely serve as the primary milk source before baby's first birthday. Be careful when using commercial infant formula to prepare according to the directions on the package. Do not water down formula as this can lead to malnutrition in your infant.

> Apart from breast milk and commercial infant formula, no other substitutes can safely serve as the primary milk source before baby's first birthday.

Cow's milk based formula is the type of formula most commonly recommended by health authorities. The cow's milk used in formula has been altered significantly to make it nutritionally closer to human milk. It has less protein, more carbohydrate, less saturated fat, and more unsaturated fat than is found in whole cow's milk. Vitamins and minerals are adjusted to better match breast milk. Regular cow's milk is not recommended during the first year of life. There are several important reasons for this. First, the infant's gastrointestinal system is often sensitive to cow's milk protein, resulting in blood loss in the stool. In addition, the amount of iron in cow's milk is low and iron absorption is only about 10 percent (compared to 50 percent from breast milk). Thus, the use of cow's milk can greatly increase the risk of iron deficiency. In addition, cow's milk contains higher amounts of protein, sodium, potassium, phosphorus, and chloride than the immature kidneys of an infant can handle. Finally, cow's milk contains insufficient essential fatty acids, zinc, niacin, vitamin C, and vitamin E.[18]

For families that do not include dairy products (e.g., plant-exclusive or vegan families) or for infants with certain medical conditions (galactosemia and rare hereditary lactase deficiency), soy formula is typically recommended. Although there has been considerable controversy about the safety of soy formula, the AAP considers it safe for term infants.[19] One of the concerns about soy formula is that it contains soy isoflavones that have a similar structure to estrogen. Some fear that soy isoflavones will have estrogenic effects in babies; however, human studies have found little or no difference in sexual development, thyroid function, brain development, or the immune systems of babies fed soy formula.[20, 21, 22] Another concern is that soy formula is higher in aluminum than breast milk or cow's milk formula.[23, 24] Aluminum may negatively impact bone health as it competes with calcium for absorption. While healthy, full term infants do not appear to be at increased risk, preterm infants weighing less than four pounds (1800 grams), and those with compromised kidney function are at greater risk. For these babies, soy formula is not recommended. Finally, soy formulas are not generally considered a good choice for babies who are allergic to cow's milk protein, as an estimated ten to fifteen percent of these babies may also have an allergy to soy protein. For these infants hydrolyzed and hypoallergenic formulas are typically suggested.[23] In addition, for infants with congenital hypothyroidism, soy formula is contraindicated as it may negatively affect thyroid function.[22] In addition to hydrolyzed formulas, there are a variety of specialized formulas on the market, including those for premature infants, for reflux, fussiness, and with the addition of probiotics. While certain formulas may be indicated for specific conditions, it's best to consult with your pediatrician if you suspect your infant needs a specialized formula. Additionally, most infant formulas are fortified with DHA (docosahexaenoic acid) and ARA (arachidonic acid), and organic options are also available.

When you look at the ingredients on formula, it can be a little disconcerting. For example, one of the most popular soy formulas lists corn syrup solids as the first ingredient, followed by vegetable oil (including palm, coconut, soy, and sunflower oils), soy protein isolate, and the entire spectrum of nutrients. Health conscious parents who are wary of processed foods may be put off by such an ingredient list. Despite any concerns you may have about these added ingredients, rest assured, commercial infant formula is the safest type of formula for your baby. Regardless, some parents are compelled to search for more natural, homemade alternatives. A ready supply of homemade "formula," recipes are available on the internet. Steer clear. These alternatives do not have the necessary balance of nutrients to support the growth and development of infants. For example, they may contain insufficient iron or more sodium than your baby's kidneys can handle. Reports of gross malnutrition in infants have been traced to such beverages.[25, 26] In some cases, formula recipes use unpasteurized raw milk that may contain harmful bacteria such as E. coli and listeria.[27] There is no gentle way to say this—homemade infant milk can be a formula for disaster. In addition, fortified or unfortified soy, rice, oat, coconut, almond, cashew, pea, hemp, and other non-dairy milks are not suitable as primary milks for babies during the first year of life.

Table 8.1: Infant Milks in a Nutshell

MILK	RECOMMENDATION	NOTES
Human Breast Milk	Most healthful milk for infants. Select as first choice, if possible.	Ensure adequate nutrition for the nursing mother, sufficient fluids, a reliable source of vitamin B12 and a DHA/EPA supplement. Continue with prenatal vitamin or multi-vitamin/mineral supplement. Add vitamin D drops for baby. Pasteurized breast milk from a reputable milk bank may be an option for some parents, although accessibility and affordability are issues. Internet-based or informal breast milk sharing is not advised.
Commercial Infant Formula	Only suitable replacement for human milk.	Select iron-fortified cow's milk-based formula for dairy consumers. Select iron-fortified soy-based infant formula for non-dairy consumers. Select a formula with added DHA. Use of specialty formulas such as hydrolyzed or hypoallergenic formulas should be discussed with your health care provider.
Homemade Infant Formula	NEVER use homemade infant formula.	Homemade formula: • Does not provide balanced nutrition for infants. • May contain harmful ingredients. • May be a source of harmful bacteria.

Cow's Milk	Do not use for infants under 1 year of age.	Cow's milk can increase risk of iron deficiency.
Non-dairy fortified and unfortified beverages	Do not use as a primary milk for infants under 1 year of age.	Plant milks provide inadequate nutrition and are not appropriate as primary milks for infants.

Months Six to Twelve...Introduction to Solid Foods

Krista was already thinking about the process of starting solid foods when Erik was just two months old. She knew that experts advised no solid foods before six months of age. She learned from her mom that thirty-one years ago, when she was a baby, the advice was not that different—solids were considered safe to introduce between four and six months of age. She received her first solid food, infant rice cereal, at five months. Her mom said that rice cereal was encouraged because of the added iron and the low potential for allergy. After she had been on the rice cereal for two weeks, her mom began providing a variety of pureed foods, one at a time. Slowly, mashed and lumpy foods were introduced, followed by pieces of soft food like banana and steamed vegetables. Although she had several friends that used a similar feeding regimen, Krista was intrigued by a more contemporary trend called "baby-led weaning," and decided to give it a try.

Baby's First Graduation...Starting Solids

Up until about six months of age, most of your baby's nutrition needs are met by breast milk or commercial infant formula alone. However, at about six months, milk is no longer sufficient to supply the calorie and nutrient needs of most infants. Around this time, the introduction of solid foods or complementary feeding is recommended. This is a very gradual process in which the baby transitions from mostly breast milk or formula at six months of age to mostly solid foods somewhere between one and two years of age. This period is critical for the development of food preferences and eating behaviors, and it can set the stage for a lifetime of healthy eating.

A key nutrient of concern at this stage is iron. By four to six months of age, your baby's iron stores start to decline. For this reason, iron-rich foods such as iron-fortified infant cereal are recommended as the first solid foods. Although the American Academy of Pediatrics recommends that breastfed babies receive an iron supplement (1 mg/kg per day) beginning at four months of age until baby meets the RDA with solid foods, not all pediatric authorities agree, so work with your pediatrician to determine if iron supplementation is appropriate for your baby. For more information on iron, see Chapter 5.

It is important to recognize that breast milk or formula remains a major component of your baby's diet until at least age one, and often to two years of age and beyond. From about six to eight months, breast milk will provide about 80 percent of your baby's calories, from nine to twelve months, it will supply about 50 percent of calories, and from one to two years, about one-third of the calories.

When Is Baby Ready for Solids?

Not all babies are ready for solids at exactly six months—some may be slightly older or slightly younger. This depends on your baby's rate of development. Signs of readiness include:

1. **Good head control.** Baby will be able to hold his head up for some time.
2. **Ability to sit up in a highchair.** Baby will sit in a highchair or feeding seat with little or no support.
3. **Interest in food.** Baby will show signs of interest in the food you are eating. He will open his mouth and lean forward when food is offered.
4. **Sustained hunger between milk or formula feeding.** Baby will be less satisfied after a milk feeding, and the intervals between feeds will begin to shorten.
5. **Can move food into her throat and swallow it.** When baby pushes the food back out of her mouth and it dribbles down her chin, she may not be ready for solid foods. Try again in a week or so.[28]

While it might be tempting to delay the introduction of solid foods beyond six months, it is not generally advisable. As previously mentioned, your baby needs the calories and nutrition by this age. In addition, this is a critical period for adapting to various food textures and tastes. By eight months of age, you will want to have introduced your baby to a variety of pureed, mashed, lumpy, and chopped foods. If different flavors and textures are not introduced by this time, your baby may have difficulty accepting them by a year of age and can become very selective or picky in their food preferences.

Is the Order of Introduction of Solid Foods Important?

While you do not need to offer solid foods in any special order, it is helpful to begin with a food that is high in iron, such as fortified infant cereal. Some experts suggest meat as a first food to enhance iron status, but fortified infant cereal is a safer, more concentrated source. The RDA for seven- to twelve-month-old infants is 11 mg iron per day (more than an adult male!). This is extremely difficult to achieve in any diet that does not include fortified foods. To illustrate this point, 11 mg of iron can be obtained from six tablespoons of iron-fortified infant cereal, thirteen tablespoons of tofu, twenty-seven tablespoons of lentils, fifty-two tablespoons of strained chicken, or seventy-nine tablespoons of strained beef.[29]

Beyond the question of iron, research does not suggest that any particular order of introduction is better for baby. While it was long thought that vegetables should be offered before fruit, there is no evidence that your baby will reject vegetables if fruit is given first. You will want to add vitamin C-rich foods soon after starting infant cereal. Vitamin C-rich vegetables and fruits will enhance the absorption of iron from the cereal.

What Method of Feeding Is Best for Baby?

Traditionally, in most cultures, baby's first foods were offered on a spoon by the baby's caregiver. More recently, there has been a trend towards a method of feeding called "baby-lead weaning (BLW)." This method of feeding provides the baby with appropriate foods that they can take in their hands and feed themselves. The goal is to give the baby more control over food intake. While it is successful in this regard, a systematic review of baby-led weaning suggests that there is insufficient evidence about BLW to determine if it provides sufficient energy and calories. Parents who use this feeding method need to receive appropriate support to ensure sufficient energy and nutrients, including iron, and details regarding choking risk.[30]

As there appear to be advantages to both methods of feeding, it may be well advised for parents to use a modified version of BLW that incorporates the best of both worlds. The goal is to ensure that complementary feeding is safe, adequate, and supports a lifelong healthy relationship with food. So, it makes good sense to feed iron-rich cereals and pureed foods with a spoon, and allow your baby to feed themselves lumpy, chunky, and finger foods (including those made with iron-fortified infant cereal—see Chapter 15, Recipes). When feeding with a spoon, be responsive to a child's hunger and satiety cues. If your baby's head turns away from a spoonful of food, stop feeding. Your baby is telling you that they have had enough.

Baby's first solid foods are best served in a dish or on a highchair tray, NOT in a bottle. While putting thinned solids in a bottle removes mess, it is a choking hazard and does not provide your baby with the exciting opportunity to enjoy the tastes, textures, and tactile experiences of eating solid foods. Expect messes—they are part of the territory when babies begin to explore food. Always supervise your baby while he is eating. Feed your little one with a baby-sized spoon, and feed slowly without distractions such as television. Put a small amount of food in a separate dish rather than feeding from the storage container in order to avoid adding bacteria to the food in storage.

What Kinds of Foods and Beverages Are Appropriate for Babies?

The primary goals in food choices for infants from six to twelve months are nutrition, variety, and safety. As you may recall, iron-fortified infant cereal is often the first food provided as babies need extra iron at this stage. At one time, authorities recommended rice-based infant cereal as the first food due to its low allergenicity. However, the FDA now advises parents against using rice cereal exclusively due to its arsenic content. While they do not go so far as to say avoid it completely, they do suggest using a variety of infant cereals such as oat, barley, wheat, and mixed cereals. Selecting organic rice products does not make them lower in arsenic. However, selecting organic baby cereals does reduce exposure to pesticides, so choose organic when you can. Our recommendation would be to use non-rice, iron-fortified infant cereals, and when brown, black, or other rice is served, prepare it in a manner that reduces arsenic content. Rinse the rice a few times, cook in plenty of water (six times more water than rice), and then drain before serving. Following this preparation method can reduce the lifetime health risks associated with the most toxic forms of arsenic by about 83 percent.[31]

Vegetables and fruits can be served cooked or raw, if soft. Hard chunks of vegetables and fruits can pose a choking risk, so be cautious with these. Vegetables and fruits can be pureed, mashed, lumpy, or served in pieces after steaming to soften. Grains can be served intact (kamut berries, quinoa, rice), or in a more processed form such as cold cereal, pasta, or toast. Provide protein and iron-rich foods such as tofu, lentils, and beans (animal products can also be provided for families that choose to include them). Nuts and seeds should be served as butters or creams and thinned to avoid risk of choking. For those who include dairy products in their diets, forgo fluid milk, selecting yogurts and cheeses, in moderation, if sufficient iron-rich foods are eaten. The only beverages recommended for babies under a year of age are breast milk, formula, and water in small amounts for babies six months and beyond. The following tips will help you to provide healthy foods for your baby:

- Keep it simple. Start with one food at a time.
- Do not add sugar, salt, or salty seasonings to the food.
- Avoid sweet beverages and juices.
- Avoid highly processed foods. Get your baby used to the natural flavors of whole foods.
- Make food from scratch when you are able.
- If you are serving commercial baby food, read the label. Many have added starches, sugars, and preservatives. In addition, many commercial baby foods contain concerning levels of heavy metals (see Table 8.2).

Does the Timing of Solid Food Introduction Affect Allergy Risk?

The prevalence of allergies has increased dramatically in the Western world, and various tactics have been suggested to mitigate this response. For many years, experts believed that early introduction to the most allergenic food would increase risk of allergic reactions. In 2000, the American Academy of Pediatrics (AAP) advised that for infants at high risk for allergy (due to family history of atopic disease) hydrolyzed formula should be used, that breastfeeding mothers should avoid eating allergenic foods such as peanuts, and that allergenic foods be delayed beyond one year of age (two to three years for more allergenic foods). The tide has turned quite dramatically with updated recommendations by the AAP in 2008 and again in 2019. The current AAP position is that there is a lack of evidence that hydrolyzed formula prevents atopic disease, a lack of evidence that breastfeeding mothers should avoid eating allergenic foods, and a lack of evidence that delaying the introduction of allergenic foods, including peanuts, eggs, and fish prevents atopic disease. The AAP adds that there is evidence that the early introduction of infant-safe forms of peanut reduces risk of peanut allergy.[32] In 2017, AAP-endorsed guidelines for the prevention of peanut allergy were released, followed by the Canadian Pediatric Society (CPS) position statement on the introduction of peanut and other allergenic foods to babies in 2019.[33] Parents are now advised to introduce allergenic foods (in an age-appropriate manner) early—around six months of age (but not before four months of age), when other solid foods are started. This is especially important for infants at risk for allergy (e.g., those with a family history of allergy or who have symptoms of atopy such as eczema). Age-appropriate "peanut" options would be smooth peanut butter diluted with water or breast milk or mixed with a previously tolerated food such as pureed fruit or vegetables. For older infants, smooth peanut butter could be spread thinly on a piece of toast or cracker. If your baby tolerates the allergenic food, offer it a few times a week to help maintain tolerance. For infants at very high risk (e.g., those with severe eczema), allergy testing is often advised prior to feeding peanuts. A referral to an allergist should be considered and she may perform a skin-prick test or IgE blood test in order to help determine whether it is safe to introduce peanuts at home or under medical supervision in the doctor's office.[32, 33]

While experts used to advise waiting three to five days between each new food introduction, this is no longer thought to be necessary. However, do introduce new foods one at a time so you can observe whether a food causes a reaction such as hives, swelling, redness, or rashes.

Additional Points for Pint-Sized Plant Eaters

To ensure optimal nutrition for babies raised on plant-exclusive or plant-predominant diets, ample macro- and micronutrients are required. While fiber is also important for babies, we don't want to overdo fiber, as it can quickly fill small bellies before adequate calories are consumed. For sufficient calories, use full-fat soy foods, such as tofu and soy yogurt. Include avocados, nut and seed butters and creams, beans and bean spreads, starchy vegetables, and grains. You may wish to select some refined grain products (such as pasta) in addition to whole grains to help moderate fiber intake. While raw foods are a healthful part of the mix, cooking does help to increase caloric density and digestibility.

Table 14.1 provides sample menus for six- to eight-month-old babies and nine- to twelve-month-old babies. Most infants will gradually transition from all liquid meals, adding one meal of solid foods at a time. Some babies will be eating three solid meals within a month of starting solids, while for others, it may take two or three months. By nine months of age, babies will usually be eating three meals a day and will begin to have one or more solid food snacks.

Be sure to continue to supplement with 400 IU of vitamin D per day for infants receiving breast milk. Breast milk (or formula) will provide sufficient vitamin B12, iodine, and DHA/EPA, assuming the mother's intake is adequate.

Averting Harm…Baby Food No-No's

There are some foods that are best avoided as they are potentially harmful to your baby. Table 8.2 provides a summary of these foods. Other foods, while not entirely off limits should be restricted. For example, babies have no need for fruit juice. It is preferable to feed whole fruits which provide more nutrients and fiber. Water is the only other beverage recommended for babies between six months and one year of age. Conventional oat and wheat products may contain glyphosate (from the herbicide, Roundup). While this does not mean you should never allow your baby to eat non-organic wheat, barley, or oat products, stick to organic when you are able. For more information see the section on grains in Chapter 6.

While non-dairy milks are not harmful for a baby when added to mashed potatoes, cereal, or prepared foods, they must NEVER replace breast milk or formula in your baby's first year. They are nutritionally inadequate, even if fortified.

Table 8.2: Baby Food No-Nos

FOOD	WHY AVOID?
Unpasteurized milk and milk products	Risk of food poisoning from bacteria and other pathogens
Cow's milk	Risk of iron deficiency
Honey and products made with honey	Risk of botulism poisoning
Raw sprouts	Risk of food poisoning

Table 8.2: Baby Food No-Nos *(continued)*

FOOD	WHY AVOID?
Sugar-sweetened beverages and added sugars	Calories without nutrients Develop a sweet tooth Dental caries
Commercial rice-based baby foods	High arsenic levels
Apple and grape juice	May be high in arsenic
Protein powder	Contains a variety of heavy metals Not appropriate for infants
Processed meat	May increase cancer risk
Foods that are round, hard, or sticky: • Chunks of hard raw vegetables (steam first) • Hard fruits (grate first) • Small, smooth foods like hard candy, cough drops, nuts, and seeds • Sticky foods like nut butter or gum (thin with water or milk or spread thinly on bread, toast, or crackers—never serve from a spoon) • Foods in round or cylinder shapes like grapes (cut in half first) or tofu dogs (or other hot dogs, cut lengthwise) • Fish with bones • Popcorn	Choking hazards

Feeding your baby during the first year of life is undoubtedly a source of excitement, entertainment, and enjoyment for both you and your baby. It provides an enriching experience for exploring, learning, and sharing. As your little one becomes a toddler, food preferences and appetite may change, but you can be sure the adventure has just begun.

TODDLERS (ONE TO THREE YEARS)

I (Brenda) vividly recall my son's first potluck experience. He was two years old. It was an Easter potluck at our local toy-lending library. The potluck table was brimming with fun foods like bunny-shaped sandwiches, crackers and cheese, frosted sugar cookies, chips, and pretzels. Predictably, I brought a tray of colorful veggies and a cashew-based herb dip. My son had never experienced a potluck before so was unaware of the protocol. He looked over the potluck table and proceeded to carry the entire veggie tray to our table. He thought you picked your favorite item and ate that. I had to explain to him how a potluck worked, and he carried the tray back to the potluck table. After he finished his plate, he stayed at his little seat until everyone else was finished, then he proceeded to polish off the remaining vegetables. Another mom was so stunned at his affinity for vegetables, she asked me how in the world I managed to get him to like vegetables so much. I responded, "I am not sure that I did anything special, other than teaching him about how they grow, taking him to help me pick them out at the market, getting him to help wash and prepare them, serving them several times a day, and always being excited about eating them." She laughed, "Well, that does explain it."

When toddlers are standing on their own two little feet, running, bouncing, and leaping through the air, their nutrient needs and dietary preferences continue to evolve. It can be such fun to see them gain autonomy and delight in new textures and flavors. It can also be rather frustrating if they become picky and uncooperative at mealtimes. There is no question that nourishing toddlers can pose unique challenges. As these are more nutritionally vulnerable times, you may need to get creative. One of the things you might notice with your toddler is that growth slows (compared to the first twelve months), and his appetite will reflect this. As you will see in Chapter 9, this is normal and no cause for concern. Trust that by providing a variety of healthful foods, and in some cases, appropriate supplements, plant-based toddlers will get what their little bodies need to thrive.

At this stage it is important for parents to provide structured meals and snacks in a warm, positive, and developmentally appropriate way (seated in a high chair or booster seat at table height and with appropriate utensils, plate, cup, etc.). Additionally, parents should include toddlers in regular family meals and serve as a role model when it comes to serving and enjoying a variety of healthy foods.

As mentioned previously, after age two, the number of calories coming from fat gradually declines and calories from whole grains, fruits, vegetables, and beans gradually increases. Because children at this age tend to eat small amounts of food at one time, it's important to consistently offer nutritious foods at meal and snack times. We will discuss feeding principles in greater detail in Chapter 9, but for now we address some of the specific nutrition issues during the toddler years.

What Is the Best Milk for Toddlers?

Breast milk remains the best milk during the second year of life, and beyond. Keep breastfeeding for as long as it seems right for you and your toddler. Breast milk continues to be a valuable source of nutrition, immune protection, and comfort for your little one. Other milks can be used in food preparation, if desired. If choosing a nondairy milk, soy or pea milk are the most nutritious options. If choosing a dairy milk, whole milk is generally recommended.

Formula-fed babies can be weaned off infant formula at one year of age. The big question for many parents is what next? Is it best to transition to cow's milk, soy milk, toddler formula or other milks? The answer depends on your family's diet and how well your toddler is growing. If your family is dairy-free, a full-fat, fortified soy or pea milk are the best options, as they are high in calories, protein, and micronutrients. Other nondairy milks, such as almond, cashew, oat, or coconut do not provide adequate nutrition to serve as primary milks for your toddler, although they are safe for use in food preparation. They can be used for older children if sufficient protein is obtained in other sources. Table 8.3 provides a nutritional comparison of various milks. Note that the non-dairy milks used in this chart are all fortified. Unfortified milks will be low in calcium and will have no vitamin D or B12 and are not recommended for children or adolescents. The calcium content of fortified milks usually ranges from about 300 to 460 mg. Not all fortified milks include vitamin B12, and the amounts of vitamin D and B12 can be quite variable. In addition, the amount of added sugar in milks varies considerably. Unsweetened milks have no added sugar and are generally good choices. Original milks typically have a small amount of added sugar, similar to the amount present in cow's milk, and these are also good choices, especially for small children who need additional calories. While we encourage avoiding sugar-sweetened beverages, the amounts added are so small that they are an exception. For example, original soy milk has 5 grams of sugar per cup (just over a teaspoon), while a cup of soda has about 28 to 32 grams of added sugar (7 to 8 teaspoons). Limit intake of flavored milks, such as sweetened vanilla or chocolate (both non-dairy and dairy) as they have higher amounts of added sugars (e.g., vanilla almond milk has 16 grams or 4 teaspoons of added sugar). Read labels.

If your family includes dairy products, whole cow's milk is typically advised to age twenty-four months. After this time, lower fat options are generally appropriate. Offer about two cups of milk each day and no more than three cups. Too much milk can interfere with solid food intake and increase risk of iron deficiency. With the aggressive marketing of toddler "formulas," many parents wonder if these might be preferable to other milks. Toddler formulas are a combination of powdered milk (cow or soy), sugars, oils, and added nutrients, and they are typically higher in sodium than infant formulas. The general consensus among experts is that these products are rarely necessary and potentially problematic.[34] While the FDA strictly regulates infant formulas for composition and labeling, no such legal requirements exist for toddler formulas. This means that compositions can be quite variable. Many products are loaded with unhealthy sugar and fat, can displace much healthier foods, and can be very costly. There are some instances where toddler formulas or supplement drinks may be warranted, for example, in toddlers with medical conditions that impact intake of solid foods, those with severe allergies, or those with delayed growth. However, they are unnecessary for most healthy children. The necessary nutrients can be obtained by foods, and/or appropriate supplements, without the downsides of the toddler formula.

Table 8.3: Comparing Milks: Nutrients per Cup

MILK	Kcal	FAT (g)	PRO (g)	Ca (mg)	Vit A (mcg)	Vit D (IU)	B12 (mcg)	K (g)	Fe (mg)
Whole cow's milk	149	8	8	276	46	128	1.1	322	0.07
Soy milk, original, fortified	110	4.5	8	450	150	120	3	380	1.3
Soy milk, unsweetened, fortified	80	4	7	300	150	120	3	350	1
Pea milk, original, fortified	90	4.5	8	465	110	240	2.5	450	0
Pea milk, unsweetened, fortified	70	4.5	8	465	110	240	2.5	450	0

Table 8.3: Comparing Milks: Nutrients per Cup *(continued)*

MILK	Kcal	FAT (g)	PRO (g)	Ca (mg)	Vit A (mcg)	Vit D (IU)	B12 (mcg)	K (g)	Fe (mg)
Almond milk, original, fortified	60	2.5	1	450	150	100	0	0	0.5
Almond milk, unsweetened, fortified	30	2.5	1	450	150	100	0	0	0.5
Cashew milk, unsweetened	25	2	1	450	150	100	0	0	0.5
Oat milk, original	80	3	2	460	230	160	2.4	190	0.7
Oat milk, unsweetened	60	3	1	460	225	160	2.4	190	0.6
Coconut milk, original	70	4.5	0	460	180	80	0.9	170	0.5
Coconut milk, unsweetened	40	4	0	460	180	80	0.9	310	0.5

Note: *soy, almond, cashew, oat, and coconut–Silk™ Brand; pea milk–Ripple Brand™*

Key: *PRO = protein; Ca = calcium; K = potassium; Fe = iron; Zn = zinc*

Sources: [29, 35, 36]

Isn't Cow's Milk a Nutritional Necessity for Toddlers?

Cow's milk is not a nutritional necessity for humans at any stage of the life cycle, not even for toddlers. While it is true that cow's milk is a rich source of calcium and vitamin D (due to fortification), and these are important nutrients for growing children, fortified non-dairy milks generally provide at least as much calcium and vitamin D as cow's milk, so can be reasonable alternatives. The reason cow's milk is generally recommended in dietary guidelines and by organizations such as the American Academy of Pediatrics is because it is also a significant source of readily available protein and fat. However, cow's milk has some potential downsides, as you may recall from Chapter 1. In growing children, milk allergies and sensitivities are common, and consumption has been associated with asthma and eczema.[37] In a recent review from Harvard, the evidence was summed up as follows: *"If diet quality is low, especially for children in low-income environments, dairy foods can improve nutrition, whereas if diet quality is high, increased intake is unlikely to provide substantial benefits, and harms are possible."* [37]

What Foods Are Appropriate for Toddlers?

Your toddler can eat healthy family foods. By providing a variety of foods from each food group, with different flavors, textures, and colors, you will help to facilitate the acceptance of novel flavors and set the foundation for life-long healthy eating habits.[38] The Plant-Based Plate provides guidelines and specific serving sizes for toddlers (see Chapter 6). Include foods from four to five of the food groups listed at every meal and from at least two food groups at snack time. Let your child decide when she has had enough to eat.

There is no need to serve or purchase "kid's meals" or to be a short-order cook. "Kids meals" are notoriously unhealthy—think deep-fried chicken fingers, burgers, fries, cheese pizza, grilled cheese sandwiches, ice cream, and soda. These foods are consistently higher in fat, sugar, and salt than is appropriate for toddlers. While these items are cleverly marketed to children and to parents, it doesn't make them good choices. Marketing giants are remarkably well acquainted with buzzwords that keep parents happy—"high in protein," "calcium-rich," "low in sugar," or "all natural". Instead of "kid's meals," serve wholesome family foods and frequent family-friendly restaurants that serve healthy fare (e.g. ethnic restaurants, soup and salad bars) most of the time. The foods that will bring comfort and joy to your child over the long haul are the foods that the family shares time and time again. Those experiences will build a foundation for a lifetime of healthy eating.

The following are essential tips for getting your toddler on track to healthy eating:

- Keep added salt and sugar to a minimum.
- Minimize deep-fried foods, including deep-fried salty snacks.
- Make water and milk (breast milk, fortified soy, or pea milk, or cow's milk) your child's primary beverages. Avoid sugar-sweetened beverages. If you give juice, keep it occasional, and limit to not more than 4 ounces per day.

- Use herbs and spices, but go very lightly on strong or hot spices. If strong or hot spices are a part of your cultural tradition, keep them mild, and gradually increase as your child's palate allows.
- Structure, variety, and gentle persistence are keys to acceptance of new foods and flavors for toddlers.
- Be cautious of foods that pose a choking risk (see Table 8.2)—those identified for infants are still risky foods for toddlers. Additionally, avoid giving food if your child is seated in the back of the car on his own (especially in a rear-facing car seat) due to the potential for choking.

How Often Should I Feed My Toddler?

Children have small stomachs. To keep them well nourished, provide meals or snacks every two to three hours. Essentially, that means breakfast, lunch, and dinner with snacks in-between. While there is a strong trend to reducing hours that we are eating (time-restricted feeding), or serving just two meals a day, these eating patterns are highly inappropriate for children and can lead to failure to thrive and nutritional deficiencies. Keep a variety of nutritious food on hand—at home, on the road, and in the park. The key to a well-nourished child is ensuring that the vast majority of foods they eat are nutrient dense. Think about including foods from all food groups (vegetables, fruits, whole grains, legumes, nuts, and seeds) as snack options.

What Can I Do Make Sure My Picky Eater Gets Enough Food?

Most toddlers can be picky eaters, at least from time to time. They can also have a favorite food one day and refuse to eat the very same food the next day. Sometimes they will go for a week or more wanting only one or two foods. They may reject much of the food on their plate at mealtime but readily eat snacks. It can be rather disconcerting for parents. Rest assured that for toddlers, this is normal behavior. Even for children who may appear to eat next to nothing, they are often getting more than you imagine. For example, over the course of a day, if a child weighing thirty pounds consumes three cups of fortified soy milk, two peanut butter sandwiches, two sliced bananas, and half a cup of peas, they're getting enough calories and triple the recommended amount of protein. We will cover the topic of picky eating in greater detail in Chapter 9, but the bottom line is if they have a lot of energy and are growing well, there is rarely anything to worry about.

Is Salt Okay for Toddlers?

Yes, it is okay to use some salt in foods but do limit intake. Using salt judiciously can help take the bitter or sour edge off foods and make foods like dark greens more appealing to toddler taste buds, and it can be a source of iodine (if the salt is iodized). However, an estimated 80 percent of toddlers age one to three years eat too much sodium, which can negatively affect their blood pressure.[39] About 75 percent of snacks and meals marketed to toddlers are high in sodium (more than 210 mg per serving).[40] One study reported that over 50 percent of fast food "kids meals" and over 35 percent of sit-down restaurant "kids meals" exceeded 1,200 mg sodium. The Adequate Intake (AI) for sodium between the ages of one and three is 800 mg. The Institute of Medicine also suggests a cut off called the Chronic Disease Risk Reduction Intake CDRR, which is 1,200 mg for the age group.[41] This means that intakes should be reduced if they exceed 1,200 mg. Read labels. Better yet, control sodium by preparing foods as much as possible at home.

Is Sugar Okay for Toddlers?

Sugar is best avoided or minimized in the diets of toddlers. As you may recall from Chapter 4, the American Heart Association recommends no added sugar for toddlers younger than two years of age. For those over two years, a limit of six teaspoons a day is suggested.[42] Including a couple of tablespoons of maple syrup in a batch of healthy muffins is not the issue—highly processed foods are. Try using fruits and dried fruits to replace sugar, when possible. Otherwise, keep sugar use to a minimum and completely avoid sweet drinks.

Is Fat Okay for Toddlers?

Yes, fat is more than okay, it is an essential part of a toddler's diet and is critical for both brain development and optimal growth. Low-fat diets are inappropriate at this stage. Toddlers should receive about 30 to 40 percent of their calories from fat (40 percent for one-year-olds, decreasing gradually to about 30 percent by three years of age).[43] Rather than trying to reduce fat in your toddler's diet, focus on ensuring the fat he does eat is healthy fat. The most nutritious fat comes from high-fat, whole foods such as nut and seed butters, nut and seed cheeses and yogurts, avocados, tofu, soy milk, and soy yogurt. While concentrated fats and oils can be used, remember that these are foods with a lot of calories and few nutrients. They can crowd out foods that provide iron, zinc, calcium, and other essential nutrients, so use them judiciously. For dairy-consuming families, full-fat milk, yogurt, and cheese can also be used.

CHILDREN (FOUR TO TWELVE YEARS)

Tabitha had been a curious and enthusiastic eater pretty much since she started eating solid foods. By the time she was one, she was successfully feeding herself most meals and snacks. When she started attending full-day kindergarten, her parents, Sandra and Neil, decided that rather than purchasing lunch from school, they would pack lunch from home. Tabitha was excited to pick out a new lunch box and loved the idea of eating lunch with her friends. After a couple of weeks of school, Neil noticed that Tabitha's lunch was coming home uneaten. He made sure to pack her favorites which usually consisted of leftovers from dinner. When he asked Tabitha why she wasn't eating her lunch, she reluctantly told him that her lunch seemed so different from everyone else's and that someone at her lunch table told her that her chickpea stew "was weird and smelled funny." She wanted her lunch to be like the other kids. That night when Neil tucked Tabitha in, they talked about the kinds of things she might prefer to have in her lunch and how they might make them more fun. With a little bit of trial, error, and reassurance, Tabitha's lunch time issues improved. A sandwich or wrap seemed to be her new favorites and the fun fruit shapes in her lunch box were the envy of everyone at the lunch table.

At this stage, children continue to grow at a slower, steady rate. Just as with the toddler years, school-age children require a variety of healthy foods in the form of three meals and one to two snacks per day. Children are able to be more involved with food prep and cooking. Some common concerns at this age include outside influences around food (from friends to food marketing), more meals eaten outside of the home (school, playdates, after-school activities), and a trend towards decreased consumption of foods such as fruits and vegetables and increased consumption of sugar-sweetened beverages, fast foods, and heavily processed foods. Layered on top of that is the emergence of body image concerns that can surface at this time. Following are the answers to common questions about childhood nutrition that parents contend with.

How Do I Get My Child Excited About Eating Healthy Foods?

There are many things you can do to foster excitement about healthy, delicious food. The following tips will get things moving in the right direction. The younger you start, the better.

- Get excited yourself. Make a fuss about the season's first asparagus or peaches.
- Use food as a conversation starter. Talk about how a food is grown, where it comes from, what cultures most enjoy it.
- Bring your children to the market or grocery store. Let them help pick out the vegetables and fruits. If they are available to you, farmers markets are a great way to introduce children to seasonal produce.
- Get your kids cooking no matter what their age. Children love to pour, stir, and shake.
- Make mealtimes enjoyable.

What Do I Do If My Child Doesn't Eat Enough Vegetables and Fruits?

Do all of the above—lead by example; get children involved in purchasing and preparation; teach them about the foods. Beyond that, make these foods attractive and accessible. Serve the freshest produce possible. Peas in the pod from the farmer's market are hard to resist! Use vegetables as decorations—to make faces, butterflies, flowers, etc. Grate, spiralize, or slice very thinly. Keep cut up fruits and vegetables handy. When children are hungry, serve up a plate of veggies and dip and cut up fruits. In the summer, frozen grapes or berries are a welcome treat. There are also many ways to use vegetables and fruits in favorite foods:

- Add to smoothies
- Puree in soups
- Add to spaghetti sauce
- Use fruit in pancakes and desserts
- Use vegetables in muffins (e.g. carrots, beets, or zucchini)

Is It Okay to Let My Child Have Candy, Salty Snacks, and Soda?

Yes, it is okay for your kids to have these foods from time to time, but it is best if they are not part of the daily diet. These foods provide a lot of calories with very little nutritional benefit. For example, an eight-year-old child needs about

1,600 calories per day. If a child eats 400 calories worth of snack food with little nutritional value, it may be challenging for them to meet needs for micronutrients, protein, and essential fatty acids. Excessive intakes of highly processed foods have also been associated with learning problems and overweight and obesity in children.[44, 45]

In your home, instead of serving sweetened beverages as a treat, serve soda water with a little unsweetened fruit juice such as blueberry or pomegranate. Freeze juice in fancy ice cube shapes to make it even more appealing. Dish up popcorn or kale chips in place of other salty snacks. Make homemade frozen fruit treats, like nice cream or frozen chocolate-covered bananas instead of ice cream bars. There are healthy recipes for many favorite children's snacks. On the other hand, don't make a big deal when candy, frozen treats, or salty snacks are served. Forbidding candy and other highly processed food has been known to backfire. Being overly restrictive with these types of foods not only makes them more appealing, but it can lead to sneaking and an unhealthy preoccupation with these foods.

How Can I Protect My Child Against the Perils of Aggressive, Child-Targeted Food Marketing?

Marketing tactics have been shown to be highly effective, enticing children to plead for the advertised food.[46] Millions of dollars are spent convincing children and teens that they would benefit from eating or drinking unhealthy products that could have serious adverse health consequences. Children and youth are targeted through movies, television, video games, the internet, and social media. Kids are targeted at home, at school, in stores, sports facilities, and restaurants. As much as 90 percent of food and beverages marketed on television are highly processed with added fat, sugar, and salt.[47] As a parent, what do you do to prevent the adverse impact of all this food advertising? First, consider supporting or promoting legislation that would restrict this type of advertising to children. Such legislation is reasonable and has been successfully carried out in some areas. For example, in Quebec, Canada, a ban on advertising goods and services to children under the age of thirteen was put in place in 1980. Quebec children have the highest vegetable and fruit intake and the lowest obesity rates among six- to eleven-year-olds in Canada.[47] Similar regulations have been put into place in the United Kingdom,

Norway, Sweden, Brazil, and Mexico. Here are some other steps parents can take to help protect their children.

- Limit your child's screen time and try to select programming that is ad free.
- Enjoy regular family meals and prepare foods at home when possible.
- Purchase fewer highly processed foods.
- Talk to older children about identifying marketing techniques and show how they can mislead and hoodwink shoppers.
- Involve your children in food purchasing and preparation.

How Can I Make My Child's Plant-Based Lunch More Nutritious and Appealing?

Many parents struggle with coming up with ideas for a nutritious and fun lunch box for children. Talk to your child about what are his most and least favorite lunch box items. Get him involved in selecting lunch foods and preparing them. The following Top 10 Lunch Box Tips will help to transform school lunches from ho-hum to hooray!

Top Ten Lunch Box Tips

1. **Go for variety. Include something from every food group.** Kids like a little bit of lots of different foods. An example would be a whole grain wrap with tofu, "cheezy" cashew spread and veggies, carrot and celery sticks, berries, and an energy ball or oatmeal cookie.
2. **Make it colorful.** Color provides eye appeal and nutrition (when it comes from real food!). Include plant foods in all the colors of the rainbow— green, red-pink, orange-yellow, purple-blue, or white-beige (e.g., pea pods, red pepper strips, cauliflower florets, mango cubes, and blueberries).
3. **Keep to child-sized portions.** Large servings can be overwhelming for little bellies. Include small portions of several foods. Select small apples, bananas, or other whole fruits, and cut up larger fruit into more manageable pieces (orange sections, watermelon cubes).
4. **Use small containers or a bento box.** Kids love little compartments, which have the added advantage of keeping wet foods wet and dry foods dry. Make sure the container is leak-proof. Most boxes have three to five

compartments—a main dish section and two smaller sections for veggies and fruits. If you don't have a bento box, use several small containers.

5. **Make a few fun shapes.** If you have the right tools on hand, brightening up a lunch box with fun shapes can be a snap. Specialty vegetable cutters are inexpensive and easy to use. Turn melons into flowers, carrots into hearts, and zucchini into stars in seconds. Save the extra bits for soups, salads, and breakfast bowls.

6. **Use leftovers.** Leftover pasta makes a terrific pasta salad. Baked tofu or veggie burgers can be used in a wrap or sandwich or served as is with leftover rice. In the winter, send a thermos of hot soup.

7. **Mix it up!** Pack breakfast items for lunch (granola, and berry parfait or whole grain waffles) or several "snack" items to make a full lunch (e.g., hummus and crackers, edamame, veggie kabobs, olives).

8. **Use plant-based versions of kid's favorites.** Plant-based kids might appreciate having lunch items that look like everyone else's. Tofu salad sandwiches can look like egg salad sandwiches, veggie "meats" can replace lunch meats in sandwiches and wraps, veggie pepperoni can replace regular pepperoni on pizza, cheezy cashew sauce can replace cheese sauce on macaroni.

9. **Try out unfamiliar foods before sending them to school.** School lunches are not the best time to test an unfamiliar food on your unsuspecting child. Try new foods at home, on weekends, or at the dinner table first.

10. **Include something fun.** When you make treats such as cookies and balls using healthy ingredients, with a little or no added sugars, they can be a nutritious and welcome addition to a child's lunch box. Include some black bean brownies, chickpea peanut butter cookies, homemade energy balls. Even non-food items such as a note from mom or dad or a few stickers can add enjoyment to a lunch box.

ADOLESCENTS (THIRTEEN TO EIGHTEEN)

Calvin was a typical teenage boy. At fifteen years old, he was already almost six feet tall and seemed to have hollow legs as far as his appetite was concerned. Although his parents were health-conscious, plant-predominant eaters, he was not on the same wavelength. Calvin usually made a mad dash out the door in the morning without time for breakfast and would live on fast food and soda at school. When he got home, he would microwave a frozen mini pizza, or make a few slices of toast, and be off again to go skateboarding or play basketball. Although he was usually willing to eat whatever his parents prepared for dinner, if he wasn't around, he would opt for a fast food meal with his friends. His parents wondered how he could possibly focus at school with such unhealthy food as his primary fuel. They also wondered what they could do to help Calvin develop healthier eating habits.

Adolescence is a period of remarkable growth and change—it heralds the transition from childhood to adulthood. This involves accomplishing some major tasks—developing a personal identity, achieving autonomy, getting comfortable with one's physical body and sexuality, accepting greater responsibility, developing more mature relationships, acquiring one's own set of values, and preparing for further education, careers, and partnerships. It is an intense period of intellectual, social, emotional, and physical change that is centered around puberty. It can be tough for parents to see their young child begin to separate and move towards autonomy. If adolescents are given the opportunity to gradually increase their independence, hand in hand with more responsibility, this stage can also bring a degree of freedom and joy for parents.

Unique Nutritional Needs

The unique emotional and physical changes of adolescence along with emerging issues around peer acceptance and body image can influence teens nutritional status and eating. The human growth rate is the second fastest during adolescence, surpassed only by infancy.[48] The rapid physical growth experienced at this stage of life creates the highest demand for energy of our lives and increased needs for certain nutrients. During this period, adolescents achieve the final 15 to 20 percent of their adult height, gain about 50 percent of their adult body weight, and accumulate up to 40 percent of their adult skeletal mass.[49] Moderately active teenage girls need about 2,000 calories daily, while active girls need closer to 2,400 calories daily.[50] Moderately active teenage boys need about 2,200 to 2,800 calories daily, while active boys need 2,600 to 3,200 calories daily. Those who are engaged in competitive sports can require upward of 5,000 calories each day.

When it comes to food choices, teens are in the driver's seat most of the time, as they so often eat outside the home. But even as they strive for independence, teens need ongoing structure and support around meals. Parents can continue to encourage teens to be a part of shopping, meal prep, and of course clean-up. Often teens can take on the responsibility of making the family meal once a week or even once a month. Learning to purchase and prepare healthy, delicious food is one of the most valuable gifts a parent can give a child. Family meals provide one of the best opportunities to draw teens out of their rooms and connect with the rest of the family.

Some of the specific considerations for adolescent nutrition include:

- Skipping of meals
- Dieting and disordered eating (Chapter 11)
- Adolescent-specific health issues
- Gaining competency and independence around shopping and cooking
- Maintaining family connections with a focus on family meals (Chapter 12)

How Do Adolescents Do?

The biggest nutritional challenges for teens are eating too few vegetables, fruits, whole grains, legumes, and calcium-rich foods, and too much fast food and sugar-sweetened beverages.

One analysis of American teens reported that that only 0.9 percent of teens meet the recommendations for fruit and vegetable intake.[51] Over half of the fruit consumed was either fruit juice or fruit with added sugar, and over 50 percent of the vegetables consumed were either fried potatoes or a tomato product (pizza, pasta sauces, salsa). Less than 4 percent of vegetables consumed were dark green vegetables.

The Dietary Guidelines for Americans recommend that at least half of the grains consumed be whole grains. Teens consume mostly refined grains and average less than one serving of whole grains per day.[50] Whole grains, in addition to other whole plant foods, are key sources of dietary fiber. Average intakes for teens are less than half the recommended intakes and nine out of ten children fail to achieve the IOM's recommendation for fiber intake.[52]

Eating patterns developed during adolescence often spill over into adulthood and have a dramatic impact on future risk of disease and quality of life.[53] It is estimated that over one third of teens eat fast food on any given day and two thirds get at least 25 percent of their calories from fast food.[54] Teens who eat fast foods more than twice a week (compared to less than once a week), have a greater risk of weight gain and insulin resistance.[55] Although intakes of added sugars have declined in recent years, teens average over twenty-two teaspoons per day. Sugar sweetened beverages alone make up about 10 percent of calories in teen diets. A scientific statement from the American Heart Association (AHA) recommends that children and adolescents ages two to eighteen consume no more than one 8 ounce serving of sugar-sweetened beverages per week and no more than six teaspoons of added sugar per day.[42]

How Do Plant-Based Teens Compare?

The evidence comparing the diet quality of vegetarian versus nonvegetarian teens is limited. However, one study near Seventh-day Adventist universities in Michigan and Southern California assessed the diet quality of 534 vegetarian and nonvegetarian students twelve to eighteen years of age.[56] Vegetarian teens were defined as those who consumed meat, meat derivatives, poultry, and fish less than once per week. Overall, teens in this study (whether vegetarian or nonvegetarian) had better diets than that of the general US adolescent population. The vegetarians ate significantly more fruits, vegetables, legumes, nuts and nut butters, and grains, and significantly less sugar-sweetened beverages, coffee, and tea than the nonvegetarians. In addition, about half of the vegetarian teens consumed less than 10 percent of calories from saturated fat, compared to only about a quarter of the nonvegetarian teens.

Adolescence: Questions, Queries, and Quagmires

During the teen years, changes in sex hormones, stress hormones, and growth hormones affect brain function, mood, and the physical body. Concerns about body weight—including both overweight and underweight are particularly upsetting for teens. This is also the age where individuals are at the greatest risk for eating disorders such as anorexia nervosa, bulimia nervosa, or binge eating disorder (see Chapter 11 for further information).

Plant-based teens may be worried about protein for growing muscles, calcium for ever-expanding bones, and iron for menstruating girls. Parents may wonder how they can better support their teens in making healthy food choices, especially at breakfast time. Competitive teen athletes may be uncertain about how to tweak their plant-based diet to optimize their performance. Acne, which can throw a curve ball into the lives of active teens, may be quite favorably affected by healthy plant-based eating. Let's dive into the questions, queries, and quagmires of adolescent nutrition.

Can Rapidly Growing Teens Get Enough Protein from Plants?

Absolutely! Factoring in the reduced digestibility of plant proteins, the average plant-based teenage girl needs about 53 grams of protein per day, while the average plant-based teenage boy needs about 60 grams of protein per day. These intakes are easy to achieve on almost any healthy diet. (see Chapter 4, the section on Protein, for further information). However, it is possible for a teen to consume insufficient protein if the diet is mostly fat and sugar—typical of a potato chip and soda diet. It is important that plant-based teens consume legumes or legume-based foods (e.g., tofu, tempeh, and protein-rich veggie meat replacements), nuts, and seeds to ensure sufficient protein intakes. The use of soy or pea milk instead of other non-dairy milks also helps boost intakes.

How Can Teens Who Do Not Drink Cow's Milk Get Enough Calcium?

As you may recall, teens need about 1,300 mg calcium per day because of the substantial demands associated with growing bones. It can be challenging to get this much calcium without dairy products or calcium-fortified foods. Including two to three servings of fortified nondairy milk alternatives provides 300–450 mg calcium per cup and can help ensure sufficient intakes. (Note that on a food label, the DV for calcium is 1,000 mg, so if one serving of nondairy milk provides 30 percent of the DV, it has 300 mg.) Teens can also incorporate other good sources of calcium such as tofu, low-oxalate greens, chia seeds, beans, hummus, almonds, oranges, and figs on a regular basis (for more information on calcium, see Chapter 5).

Are Teenage Girls Prone to Iron Deficiency on Plant-Based Diets?

Once a girl begins to menstruate (regardless of age), iron needs increase by about 2.5 mg per day. To boost iron status, ensure a variety of iron-rich foods in the daily diet (e.g., tofu, lentils, beans, nuts, seeds, and iron-fortified foods), and include vitamin C-rich foods along with iron-rich foods to enhance absorption (for more information, see Chapter 5). It can be helpful to include a multivitamin with iron for girls who have difficulty meeting the recommended intakes from food alone.

How Can I Support My Teen in Making Healthy Food Choices?

Teens are independent eaters—which means they make their own food choices much of the time. Recall Calvin's story, and the concern his parents had about his poor eating habits. Calvin had three habits that are all too common among teens—skipping breakfast, eating highly processed and fast foods as staples, and drinking sugar-sweetened beverages. Here are some simple steps that parents can take to help their teens turn the tide:

1. **Skipping Breakfast.** Teens tend to skip breakfast because an extra fifteen minutes in bed takes priority. Some teens are just not hungry first thing in the morning. Parents can help to facilitate healthy breakfast choices by putting out some fast and easy options such as cereal, soy milk, fruit, toast, nut butter, or whatever your teen enjoys. If your teen tends not to be hungry first thing in the morning, have a little breakfast "grab and go meal" ready—a muffin, some nuts, and a piece of fruit, or a green smoothie.

2. **Eating Highly Processed and Fast Foods.** The most important thing you can do to reduce intake of highly processed and fast foods is to have your fridge and pantry loaded with healthier alternatives. Teens want food fast even if it is not fast food. If instead of chips and candy bars, you stalk up on roasted nuts, seaweed snacks, roasted chickpea snacks, homemade baked goods, cut up fruits and vegetables, hummus, and healthy energy bars, chances are good your teen will eat them. Keep some almost instant meals like frozen bean burritos in the freezer. While you can't control the choices made outside of the home, you can have healthy options available that make it easier for your teen to meet his nutritional needs.

3. **Drinking sugar-sweetened beverages.** Don't keep sweet drinks in your house. Make water the go-to beverage. Keep some soda water and frozen juice cubes on hand for fizzy drinks. Unless your teen is a competitive athlete, there is no need for sports drinks.

Can Competitive Athletes Thrive on a Plant-Based Diet?

Adolescent athletes have unique nutritional requirements, with the demands of training and competition on top of the usual requirements of growth and development. Many teens are fueled by "Western-style diets," rich in processed foods and fast foods. Such diets tend to be calorically dense, but not very nutrient dense. Many are low in vegetables, fruits, whole grains, and legumes, and are not optimal fuel for athletes. Plant-based diets, are, on the other hand, nutrient dense, but often significantly less calorically dense, so planning is required to ensure sufficient energy for active teens. Inadequate energy intakes can negatively affect bone health, hormones, and performance. Adolescent athletes may engage in unhealthy strategies to control body weight or shape, or to achieve extreme leanness. Teens engaged in competitive sports have high energy needs so are particularly vulnerable to adverse consequences of low energy intakes. Restrictive eating in athletes can lead to a syndrome known as Relative Energy Deficiency in Sports (RED-S). The syndrome, driven by relative energy deficiency, can result in significant changes in protein synthesis, metabolic rates, menstrual function, bone health, immunity, and cardiovascular health.[57] Nutrition for adolescent athletes takes careful planning. Plant-based eaters have some special considerations. Using the Plant-Based Plate will help to ensure nutritional adequacy. Chapter 14 provides a sample menu for plant-based adolescent athletes.

If there is a teen athlete under your roof, you can support their athletic goals by promoting some basic dietary guidelines:

1. **Ensure adequate energy intake.** Growth, development, and expected gains in athletic performance will be the best indicators of caloric adequacy. Because athletes require more calories, more emphasis on calorie-dense plant foods is appropriate. For example, teen athletes can enjoy a higher volume of energy-dense foods such as avocado, nuts, seeds (and their butters), tofu, and starchy foods such as potatoes, pasta, breads, and cereals. Including some refined grains can help boost energy intakes. Be sure to have plenty of snacks on hand, at home, at school, and at practice—energy bars, healthy baked goods, trail mix, stuffed dates, and smoothies are all great choices.

2. **Push protein to about 1.4–1.6 grams per kilogram body weight.**[58] This amounts to about 80 to 90 grams of protein for a 55 kg (121 lb) athlete, and 100 to 110 grams of protein for a 70 kg (154 lb) athlete. Because of the increase in calorie intake, this target is not so difficult to achieve.

Ensure excellent protein sources with every meal and snack—soy milk, tofu, tempeh, veggie "meats," lentils, beans, peas, seeds, nuts, and whole grains are all good choices. Plant-predominant eaters can further boost protein intakes with animal products. Protein powders can rapidly boost protein intake but are generally unnecessary, and potentially harmful (see page 88 for further information).

3. **Include moderate amounts of healthy fat.** Athletes need healthy fats. Fats from nuts, seeds, avocados, and soy foods are the most nutrient-dense and should be the primary fat sources. Oils such as avocado, flax, hemp, or olive oil can help to add calories for teens that have difficulty meeting energy needs.

4. **Ensure sufficient iron.** Iron deficiency is relatively common among athletes and is associated with reduced athletic performance.[58, 59] Both males and females can develop iron deficiency due to increased iron demand associated with intense physical activity, elevated iron losses through sweat, gastrointestinal blood loss, hemolysis (rupturing of blood cells), and reduced iron absorption. Menstrual losses and lower total iron intake make female teens more susceptible to iron deficiency. Plant-based athletes need to include plenty of iron-rich plant foods in the diet (see Chapter 5 for more information). Athletes are well advised to include vitamin C-rich foods with iron sources. Including a multivitamin with iron will also help to prevent iron deficiency.

5. **Include rich sources of calcium and vitamin D daily.** Adolescence is a period of rapid bone growth, so calcium needs are higher than at other stages. While physical activity can positively impact bone density, females who train vigorously can develop irregular menstruation, which can adversely impact bone health.[58] Athletes who exclude dairy products are advised to include at least two to three servings of calcium fortified non-dairy milk per day. Vitamin D can also fall short for many teens. Including a vitamin D supplement providing at least 600 IU vitamin D, or a combination of a multivitamin with vitamin D and some vitamin D-fortified foods, can help to ensure optimal vitamin D status.

6. **Drink appropriate and sufficient fluids.** Teen athletes need to stay well-hydrated during training and competition. For active teens engaged in

sports or other physical activities, water is the preferred beverage to maintain hydration. For competitive athletes, sports drinks are appropriate
during prolonged, vigorous physical activity. Caffeinated energy drinks are
not recommended.[58] Be selective with sports drinks, as many are simply
sugar, artificial color and flavor, and electrolytes. Some coconut water-
based or fruit juice-based sports drinks avoid the use of artificial flavors
and colors. Read the label.

7. **Take a multivitamin-mineral supplement.** While well-planned plant-
exclusive diets provide ample amounts of most nutrients, some vitamins
such as vitamins B12 and D, and minerals, such as iron and zinc, can fall
short. Including a multivitamin with these nutrients helps to ensure adequate intakes.

How Do Plant-Based Diets Impact Acne Risk?

Few things can derail a teen's emotional well-being like acne. Acne can alter
how a teen sees himself and how he imagines others see him. It can erode self-
esteem, triggering despair and depression. Acne is initiated by the onset of
puberty in an estimated 85 percent of those aged twelve to twenty-five years.[60]
The surge in hormones called androgens (which increase in both boys and girls
during puberty) can enlarge and stimulate oil glands in the skin, particularly
around the nose and on the neck, chest, and back. Risk is elevated in populations
consuming Western-style diets rich in added sugars, fast foods, refined grains,
and high-protein, high-fat dairy products. Highly processed foods also tend to
have a high glycemic index, which further exacerbates the problem.[60] One large
meta-analysis of over 78,000 children, adolescents and young adults reported a
positive association between dairy and acne, with a 41 percent increased risk in
those consuming one glass of milk per day and 43 percent in those consuming
two or more glasses per day compared with those consuming less than one glass
of milk per week.[61] Conversely, risk is averted in populations eating low meat
diets, free of dairy products and refined grains.[62] Other dietary factors that may
be protective are fiber, omega-3 fatty acids, antioxidant-rich foods, and vitamin
A.[63] So, plant-based teens may well be at an advantage where acne is concerned.

FROM TODDLERS TO TEENS —
COMMON QUESTIONS AND CONCERNS

Is Soy Safe for Children?

Yes, soy is not only safe for children but it is an excellent addition to a child's diet, particularly children who are plant-based. Soy foods have some impressive benefits:

- They are more concentrated sources of high-quality protein than are other legumes. Soy foods are also rich sources of iron, zinc, calcium, potassium, riboflavin, and both essential fatty acids.
- Some products such as tofu, soy milk, and soy-based veggie meats are lower in fiber, so the protein digestibility is similar to that of animal products.
- They contain isoflavones that can exert weak estrogenic effects or antiestrogenic effects. This may turn out to be an advantage for girls, as soy intake in childhood and adolescence reduces lifetime breast cancer risk. Although concerns have been raised about potential feminizing effects in boys, several dozen studies have found no effects of soy protein on male hormones.[72]
- While we don't know how much soy is safe to consume, experts suggest one to two servings per day for children and two to four servings per day for teens or adults. This is the amount typically consumed by people in two of the Blue Zones—Okinawa and Loma Linda. Purchase organic soy products, if possible, to minimize pesticide exposure.

Are Raw Food Diets Recommended for Children?

Raw food diets are not generally recommended for children. In addition to concerns about several micronutrients, the diet can be too bulky to provide sufficient calories.[73] Cooking helps to make foods more calorie dense, so it is easier to consume a greater number of calories with a smaller volume of food. Many raw food diets eliminate legumes, which are important sources of protein, iron, and zinc for children.

Are Probiotics and Prebiotics Recommended for Children?

Probiotics are supplements or foods that contain viable microorganisms that can alter the population of microflora in the gut. *Prebiotics* are supplements or food that contain nondigestible carbohydrates that stimulate growth and activity of probiotic bacteria. In other words, prebiotics feed probiotics.

Probiotic supplements are extremely popular for people of all ages. Many parents wonder if it is wise to provide a daily probiotic supplement to their children. While there are some circumstances for which a supplement may be warranted, daily use is not recommended. Most children can maintain a healthy gut microbiota by consuming a prebiotic-rich, plant strong diet. If you think your child might benefit from a probiotic supplement due to atopy, constipation, gastrointestinal disorders, or following a course of antibiotics, discuss with your pediatrician before supplementing.

Prebiotics are types of fiber that are fermented by intestinal microflora and stimulates the growth and activity of that microflora. While all prebiotics are types of fermentable fiber, not all types of fiber are fermentable prebiotics. Prebiotics are plentiful in breast milk, and breastfed children tend to have a robust colony of beneficial bacteria in the digestive systems.[74] Other concentrated sources of prebiotics are legumes, vegetables (e.g., onions, leeks, garlic, savoy cabbage, and Jerusalem artichokes), fruits (e.g., bananas, watermelon, and grapefruit), grains (e.g., barley and oats), and nuts and seeds (e.g., almonds, pistachios, flax and chia seeds). Although prebiotics are added to supplements and processed foods, it is best to get them from whole plant foods, for children and adults alike.

There is another way of safely introducing probiotics into your child's diet, and that is by using food-based probiotics also known as fermented foods. These are not only safe for infants (once solid foods have started) and children, they may be highly beneficial. Fermented foods can contribute to healthy gut flora, aid digestion, support immune function, and enhance the nutritional content of the foods. Providing fermented foods at an early age appears to dampen the desire to eat sweets. Fermented foods have been shown to be more effective in restoring a healthy gut microbiome than probiotic supplements.[75] Plant-based fermented foods, such as vegetables (e.g. sauerkraut, kimchi), non-dairy yogurts, miso, and fermented nut cheeses are all reasonable choices. Fermented vegetables can be very high in salt, so keep intake moderate. If you are fermenting foods at home, follow good sanitary practices—washing hands, produce, utensils, cutting surfaces, and containers. Generally, fermentation kills pathogens, so if contamination occurs, it is generally from poor handling practices after the food is fermented. Kombucha, a fermented, tea-based beverage, does contain a very small amount of alcohol (<0.5 percent for commercial products), so is best minimized, especially for small children. Homemade kombucha can be higher in alcohol so is best reserved for adults.

FOOD SAFETY

Are Pesticides in Our Food Dangerous for Children?

Pesticides are chemicals designed to kill living organisms like insects and rodents, hence they are inherently toxic. Low-level exposure from eating foods that are sprayed with these chemicals may negatively affect cognitive function, behavior, and cancer risk.[76] The adverse effects of pesticides are more pronounced in small children than in adults. This is because per pound of body weight, the level of exposure is greater.

Should I Stick to Organic Foods?

While the benefits of eating fruits, vegetables, and other plant foods consistently outweigh the risk, when you can, choose organic. This significantly reduces exposure, although it does not completely eliminate it.[77] Among the best resources for parents is the Environmental Working Group (EWG) Shopper's Guide to Pesticides in Produce, which is released every spring. The idea behind the guide is simple: identify the products that are the most concentrated sources of pesticides, and the products that are the least concentrated sources. This allows consumers to save money purchasing conventional produce that has low pesticide levels (called "The Clean Fifteen") while protecting their families by purchasing organic versions of the most concentrated pesticide sources (called "The Dirty Dozen"). For example, between 2018–2020 strawberries topped the Dirty Dozen list. Strawberries are also a favorite fruit among children, so parents are well advised to purchase organic strawberries. Pineapples are in the top three Clean Fifteen list, so conventional versions of these are fine. Purchasing only organic products from the dirty dozen list will go a long way towards minimizing pesticides in your child's diet. As a bonus, organic produce has higher levels of antioxidant phytochemicals than conventional produce.[78]

How Do I Minimize Exposure to Heavy Metals?

Heavy metals such as arsenic, cadmium, lead, and mercury can contribute to deficits in intelligence, and increase risk of cancer, heart disease and diabetes. Tests of 168 baby foods found heavy metals in 95 percent of the products tested.[79] There are several steps parents can take to reduce heavy metal exposure in their children:

- Minimize rice-based snack foods, cereals, and sweeteners.
- Avoid hijiki seaweed.
- Avoid commercial teething biscuits and fruit juices.
- Avoid high mercury fish including shark, swordfish, king mackerel, marlin, orange roughy, bigeye tuna, and tilefish. For those who eat tuna, white or albacore tuna contains more mercury than light tuna.
- Avoid candies imported from countries that do not regulate food.

Are Persistent Organic Pollutants (POPs) an Issue for Children?

POPs such as PCBs, DDT, and dioxins are chemicals that remain in the environment for decades. These chemicals can cause birth defects, disrupt hormones, impair brain function and learning, increase cancer risk, and cause immunological disorders.[80] Plant-based eaters are at a huge advantage where POPs are concerned as they move up the food chain (plants are at the bottom of the food chain, then smaller animals, and the largest, most carnivorous animals are at the end; as you move up the food chain, POPs accumulate). Over 90 percent of human exposure comes from food, particularly food of animal origin, such as meat, dairy products, and fish.[81]

How Can I Minimize Harmful By-Products Produced in High-Temperature Cooking?

Chemicals formed in foods when foods are cooked at high temperatures can have multiple adverse health effects and are potential carcinogens.[82, 83, 84, 85] Common examples include heterocyclic amines (HCAs), polycyclic aromatic hydrocarbons (PAHs), advanced glycation end-products (AGEs), and acrylamide. HCAs are found exclusively in animal products, so are not an issue for people who are exclusively plant-based. PAHs are found in all foods that are significantly darkened or blackened. AGEs are found in foods cooked with dry heat but are especially high in processed meats. Acrylamide is most concentrated in starchy foods rich in the amino acid asparagine, and potato products (both regular and sweet potatoes) are particularly plentiful sources. Potato chips and french fries top the list. The best ways of minimizing these compounds is to avoid fried foods and use moist rather than dry cooking methods more often. In practical terms, this means steaming, boiling, or stewing instead of frying, grilling, or baking at high temperatures. While air frying is preferable to oil frying, it still produces acrylamide, so more occasional rather than daily use is advised.[86] Minimize ultra-processed foods.

Should I Be Concerned About Plastics and BPA?

BPA disrupts hormones and can impact reproduction, brain structure, behavior, and cancer risk.[87] Exposure in childhood has also been linked to obesity and early puberty.[88] BPA is found in plastics, which are usually clear and hard, marked with the recycle symbols 3, 6, or 7. Try to reduce exposure where possible by minimizing pre-packaged food and opting for glass or paper instead of plastic. Use glass for storage and reheating as well. Minimize use of cans or look for cans with BPA-free liners.[88]

While all of this may seem overwhelming, and even frightening, it is important not to be overly rigid. This only creates anxiety, and that is not good for you or your child. Make the best choices you can when you can. Beyond that, don't stress about fine details and enjoy your food. Your take-away points are:

- **Select organic foods when you are able.** Get familiar with the EWG's dirty dozen and clean fifteen, so you can better minimize pesticide exposure.
- **Be aware of the key sources of heavy metals.** Limit use of foods high in heavy metals such as large, predatory fish, rice-based snacks and cereals, and hijiki. Cook rice in a large amount of water to reduce arsenic content.
- **Use moist cooking methods most often.** When cooking with dry heat, keep temperatures moderate. Avoid blackening foods.
- **Limit use of plastic food containers and BPA-lined canned goods.** While it is almost impossible to completely avoid plastic, select glass or steel storage vessels when you can.

SUPPLEMENTS AND LAB TESTS

Does My Plant-Based Child Need a Multivitamin Mineral Supplement?

The need for supplements in plant-based children depends on many factors —the overall quality of the diet, the use of fortified foods, the child's health and digestion, and whether or not animal foods such as dairy, eggs, or fish are included in the diet. Providing a variety of nutritious foods is the most important step we can take to ensure nutritional adequacy. However, a good quality multivitamin mineral supplement can help to ensure sufficient intakes of nutrients that may fall short, such as vitamin B12, vitamin D, iodine, iron, and zinc. Multi-vitamin mineral supplements can also give you peace of mind when your toddler seems uninterested in food, your child wants only peanut butter sandwiches, or your teen makes a habit of missing meals.

Liquid multivitamins are generally recommended for children twelve through thirty-six months of age, to reduce risk of choking, while chewable vitamins are suitable for children three years of age or more. Adult multivitamin mineral supplements are appropriate for teens. There is some concern about preformed vitamin A and folic acid in supplements, so be sure not to exceed upper limits for those nutrients (see Chapter 5). While organic, whole food supplements are a great option, they are significantly more costly.

Does My Plant-Based Child Need Other Supplements?

For plant-based children, vitamin B12 and vitamin D supplements are advised if the child is *not* taking a daily multi-vitamin mineral supplement containing the recommended amounts of these nutrients. Vitamin B12 can be taken daily or twice a week (see Chapter 5, page 102 for appropriate amounts). Children above the age of one year need 600 IU of vitamin D, which can be obtained from a combination of food (including fortified foods) and sunshine. However, many children require a vitamin D supplement, especially those with darker skin or who are living in cooler climates. One other supplement that deserves consideration is DHA/EPA for those who do not consume fish. For suggested amounts, see Chapter 4, page 80. The following is a summary of recommended supplements.

Table 8.4: Supplement Summary

Supplement	Infants (0–12 m)	Toddlers (1–3 y)	Children (4–12 y)	Adolescents (13¹–18 y)
These supplements are recommended, but not essential.				
Multivitamin	None	Daily	Daily	Daily
DHA/EPA²	From breast milk or formula	70 mg/day	90–120 mg/day	110–160 mg/day
These supplements are conditionally essential. A supplement is necessary if intakes are insufficient from food and/or a multivitamin. Recommended intakes can be adjusted, according to the amount obtained from food and supplements.				
Vitamin B12	From breast milk³ or formula	10 mcg daily *or* 250 mcg 2x/wk	25–50 mcg daily *or* 500–750 mcg 2x/wk	100 mcg daily *or* 1,000 mcg 2x/wk
Vitamin D	400 IU/day	600 IU/day	600 IU/day	600 IU/day

1. In this chapter, thirteen-year-olds are grouped with adolescents, while they are grouped with nine to thirteen-year-olds in the DRI. Vitamin B12 recommendations for this age could be 50 mcg daily or 750 mcg weekly, however higher intakes as indicated are safe.

2. For more precise DHA/EPA amounts, see Chapter 4, Table 4.4.

3. Infants of mothers who do not ensure a consistent, reliable source of vitamin B12 should receive a supplement of 1 mcg twice daily or 5 mcg once daily.

Should My Child Get Lab Tests to Check for Potential Nutritional Deficiencies?

Lab tests are not typically ordered for children unless your physician feels it is necessary. The exceptions are iron and blood lipids. The AAP suggests universal screening for anemia at about one year of age.[89] A complete blood count (CBC), which includes hemoglobin and serum ferritin (a measure of iron stores), is commonly used to assess iron status. In 2011, the AAP endorsed the National Heart, Lung and Blood Institute (NHLBI) guidelines advocating universal age-based lipid screening between nine and eleven years, and again between seventeen and twenty-one years.[90] Selective screening is also suggested beginning at age two years for children with risk factors based on family history, high-risk conditions, or obesity.

The AAP recommends a risk assessment for lead poisoning at six, nine, twelve, and eighteen months, and at three, four, five, and six years. A blood test is only ordered if the assessment comes back positive.[91]

Other tests that your doctor may want to run on your plant-based child include vitamin B12 and vitamin D. Vitamin B12 and vitamin D tests are not needed for those eating sufficient fortified foods and/or taking supplements. If tests are deemed necessary, serum B12 and serum vitamin D are commonly run. However, serum B12 is a less reliable indicator of B12 status than MMA and homocysteine, so these additional tests are recommended. While iodine status is not typically measured directly, thyroid hormone tests may be ordered, if indicated.

This concludes the Care section of this book. You are now thoroughly versed in macronutrients, micronutrients, designing a healthy plant-based diet, and the unique nutritional requirements of pregnant and lactating mothers, infants, toddlers, children, and adolescents. Next, we move on to Confidence. In this section, we address the practical aspects of navigating the nutrition trials and tribulations of today's world. We explore the dynamics around the dinner table, and how parents can create an environment that nourishes a child's body and spirit. We provide the essential ingredients for managing some of the toughest food-related issues parents face, including picky eating, childhood obesity, and disordered eating.

Part III

CONFIDENCE

Confidence is about supporting parents in a way that positions them to be the experts of their family's nutrition. This section addresses many of the concerns families face at and around their dinner tables. A health-promoting diet requires a nurturing environment as well as support and guidance from parents to be fully realized. From picky eating to childhood obesity, disordered eating, and more, we will explore the idea that *how* we feed our families matters as much as *what* we feed our families. As parents ourselves, we understand all too well the challenges families face around their dinner table and hope that a thoughtful conversation around these topics will introduce greater joy and confidence at mealtime. We will review feeding principles and concepts (picky eating and when to worry), the importance of family meals, and pediatric weight-related issues, and end with a conversation on how to weave all of these concepts into a plant-leaning diet for your family.

Chapter 9

Principles of Feeding: Setting the Table

"The secret to feeding a healthy family is to love good food,
trust yourself, and share that love and
trust with your child."

—*Ellyn Satter*

Sonya and her four-year-old son, Leo, stopped at a local restaurant for lunch after a morning at the park. They had had a wonderful time, but she could tell that he was tired and hungry. It was close to nap time and she was anxious to get home. When Leo's plate arrived, he was eager to eat. He got his favorite—spiral pasta with red sauce. It came with a side of broccoli and a chocolate chip cookie. Sonya quickly took the cookie from his plate and set it next to her own so that Leo wouldn't eat it immediately. He ate the pasta with enthusiasm, tried a piece of broccoli, and then went back to the pasta. He began to whine for the cookie that had been abruptly taken from his plate. Sonya's frustration was mounting, and she feared that a meltdown was imminent. After quite a bit of prompting to eat the rest of the broccoli (and Leo's frank refusal to do so), Sonya finally conceded and said, "One more bite of broccoli and you can have the cookie."

Nearly every parent we know has been witness to or participated in a similar conversation with their child. You can replace both the broccoli and the cookie with your choice of food, but it essentially reads, one more bite of the food "I" want you to eat, and you can have the food "you" want to eat. In the moment it seems like a winning strategy because you both get what you want, right? In reality, however, these sorts of interactions around food and with our children perpetuate struggle, build tension around mealtimes, and have the potential to create an unhealthy relationship with food. The focus of this chapter is to provide you with the information and tools necessary to set up a healthy environment around, and a better quality of, feeding. The guiding principles provided in this chapter will position parents to become the experts in feeding their children, bringing greater peace and connection around the dinner table. A good feeding relationship is like fertile soil that allows healthy eating habits to flourish.

> A good feeding relationship is like fertile soil that allows healthy eating habits to flourish.

THE SECRET

Not to disappoint you, but there is no secret five- or even ten-step process we have to offer that will bring immediate peace, joy, and compliance around mealtimes. No tricks or treats, and certainly no magic bullet. What we can offer you is information on what the research suggests works when it comes to fostering a healthy, positive, and nurturing feeding relationship. The real secret is that there is no greater expert on feeding your family than you.

As parents, more than anything, we want our children to thrive. We work tirelessly to ensure their optimal growth, development, and happiness. Despite our best intentions, however, busy schedules, picky eating, limited resources (perhaps, time, money, or patience?), and the pressures that pervade our daily lives all seem to collectively conspire against our well-intended efforts at our dinner tables. The simple act of feeding our children has become incredibly complex, and for many families, entirely chaotic. Many factors may influence the quality of feeding within a given family. The quality of feeding refers both to the food (nutrition, quantity, variety, etc.) as well as the dynamic feeding relationship between child and caregiver. We recognize that for families that are experiencing food insecurity, many of these principles may be out of reach, and the most pressing concern is simply getting enough to eat and choosing dependably filling and satisfying food.[1]

FEEDING STYLES AND PRACTICES

Feeding styles and practices play a critical role in shaping children's eating behaviors and habits. In order to foster a positive feeding relationship so that our children are able to feed themselves in a way that is nourishing, satisfying, and healthy, as parents, we need to provide adequate structure and support, while at the same time offer enough autonomy and independence so that our children are able to eat with competence and confidence.

Feeding styles can be categorized in a way similar to parenting styles. Four broad categories of parenting are defined by the balance of both expectation and responsiveness (some refer to this as support or warmth).

- Authoritative (high expectation, high level of responsiveness)
- Authoritarian (high expectation, low level of responsiveness)
- Permissive (low expectation, high level of responsiveness)
- Uninvolved (low expectation, low level of responsiveness)

Although we likely have some of these traits in certain situations and there can be overlap, we tend to gravitate toward one general approach. In terms of feeding practices, these categories are defined as responsive, controlling, indulgent, and neglectful.[2] A responsive style of feeding is the preferred approach; the parent places appropriate expectations on the child *and* responds to the child's needs in order to foster a sense of autonomy and competence with sufficient structure, support, and warmth.[3,4] When you consider that a controlling style would insist that children eat as the parent demands with little concern for the child's wants and needs, an indulgent style would completely yield to the child's wishes without setting any expectations, and a neglectful approach would leave the child fending for himself, it's clear why a responsive approach would help to not only improve overall diet quality but also to help strengthen the connection between parent and child. Let's take a look at what that structure (expectation) and support (responsiveness) look like from a feeding perspective.

Ellyn Satter, a registered dietitian and family therapist, is widely regarded as one of the preeminent experts on childhood feeding. She devised a model of feeding centered around a division of responsibility (DOR). The shorthand version is that when it comes to the feeding relationship, parents are responsible for the *what, when,* and *where* of feeding (we will have pasta, bread, and salad at 6:30 at the kitchen table) and children are responsible for the *whether* and *how much* of eating. Satter explains that, "the feeding relationship is the complex of interactions that take place between parent and child as they engage in food selection, ingestion, and regulation behaviors. Feeding is a reciprocal process that depends on the capabilities of both parents and children. Optimal feeding interactions depend on emotionally healthy, sensitive, and responsive parents and on children who are able to achieve a minimal level of communication and stability. As a guide for parents during the feeding process and a support to this reciprocal interchange, a division of responsibility in feeding is recommended. Parents are responsible for what children are offered to eat; children are responsible for how much they eat. Parents choose appropriate food, provide structured meals and snacks (after the first year), and ensure a pleasant eating environment. Children decide how much and even whether they eat what parents put before them. In this way, adults give children concrete and repeated experiences of being able to behave autonomously without being abandoned, of being supported without being intruded upon."[5]

This DOR starts in infancy. During this critical phase of feeding, the focus is on allowing the infant to gain a sense of regulation and stability as well as attachment and bonding to the caregiver. During the first few months of life, parents are responsible for the *what* (breast milk or formula), but baby is essentially responsible for the *when, where, and how much*. Infants should be fed on demand and parents can be alert to the cues of hunger and satiety. It's about being attentive and responsive to baby's cues around feeding and letting baby know that he will be reliably and lovingly fed.

Moving forward, as solid foods are introduced at around six months of age, parents can begin to create a dynamic and responsive feeding environment. Once signs of readiness become apparent, solid foods, in pureed form for traditional complimentary feeding and soft, finger foods where a baby-led weaning approach is used, are introduced (see Chapter 8 for more details). During this window of time, it is critical for parents to be engaged and create a positive environment but not be forceful or overwhelming in their approach.

Although there is some data to suggest that babies can be exposed to different flavors through amniotic fluid and breast milk,[6] many experts hypothesize that the effects of the development of food and flavor preferences may be the greatest as complementary feeding begins. Up until this point babies have only had breast milk or formula, and the acceptance of a variety of solid foods is essential in consuming a diet that supports growth and health.[7] Early exposure (from six to twelve months of age) to both a variety of flavors and textures, including having the same foods prepared in different ways, have both been shown to be linked to childhood and adult food preferences and dietary range.[8] Parents often greet this new phase with enthusiasm and curiosity. Many cultures even celebrate the milestone with special rituals and ceremonies. It can be an exciting time for both baby and parent. However, misconceptions around normal development and growth can create unnecessary stress and conflict. Babies (and even adults!) have different temperaments around food. Some are enthusiastic and curious, while others may be more cautious. We will discuss this a little later in the chapter when we address picky eating, but for now, it's important to keep a few key things in mind, even from the start of feeding:

- Children may require repeated exposures (sometimes upwards of fifteen) to foods in a pleasant, neutral environment for different foods and flavors to be accepted. It's important to note that a "negative" or forceful food exposure can make future exposures more challenging.
- During the second half of the first year of life and up until puberty, children's growth velocity (the rate at which they grow), naturally slows down; many parents can misinterpret this normal progression of growth as poor growth and this can lead to anxiety and pressure around feeding.
- Knowing your baby's temperament can help guide your approach and pace; it's not good or bad, just useful information.

Older infants between the ages of eight and twelve months will become increasingly interested in gaining independence around food. Most children at this age are beginning to self-feed. As children approach the toddler years, many fallacies around "normal" feeding can create anxiety, frustration, and even the beginnings of feeding difficulties. Feeding at this stage is supposed to be somewhat inconsistent (a very small breakfast or seemingly low appetite on one day followed by a more vigorous intake the next) and messy. As children develop grasping motions, gross and fine pincer grasps, and even language, their capabilities will change. Knowing that the mess and inconsistency are a normal part of feeding and development can offer parents reassurance.

As children enter the toddler years, they continue to work towards gaining more autonomy around nearly everything they do, including eating. In our (Reshma) house we called this the "me do phase." Whether it's getting dressed, buckling up their car seat, or eating breakfast, children are wanting to do more and more for themselves. Many parents have expressed frustration over the fact that their baby "used to eat everything put in front of her" and now seems more selective and opinionated about the foods being offered. In addition to the quest for independence, the toddler years are also a time marked by suspicion of new, and at times even previously accepted, foods. This is a perfectly normal and expected stage of development and precisely when the DOR is truly put to the test.

As parents, we can continue to provide structure and support (scheduled meals and snacks) without pressure while also creating opportunities for independence. In a way it's sort of like allowing your toddler to play in the yard, knowing that there is a fence to keep him away from traffic and your presence for appropriate supervision. He is free to roam, explore, jump, dig, and twirl, but you will ensure that he doesn't climb to an unsafe height and washes his hands when he comes inside. In the instance of feeding, you may have a regularly scheduled snack and offer a choice of blueberries or strawberries to go with his yogurt. Alternatively, you may offer a lunch of soup, sandwich, and apple slices without worrying too much about how much of each he eats, knowing that he will have many opportunities to try and enjoy new foods. If consuming enough quantity and variety becomes an ongoing problem, the issue may need to be further explored. In most instances, however, children just need our continued guidance, support, and patience.

During the preschool and school-age years, children will gain more independence, but you may still see a reluctance to try new foods. Although this generally improves with age, for some children, this cautious approach may persist. Adolescence is a time when children are likely eating more meals away from home and are also preparing some meals and snacks on their own. Throughout the stages of development, it is important to include children in the process of meal planning, grocery shopping, cooking, and of course clean-up. Part of the process of feeding includes preparing kids to nourish themselves when they are out in the world without our supervision and support.

One of the main areas of concern for parents is the worry that, if they allow their child to decide how much and whether they will eat certain foods, their child will not eat a balanced and nutritious diet. This can certainly be an issue worth addressing as we will see when discussing picky eating and "when to worry," but in general, the research supports the idea that when children are offered a variety of nutritious foods, they will meet their general dietary requirements over the course of the day(s). It's our job to provide them with a variety of foods to support balanced nutrition, health, and enjoyment; it's our children's job to do the rest. Here is a summary of what the research supports:

- Exposure to a variety of foods and positive role-modeling have both been shown to be significant factors in the acceptance of new foods by children. If parents eat a limited diet, they are less likely to offer these foods to their kids. If children see their parents enjoying a variety of foods, they are more likely to try and enjoy them as well.
- Pressure to eat, in the form of verbal prompts ("eat your peas"), incentives/rewards ("and then you can have a cookie"), and even praise ("what a good boy you are for finishing your lunch") can all undermine our children's natural ability to eat with competence and also diminish their acceptance of new foods and flavors.
- Overly restricting food (and especially foods deemed by parents to be "bad") has actually been linked to increased consumption of these foods and excess weight gain in children.
- A responsive feeding style has been associated with higher intake of fruits and vegetables in children.
- Hands-on activities such as garden programs and cooking, as well as a focus on eating enjoyment, can have a positive impact on nutrition.[9]

Research suggests that "maladaptive feeding practices often derive from a parent's anxiety about the health and wellbeing of their child; the belief that their child is unable to self-regulate, is perceived to be underweight or overweight,

Research suggests that "maladaptive feeding practices often derive from a parent's anxiety about the health and wellbeing of their child; the belief that their child is unable to self-regulate, is perceived to be underweight or overweight, or over responsive to food."

or over responsive to food." [10] Pressuring kids to eat more of certain foods actually causes them to eat less. Restricting kids from eating less of other foods causes them to want to eat more of them. Using foods as incentives or rewards, not only heightens the value of that food (thereby diminishing the value of the food you are trying to get your child to eat!), but can also impede normal development of self-regulation around eating. Both parental feeding practices (exposure, modelling, pressure to eat, use of restriction, rewards, and using food to soothe) and parenting and feeding styles can have a significant impact on children's food preferences and intake.

Here are some guiding principles that sum up the general feeding practice framework:

- Approach feeding with warmth, responsiveness, and support while also maintaining a sense of structure and expectation.
- Let your child's developmental stage and temperament guide your approach and pace.
- Offer children a variety of foods in a neutral, pleasant environment.
- Be a role model. Allow your children to see you eating and enjoying a variety of foods. When your child sees you slurping a juicy mango or diving into a bowl of lentil soup, she is more likely to want to try it herself, no prompting required.
- Notice when you are feeling anxious about feeding and explore what the underlying fear might be (He will eat too little? He will eat too much? He will not eat what I want him to eat?) and remember that you are in it for the long haul. Try shifting the worry from a single meal, food, or even ingredient into wondering about how you might support your child's overall eating.
- Pressure (to eat or not to eat) generally backfires. Avoid it.
- Praise can also be a form of pressure for some children. It's sneaky so be on the lookout.
- Bribing, arguing, and negotiating may provide a short-term fix, but the long-term price of disconnection (both in terms of your child's internal regulation and in terms of your relationship with your child) is hardly worth it.

Before we move on to the topic of picky eating (which is on many parent's minds), we offer this beautiful sentiment from Satter: "Enjoyment of food and reward from eating are essential to having eating and feeding turn out well. When the joy goes out of eating, nutrition suffers."[11]

THAT ALL SOUNDS GREAT BUT ...
PICKY EATING AND MORE

We've painted a picture of eating and feeding where parents provide enjoyable, nutritious food in a reliable and pleasant way, without pressure, force, or anxiety, and children regularly and happily eat. Many of you may be thinking, that sounds very nice and all, but have you been to my house? In fact, for some families, mealtime is a regular struggle and parents face real feeding difficulties. It is not our intention to eliminate all of the challenges around feeding but, rather, to provide a framework of how to approach difficulties and a guidepost for when to worry or look for more support.

It is estimated that more than 50 percent of parents report that at least one of their children eats poorly, ranging from a mild to severe problem. This would represent about 25 percent of all children. The fears generally fall into three categories: eating too little (limited appetite), eating a poor variety of foods (selective intake), or showing a fear of eating. The authors of a 2015 article in *Pediatrics* define these categories in the following way:

- **Neophobia:** As mentioned previously, the rejection of foods that are new or unknown to a child is a typical aspect of development and generally resolves with repeated exposures. Extreme reactions are often given the term neophobia. This can be confusing nomenclature because some researchers describe neophobia as an aspect of typical development while others use it to describe a more extreme version of the normal developmental phenomena of being skeptical of new foods. Either way, for the majority of children, a fear or reluctance to accept new foods is perfectly and typically normal. Repeated exposure in a pleasant environment, without pressure or force, is key.
- **Picky eating:** A term that has inconsistent definitions and meanings in different countries and among different researchers. Some describe it as

"fussy" children with a poor appetite and others view it as a form of sensory disturbance; however, it is generally perceived to be a mild or transient problem. Although it is not considered a "medical condition," it can be significant enough to warrant attention and require intervention.

- **Feeding disorder:** Signifies a severe problem that results in substantial organic, nutritional, or emotional consequences. One category of feeding disorders, avoidant/restrictive food intake disorder (ARFID), has defined criteria in the American Psychiatric Association's *Diagnostic and Statistical Manual of Mental Disorders, Fifth Edition* (DSM-5).
- **Feeding difficulty:** An umbrella term that suggests there is a feeding problem of some sort. In essence, if the parent says there's a problem, there's a problem.[2]

According to the authors, roughly 75 percent of children fall into the "normal" category of feeding behaviors, and of the 25 percent of children identified by parents as having some form of a feeding difficulty, only 1 to 5 percent meet the criteria for a feeding disorder. The remaining >20 percent are "normal" children that have either a mild feeding difficulty that can be easily treated or is related to parental misperception (as in the instance when a parent feels the child is not growing adequately but a review of the growth chart can offer reassurance).

While a discussion of the top category of feeding challenges, feeding disorders, is beyond the scope of this book, we did want to provide some guidance on "when to worry." An excellent, thoughtful, and practical resource for parents looking for more information around significant feeding problems is *Helping Your Child with Extreme Picky Eating* by Katja Rowell, MD, and Jenny McGlothlin, MS, SLP. In addition to providing parents with strategies to manage their child's feeding difficulties, the authors offer a compassionate and reassuring approach.

WHEN TO WORRY

We want to begin by acknowledging that when parents sense there is a problem with feeding, it's generally worth exploring. If your child is growing and developing well, is eating a variety of foods, and mealtimes are (for the most part!) enjoyable for both you and your child, then feeding is probably going quite well. If, however, there are physical/medical problems or an excessive amount of stress, anxiety, or upset at mealtimes, a feeding difficulty exists. If a parent or child is struggling with feeding and mealtimes, it should be addressed. More often than not, simple measures can be taken to deal with the issue, and the problem exists in one of two categories: "normal" children with concerned parents (as mentioned previously, generally due to a misperception of typical growth and development or frustration with temperament) or children with mild, but recognizable and treatable conditions. The following list can provide some guidance on when a more serious feeding problem might be present:[2, 12]

Physical/medical:

- Poor growth
- Nutrient deficiencies
- Difficulty or pain with eating and swallowing (reflux, allergies, eosinophilic esophagitis, constipation)
- Concerns of choking, gagging, or aspiration
- Persistent vomiting or diarrhea
- Chronic cardiac or respiratory symptoms
- Sensory challenges
- Developmental delay

Social/behavioral:

- Mealtimes that are excessively long
- Food refusal lasting > one month
- Stressful mealtimes
- Lack of appropriate, independent feeding
- Failure to advance textures
- Extreme dietary limitations
- An abrupt change in eating after a triggering event (for example following a stomach flu or choking episode with a particular food)

If you suspect that your child is experiencing a feeding difficulty, the first step can be to consult with your child's pediatrician. A dietary history, understanding of the specific feeding challenge, and a review of your child's overall growth and development can help to define the problem and offer either reassurance or a plan of action. If an underlying medical problem is suspected, the appropriate tests and referrals should be explored. If the problem appears to be more social or behavioral, an evaluation by a feeding specialist may be warranted. While it may be tempting to ignore, downplay, or dismiss feeding challenges, left untended, they can grow in severity and result in persistent, more difficult to manage problems.

For more severe feeding issues, a thorough evaluation and appropriate referrals are warranted. For milder difficulties, interventions may still be warranted
depending on the degree of distress for parent and child. You can work towards
unwinding any disruptive, counterproductive, or even potentially harmful habits.
Return to the concepts of DOR and work to integrate them into your mealtimes.
Before even addressing any specific food/nutrition issues, you can begin by trying
to create more structured, calm, and pleasant mealtimes. If the deleterious habits
and routines (forcing, bribing, pushing, or restricting) have been going on for
some time (and especially with older children), an open and honest conversation
with your child might be necessary to lay out the new path forward. Your child
may initially be mistrusting. That is to be expected. Have patience and gently move
forward. Often times, these patterns have been going on for years and years. It's
unreasonable to think that a quick five-step process and a week or two of effort
will solve them. If the struggle of feeding has been going on for quite a while, it
may take some time to get to the other side. In addition to the prior book recommendation on extreme picky eating, another excellent resource is Ellyn Satter's
seminal work *Secrets of Feeding a Healthy Family*. Chapters 1 through 7 cover the
broad categories of How to Eat and How to Raise Good Eaters. While we diverge
on some of the nutrition information (for instance her position that plant proteins are "incomplete proteins"), the overall concepts on eating and feeding are
invaluable. If you sense that feeding in your home could use a little "tweaking,"
this is an excellent place to start.

Many experts (and non-experts!) offer a variety of approaches when it comes
to managing feeding difficulties. It can be confusing for parents to know what
approach will work without causing further harm. No two parents and no two
children are alike. What may work for one child (try one bite and if you don't
like it you don't have to have anymore) can be cause for a meltdown in another.
In general, you can gauge the effectiveness of your intervention by your child's
response.[13] If a particular approach (you must try at least one bite) is increasing
anxiety and stress, it's worth reconsidering. One of my (Reshma) children is often
skeptical of new foods. However, he will generally try a bite (even if it's very tiny!)
of a new food without protest. He does not seem stressed or anxious. Sometimes
he discovers a new food he enjoys and sometimes he does not move beyond the
tasting. The "try a bite" approach works for him (and me!) so we use it often.
Trust yourself, trust your child.

THE ELEPHANT IN THE ROOM

You may be wondering how all of these strategies fit in with a plant-based approach to feeding your family. We will discuss the specifics in greater detail in Chapter 12, but we wanted to emphasize that a plant-based approach to feeding can absolutely work alongside the DOR. It's important to remember that as parents, we are responsible for the *what*. If your household already eats a plant-leaning diet, there is not much to do. Continue offering a variety of foods in a structured, pleasant way and allow your children to do the eating. If you are in the process of shifting toward a plant-based diet for your family, some additional care and steps will be required as we will review in Chapter 12.

WRAPPING UP

For now, we want to leave you with a few guiding principles and suggestions for the "how" of feeding. No one knows your child better than you. Building trust and a loving connection with your child matters more than "one more bite" of pretty much anything. If you or your child are struggling with feeding, don't be afraid to seek out support. Use providers and specialists to offer guidance, but know that you are your child's greatest advocate and will know best if something is helping or harming.

- **Create structure for regular meals and snacks.** Having a consistent routine creates the foundation for successful feeding.
- **But also be flexible. Sometimes our best laid plans can go awry.** If the situation calls for an extra snack, an earlier dinner, or a missed meal because of a birthday party, having a regular routine means that a little flexibility can (and should!) be allowed.
- **Avoid being a short-order cook.** It's exhausting for parents, undermines the DOR, lowers expectations of children, and can take away from the traditions and joy of shared family meals.
- **Have at least one item at each meal that your child readily accepts and enjoys.** This is important for the DOR to really work and can be especially helpful when you are serving something new. For instance, if you are trying a new stew, make sure to serve some favorites alongside it, such as rolls and a favorite veggie.

- **Be patient and calm when introducing new foods.** Remember, it can take upward of fifteen attempts (in a calm and pleasant setting!) for a child to accept a new food.
- **Pair familiar foods with less familiar foods.** For instance, pairing crackers with something different like the White Bean, Garlic, and Lemon Spread in Chapter 15) can ease your child into trying new foods. Your child might just lightly dip into it, politely decline, or have a second helping!
- **Shrink it.** Size matters to kids. Children often prefer things that make them feel bigger. Keep portions "toddler-sized" (see The Plant-Based Plate, Chapter 6), and use child-sized cups, plates, bowls, and utensils.
- **Engage and encourage.** Involve kids in food selection and preparation. Grow some vegetables or herbs; let your child select fruits and vegetables at the market; encourage your child to help count, measure, sift, stir, pour, or brush.
- **Keep mealtimes short and sweet.** Many children are very active and are more interested in playing games or coloring than sitting at a dinner table. Keep mealtimes to fifteen minutes (you can excuse your child from the table when the time seems reasonable). Have some fun traditions at the family table. For example, children absolutely love to toast. Say "cheers" to the sunshine, to your spouse, to a beloved pet, or to your child.
- **Be a role model.** Children learn by what they see. We don't need to have complicated conversations about nutrition with our children. Rowell and McGlothlin state this perfectly when they say, *"Adults teach nutrition by serving and enjoying the foods we want our children to eat!"*[13]
- **Try not to be sneaky.** No one likes to be tricked. The few leaves of kale you covertly mixed into their morning smoothie could backfire. If little ones detect bitterness or a less sweet version of their favorite smoothie, they will learn to distrust your offerings. A different approach could be: "I've added a secret ingredient, and I'm wondering if you can figure out what is," or allow them to throw in as many leaves of spinach as they would like and gradually work your way up. When you "sneak" things in, you may inadvertently be teaching your kids that these foods are not enjoyable.
- **Make it fun and be creative. Use fun shapes, an assortment of colors, and a sense of playfulness to make food appealing to little ones.** Additionally, turning anything into a "bar" (i.e., salad, taco, rice bowls, etc.) is a great way

to get kids to try new ingredients or combinations. It also gives them some control over the meal by allowing them to add which and how much of each ingredient. These sorts of meals are ideal for exploring the DOR.

- **Be a good listener.** If your child really dislikes something, be willing to hear him out and offer a reasonable substitute. This is not about being a short-order cook, but if there is something you can do that makes the meal more enjoyable, go for it! One of my (Reshma) kids really dislikes warm or sautéed snap peas. So, when I make a stir-fry, I try to set aside a handful of snap peas so that he can enjoy them raw.

- **Set yourself and your child up for success by menu planning, grocery shopping, and cooking in a way that supports routine, structure, and pleasure around eating** (this will be covered in Part IV). Know your family and your schedule as you take this on. For some families, it may work to have all of the meals planned for the week, for others, a slightly less structured approach may work better.

- **Provide structure, warmth, and support.** Avoid pushing, bribing, sneaking, restricting, and bargaining. Center the focus of mealtimes around enjoyment.

- **Focus on the journey.** As important as it is to fuel our families with nutritious foods, we have an even greater responsibility as parents to teach our kids how to feed themselves when they are away from our dinner tables. Pushing one more bite of greens or two more bites of anything is not the end goal. Don't forget that food and family meals connect us. Yes, food should be nutritious. But it should also be delicious and most definitely shared. It's not always easy to do, but when we focus more on the conversation than the number of bites of broccoli, everyone feels more relaxed.

- **Be kind to yourself and have patience.** We are all just learning, experimenting, and growing.

- **Make mealtime a family event.** Family meals ground us and are at the core of feeding. This last tip is so valuable that we have devoted the entire next chapter to it. See you there!

Chapter 10

Family Meals

"Is there any practice less selfish, any labor less alienated, any time less wasted, than preparing something delicious and nourishing for people you love?"

—*Michael Pollan*

Cecelia is rushing from work to pick up her youngest daughter, Lily, from soccer practice. She is wondering if the travel league soccer team, debate club, and school newspaper might just be too much. Lily seems tired all the time. She ends up bringing dinner to her room most nights so that she can eat while working on her homework. Thankfully, her son, Elijah, is getting a ride home with friends after another late night of drama rehearsals. Hopefully, he will have something for dinner at school. Unfortunately, the weekend won't offer much relief, as the children have more practices, rehearsals, and of course homework. Between shopping for the week, cleaning, and carpooling, Cecelia doesn't imagine she will have much time to relax herself.

Some things have such inherent worth that they require little in the way of evidence or support to persuade you of their value. Family meals are one such thing. Akin to reading to your child, most would easily accept the assertion that this daily ritual, practiced with love, patience, and generosity offers benefits that far outweigh any potential cost. Family meals are one of the most powerful tools that parents have in protecting and nurturing their children. Perhaps you are a family that already participates in regular family meals or aspires to do so. This chapter will offer the reassurance and support you need to press on. On the other hand, if you are a family that does not consider family meals a priority, finds them to be completely out of reach, or are not impressed by the advantages they can offer, it is our hope that this chapter will sway your position. Family meals matter. Let's learn why.

WHAT EXACTLY IS A FAMILY MEAL?

Believe it or not, there is no wide consensus on the definition of what constitutes a family meal, and researchers describe various parameters when it comes to examining and evaluating outcomes associated with family meals. These parameters include frequency (the number of meals per week), which meal (do breakfast or snacks count?), where the meal is eaten (in the car, at the kitchen table, in front of a computer), who is present (does it "count" as a family meal if not everyone is present?), and how long the meal lasts.[1] While these factors can provide useful information from a research perspective and offer guidance for recommendations at the family level, one of the most accessible definitions of family meals is provided by The Family Dinner Project and it states: "As long as there are two family members eating together, talking, and enjoying one another, that is a family dinner...The goal is not to achieve a magic number but to find as many opportunities as you can and to make the most of them."[2]

While the research on family meals references five or more meals per week as the minimum number necessary to have an effect on many of the positive outcomes we will discuss, Anne Fishel, an Associate Clinical Professor of Psychology at Harvard Medical School and the cofounder of The Family Dinner Project, explains that, "this figure may be arbitrary, and there are inconsistencies in how researchers arrive at this 'magic number'...the emphasis on the number of dinners per week skirts the influence of the quality of the mealtime experience, which may be a more powerful factor than the quantity of meals."[3] Additionally, while the emphasis of family meals is often placed on dinner, any meal (or snack!) can serve as opportunity to share and connect. Fishel also clarifies that dinner tends to be the most reliable time of day for families to come together, and that, "dinner may be the one time of the day when a parent and a child enjoy something positive together—a well-cooked (veggie!) roast or a joke—and then, that small moment can build on moments away from the table." Family meals, whether they be breakfast, dinner, or a snack, provide us with a consistent, meaningful way to connect with those we love.

WHY FAMILY MEALS MATTER

In addition to serving as a time and space to connect, family meals also offer a protective shield for our children in three broad ways: intellectual functioning, physical health, and mental health. If we could provide in a pill what regular, positive family meals can offer, every parent in the neighborhood would be lining up for a prescription. In fact, some researchers suggest that "family meals have more to do with adolescents' positive outcomes than socioeconomic status, family structure (two-parent, one-parent, multi-generational), after-school activities, tutors, or church."[4]

The research around family meals can be complicated because families that are able to participate in regular family meals may differ from families who are unable to. Many studies do correct for variables such as socioeconomic status, family structure, and race/ethnicity. Despite these challenges, numerous favorable outcomes for children have been attributed to frequent family meals. Regular, positive family meals can help to support our children in many ways. They can:

> Some researchers suggest that "family meals have more to do with adolescents' positive outcomes than socioeconomic status, family structure (two-parent, one-parent, multi-generational), after-school activities, tutors, or church."

- **Help children do better in school.** The nature and quality of meal-time conversations promote language development and literacy as well as future academic success. One study showed that "mealtime was a more richly supportive context for the use of rare words, in informative contexts, than toy play or even book reading . . . The more children are exposed to extended conversations during meals, the more chances they have to acquire vocabulary, understand stories and explanations, and know things about the world."[5]

Meal-time discussions uniquely support language and literacy development because of the specific characteristics of these conversations. Extended talk at the dinner table increases children's exposure to rare (defined as words not found on the 3,000 most common words list) and "sophisticated" words (budget, oxygen) that have been linked to children's success in participating in classroom talk and reading after grade three. The academic benefits carry through the teen years. Research from the National Center on Addiction and Substance Abuse at Columbia University (CASA), revealed that adolescents who had infrequent family meals were twice as likely to do poorly in school (mostly C's or below) than children who ate dinner frequently with their families. Children who ate regular family meals (five to seven times per week) were twice as likely to get A's than those who ate dinner less than twice per week.[6] **Family meals support kids' academic success.**

- **Help kids be healthier.** The frequency of family meals has been positively associated with higher intakes of fruits, vegetables, dark green and orange vegetables, calcium-rich foods, fiber, and several micronutrients as well as a lower intake of soft drinks in middle school and high school-age kids. These behaviors persisted through young adulthood. Additionally, children who ate regular family meals during adolescence had a stronger desire to share meals with others during young adulthood. Frequent family meals have also been shown to be protective against disordered eating behaviors; even after five years, family meals were associated with decreased use of extreme weight-control behaviors in girls.[7] In a longitudinal study of eating patterns and weight-related issues in adolescents, researchers found that girls eating five or more meals per week with their family reduced the risk of extreme weight control behaviors by a third.[8] Research also shows improved self-esteem and higher body satisfaction among overweight boys and girls. Making family meals a priority was associated with significantly decreased unhealthy weight-control behaviors among both overweight boys and girls, suggesting that a positive mealtime context can be beneficial for the psychosocial health of overweight youths.[7] Although the data are not as conclusive for the risk of overweight, some studies suggest that children and adolescents who share three or more family meals per week have a reduced risk of being overweight or experiencing disordered eating.[9] Some researchers suggest that the relationship between family meals and weight status may be dependent upon certain aspects of the family meal (types of food being served), instead of solely on the frequency of eating together.[8] In this way, a plant-based approach to feeding your family in combination with regular family meals can bolster your efforts at the dinner table. **Family meals support kid's health.**

- **Help you worry (a little less!) about your teen.** Adolescents who eat regularly with their family are less likely to smoke cigarettes and marijuana, and have a reduced risk of abusing alcohol. The effect of family meals on these high-risk teen behaviors was even stronger for younger teens (ages twelve to thirteen). The National Center on Addiction and Substance Abuse at Columbia University is a leading research organization that studies drug abuse and its ramifications on society. One of its earlier publications emphasized that "a child who gets through age twenty-one without smoking, abusing alcohol, or using illegal drugs is virtually certain never to do so. And no one has more power to prevent kids from using substances than parents. There are no silver bullets; unfortunately, the tragedy of a child's substance abuse can strike any family. But one factor that does more to reduce teens' substance abuse risk than almost any other is parental engagement, and one of the simplest and most effective ways for parents to be engaged in teens' lives is by having frequent family dinners."[6] Compared to teens who eat dinner frequently (five or more times per week) with their families, teens who eat family dinner infrequently (less than three times per week) were three and a half times likelier to have abused prescription drugs, three and a half times likelier to have used illegal drugs other than marijuana or prescription drugs, three times likelier to have used marijuana, more than two and a half times likelier to have used tobacco, and one and a half times likelier to have used alcohol. One study found that "family dinner frequency and adolescent high-risk behavior patterns were significantly inversely related. Among adolescents who reported eating frequent family dinner meals, the odds of reporting use of alcohol, tobacco, and other illicit drugs; sexual intercourse; depressive symptoms or attempted suicide; antisocial behavior or violence; school problems; binge eating or purging behaviors, and losing a large amount of weight were relatively one-half the odds of such reporting among adolescents who reported eating very few family meals."[10] **Family meals protect teens against high risk behaviors such as alcohol, tobacco and drug abuse, early onset of sexual activity, yielding to negative peer pressure, and anti-social and violent behavior.**

- **Make teens happier.** Family meals have been linked to improved self-esteem, having a sense of purpose, and a positive view of the future. A study among adolescents in New Zealand found that teens who shared in family meals five or more times during the week had greater well-being scores and lower rates of depression, thoughts of suicide, and suicide.[11] It has also been reported that teens eating regular family meals are one and half times less likely to report high levels of stress.[12] **Family meals help teens flourish.**

- **Make parents happier.** A study looking at the influence of family meals found that parents who ate frequent family meals consumed more fruits and vegetables, fathers ate less fast food, and mothers engaged in fewer dieting behaviors. Additionally, greater frequency of family meals was associated with greater family functioning and greater relationship strength (among participants with a significant other) as well as lower levels of depressive symptoms, lower stress index, and greater self-esteem among parents.[13] **Frequent family meals are associated with parental social and emotional wellbeing.**

- **Allow you to feel more connected and involved in your child's life.** The daily routine of connecting and sharing about everyday life events, be they big or small, creates effective channels of communication that build trust and intimacy. These fifteen to twenty minutes a day provide a consistent time for parents to "check-in" and tune in to the emotional well-being of their children.[14] It's a wonderful way for kids and parents to unwind and lessen the stress of their everyday lives—which seem to get busier by the day. Teens who have frequent family dinners are more likely to say their parents know a lot about what's really going on in their lives and are more likely to report having high-quality relationships with their parents.[11] Regular mealtime conversations also lay the foundation for more sensitive discussions and can be a way of identifying problems (trouble in school, difficulties with friendship, anxiety) early and before they become serious. **Family meals help families stay connected.**

- **Provide you with an opportunity to share your values and build family traditions and rituals.** Whether it's through the food that is being served or the stories that are being told, family meals provide parents with a tool to share their values and traditions. The dinner table is a place to model behavior (manners, empathy), share family stories and traditions, and learn about the world. Family mealtime is a simple, daily ritual that can support family life. In *Home for Dinner*, Anne Fishel explains that "rituals help create a shared family identity and a sense of belonging...rituals in their repetitive predictability offer stability. There is something very comforting about knowing that one part of your day is going to unfold in pretty much the same way, day after day. Rituals punctuate a world that often feels frenzied and out of control, and these semi-choreographed events are as welcome to adults as to children."[3] **Family meals allow parents to express their values and strengthen traditions.**

A 2014 article from the American College of Pediatricians concluded that, "when families regularly share meals together, everyone benefits—the children, parents and even the community. Making the "Family Table" a priority from an early age can serve as a "vaccine" against many of the harms that come to children from a hurried lifestyle."[15] Perhaps the best way to sum up the benefits of family meals is the acknowledgment from a paper published by the Emory Center for Myth and Ritual in American Life that "Eating together surely is a good thing."[16]

WHAT GETS IN THE WAY OF FAMILY MEALS?

If family meals are associated with so many positive outcomes, why don't they happen with greater frequency? About half of American families rarely have family dinner with only about 58 percent of children eating five or more meals per week (what most research recommends) with their family.[17] Over the past three decades, family time at the dinner table and family conversation in general has declined by more than 30 percent.[15] For many families there are real barriers to making family dinner happen, and it requires far greater effort than simply taking a magic pill.

One of the most common reasons cited for not having regular, family meals is a lack of time. Whether due to work or afterschool activities, families face increasing demands on their time. Over the last several decades not only have we seen a decline in the frequency of family meals but also in the amount of free, unstructured time that children have. These "lost" hours have mostly gone towards structured sports (with the unanticipated consequence of a five-fold increase of non-participating children standing along the sidelines) and homework.[16] A recent article in *The Atlantic* clarified the reality for many working adults by acknowledging, "there has also been tremendous upheaval in the structures of American life and work. Women—the people traditionally forced into meal management—have voluntarily entered the workforce in droves or been forced into it for financial reasons. Average commute times get longer seemingly every year, ensuring that working adults get home later and later. And almost all middle-class work now involves a great deal of time spent on a computer, which means millions of Americans' jobs don't end for the day when they leave the office. For many, their work never really ends at all."[18] Following a long day of work, after-school activities, and perhaps more work, it's no surprise that families struggle to find twenty minutes for dinner, not to mention the time for shopping, planning, prepping, cooking, and cleaning that family meals require. In addition to time, other barriers to frequent family meals include cost, conflicting schedules, not knowing what or how to cook, family tension (dissatisfaction with family relationships), food preferences/picky eating, the burden of meal prep/cleaning, feeling too tired, and a desire for autonomy during the teen years.[19] We think it's more likely than not that families want to reap the benefits and enjoyment that family meals can offer; they are perhaps just struggling to find a path to it.

HOW TO MAKE FAMILY MEALS HAPPEN

We want to end this chapter with a few practical strategies that can support your efforts to sustain or introduce the practice of family meals in your home. Part IV will provide many of the resources and tips that will hopefully make family meals more accessible.

- **Start with where you are.** Even though research looking at outcomes suggests five or more meals per week as the goal, it's not an all-or-none proposition. If your family is not used to having meals together, start with a goal of once or twice a week. Focus on making mealtimes pleasant so that your crew will want to come back. Work your way up in a way that seems manageable. Think of it as creating a refuge for the day, a safe space to land.

- **Keep it simple.** Don't worry about creating gourmet meals each night. A one-pot stew, pasta with store-bought marinara, even sandwiches will do. A beautiful reminder from the executive director of the Family Dinner Project: "I believe the magic can happen without perfection."[20]

- **Set the table.** It's not about fancy plates or splashy place settings, but rather, creating a calm, inviting space that signals "this is special." It can be as simple as clearing the table of clutter and bringing a welcoming smile.

- **Ask for help.** It can be a lot for one person to manage all of the work of family meals. Consider dividing up the work if possible (in our house the cook does not generally do the dishes) and recruit children to help in age-appropriate ways (setting the table, cleaning, and even cooking when they are old enough).

- **Insist on attendance.** Whoever is at home comes to the table for dinner. While it is tempting to let children eat in their rooms so that they can finish up homework to allow for a (more) reasonable bedtime or to avoid conflict by allowing everyone to retreat to their own spaces for dinner, insisting that everyone who is home comes to the table sets a clear expectation.

- **Prioritize.** Regular family meals won't happen unless you prioritize them. The average American family spends less than twenty minutes eating dinner.[21] These twenty minutes are often the only time that families have to sit, pause, and connect. Protect them fiercely. Since lack of time is the number one reason cited for not having family dinner, think about where you might "nudge" the schedule. Consider limiting the number of after-school activities, shifting the timing of dinner (this may require a "tide-me-over" snack), or setting a pause on work brought home. Creating a habit around family meals takes effort and consistency. The payoff, though, is that it becomes such an essential part of your day that you hardly consider questioning it. Just like brushing your teeth or buckling your seat belt, it becomes a thing you just do. As Ellyn Satter powerfully states, "The day to day routine of structured, sit-down family meals and snacks reassures children that they are loved and that they will be provided for—nutritionally and in all other ways."[4]

- **Be flexible.** There are times in life when everyone coming to the table is just not possible, be it a work deadline or the big play production. Maintain a sense of ritual and connection by joining your teen when she comes home late from rehearsals with a cup of tea or bedtime snack. The magic of dinner can happen over a snack.

- **Meal plan, prep, and shop.** The burden of these tasks can be enormous for any one person to take on, but without them, mealtimes are likely to be chaotic, exhausting, and frustrating. This doesn't mean you need to create complex, multi-colored graphics or find a fancy app. A simple note card will do (see Chapter 13)! Some degree of planning and prepping will go a long way to ensuring that family meals will happen. A little extra time spent on the weekends (prepping veggies, making a sauce or even a meal or two) can make a big difference during the week.

- **Cook at home as much as possible.** Research suggests that meals prepared and eaten at home are more nutritious. It is estimated that roughly 70 percent of meals in the United States are eaten outside of the home and roughly 20 percent are eaten in the car.[20] Additionally, for any parent who has ordered a "kid's meal" for their child, you know that the nutritional quality and variety of these meals vary considerably from meals made at home. Again, an occasional kid's meal is not the problem; it's the reliance of these foods on a regular basis that can undermine our efforts at home. If you are eating out with your family, enjoy the meal without added fuss or stress. Consider ordering from the "regular" menu and have children share or eat family style and remember to model the same behaviors when eating out. The more you cook at home, the more comfortable you will become. Just as with frequency of meals, start with where you are, and add on.

- **Don't be a short-order cook—serve everyone the same food.** Make one meal for the whole family, with small accommodations as needed (i.e., spice level, food allergies, size of bites, etc.). Remember the DOR from Chapter 9: you decide what, when, and where! If you start out making something different for everyone at the table, this will become your reality on a daily basis. And that's just exhausting. There is also something very gratifying about the experience of everyone at the table enjoying the same meal.

- **Invite conversation.** There can be a lot of pressure to have meaningful conversations filled with brilliant ideas and laughter at the dinner table. Add to this the one-word answers of "fine" and "okay" when asking children about their day or the bickering among siblings and you may wonder what, in fact, is so great about dinnertime conversations? These opportunities to connect don't have to be filled with fantastical stories or vocabulary lessons. Avoid placing pressure on your children or yourself. If the conversation stalls or seems tense, you can model the behavior by sharing about your day or an interesting article you read. Sometimes even sharing about a difficult moment in the day can be a way to show children how to manage feelings of hurt or disappointment. Engage in conversation with other adults at the table if they are present and try to not make the children the sole focus or topic of discussion. Additionally, avoid bringing up sensitive topics at the table. Remember, it's about creating a calm, daily respite. This may not be the best time to talk about chores left undone or a poor grade on last week's math test. Some families enjoy dinnertime conversation starters such as Table Topics and other games.
- **Share family stories.** Research shows a positive correlation between what children know about their family's history and that child's locus of control (resiliency), level of self-esteem, and perception of family functioning.[16] In addition to sharing stories, mealtimes are an ideal platform to share values (such as sustainability and compassion), create new traditions (Friday-night homemade pizza), and celebrate old ones (special holidays or celebrations).
- **Put away the screens.** Screen time during meals has been associated with distracted (or absent!) conversations, less enjoyment of the meal, and less healthy dietary intakes.[22,23] An indoor picnic with movie night can be a fun treat, but the general rule should be no screens (phones, TVs, tablets) at the table. Be firm. Be a role model. You can do this!
- **Have fun!** Not every meal is full of grace and peace. Sometimes there can be such chaos at the dinner table that we wonder why we even bothered. Picky eaters, fighting siblings, and dirty dishes can leave us feeling drained. Work to create warmth, calm, and joy at mealtimes. Try not to take things too seriously, be consistent (and persistent!), and experiment with what works best for your family.

While Lily was in the shower, Cecelia hurried to get dinner together. She warmed up leftovers, made a quick salad, and sliced up some bread. She paused as she started to put together a tray to take to Lily's room. Instead, she laid out two dinner plates and napkins at the kitchen table. She called for Lily to come to the table. To her surprise, Lily sat down without resisting or complaining and began eating. After a few moments of silence, Lily said, "Mom, you're not going to believe what happened in biology today."

Despite all of the potential advantages, family meals are not a panacea. Our children will still struggle—with school, with relationships, with food, and with health, both physical and mental. But these rituals practiced with consistency may diminish their chances of experiencing such suffering. And, if such suffering should come upon them, the foundation of family meals can be a wonderful source of ongoing support, comfort, and love. Through the food and conversations we bring to our dinner tables, we have the wonderful and fantastic opportunity to nourish our families, each and every day.

Chapter 11

Weighty Matters

"Knowing that we can be loved exactly as we are
gives us all the best opportunity for growing
into the healthiest of people."

—Fred Rogers

When David picked up his thirteen-year-old-daughter Elisa from school, he was eager to hear about her day. She was struggling with adjusting to the middle school. She signed up for a few clubs, and he was hoping that some new friendships would help her find her way. She entered the car with unexpected enthusiasm. She explained that they had a lunch-time meeting for the environmental club. They were each supposed to sign up for a project aimed at helping the school "go green." She chose to head up the meatless Monday initiative and announced that she was now vegan. Her hands were wild with animated gestures as she spoke about the toll that factory farming took on our planet and how changing what we eat could have an enormous impact on our environment. David tried to hide his concern. When he was growing up, his older sister had an eating disorder and he remembered that it started when she decided to become vegetarian. He wondered, could Elisa be heading down the same path?

Weight is a complex issue. We could devote an entire book to pediatric weight-related issues, and this chapter will fall short in addressing the breadth and depth that these topics require. We will, however, do our best to address them with evidence, care, and compassion in order to start the conversation. Weight-related concerns take center stage when it comes to pediatric nutrition. Though they may sometimes be misguided, at the core of parental concerns around weight is the hope that our children not only avoid suffering but, in fact, thrive. In this chapter, we will discuss broadly the issues of being under- and overweight (with a specific focus on plant-based diets), the role of obesity prevention in propagating a culture of disordered eating, and end with a discussion on the much argued and controversial role of vegetarian and vegan diets in relation to eating disorders.

GROWTH CHARTS ARE NOT REPORT CARDS

Growth charts are an invaluable tool for pediatricians. Trends in growth can provide information about a child's health and development, but it is only one marker of their overall well-being. The parameters of growth must always be placed within the context of the child's general health; used incorrectly, growth charts have the potential to do great harm. A few key points to keep in mind when it comes to growth charts:

- Babies born prematurely and children with certain medical conditions (such as Down syndrome) require specific growth charts. Take care that the correct growth chart is being used.
- If your child seems to be doing well but the growth chart indicates a reason for concern, request a repeat measurement. A common reason for (mis) diagnosis of poor growth is inaccurate measurements!
- Children grow in spurts. A slight shift between percentiles (up or down) is not a reason for worry in and of itself. Follow the trends and consider how your child is doing as a whole.
- While percentiles can offer information on where your child's weight and height fall compared to a representative sample, it's much more valuable to follow the trends of your child's growth instead of focusing on the specific percentile.

The authors of *Helping Your Child with Extreme Picky Eating* summarize this nicely: "Growth charts are often misinterpreted even by doctors, with harmful consequences. They are not a report card or a standardized test of your parenting, where tenth percentile is worse than fiftieth. Tenth percentile may be right where your child should be. The percentiles only tell us how big or small a child is relative to a sampling of children the same age. Humans come in a variety of shapes and sizes."[1]

The following sample growth chart [2] illustrates some of these points. (*Note: for simplicity, only the weight parameter is included, but a thorough evaluation also takes height and, for younger children, head circumference, into account.*)

Figure 11.1: Sample Growth Chart

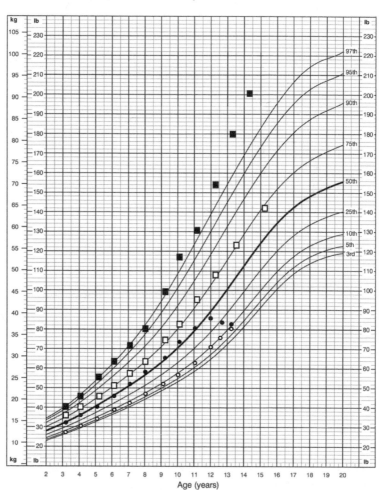

In this chart, the open shapes represent stable growth, whereas the solid shapes represent a potential for concern. The open circle represents a child growing steadily between the fifth and tenth percentiles and the open square, a child growing steadily near the seventy-fifth percentile. In both cases, if the child is doing well medically and without other areas of concern (socially, with feeding, etc.), then these both likely represent healthy growth. Both the solid dark circle and square, however, signal potential concern. In both circumstances, there is a change in the trajectory of growth. A leveling off and decline can indicate an underlying medical problem (such as celiac disease) and a progressive climb in weight beyond the typical trend for the child deserves further discussion. Assuming that the appropriate growth chart is being used and measurements are accurate, changes in growth trend that are accompanied by worrisome symptoms or concerns are a red flag that warrant attention. If your child is tracking along his curve, eating, and generally doing well, then there is often little need for alarm.

BMI IS IMPERFECT, BUT . . .

Body mass index (BMI) is a measure of a person's weight divided by height squared and is used as an indirect measure of body fat. It is an imperfect measure because it does not factor in bone structure, fat distribution, muscle mass, and, for adults, age and sex.[3] It continues to be used, however, because of its ease of use (alternatives would include MRI scans, waist to hip ratios, DXA scans, and bioelectrical impedance—all of which are less accessible and with potential downsides) and because, while imperfect, there is a strong relationship between BMI and body fat percentage. BMI correctly categorizes people as having excess body fat more than 80 percent of the time. It incorrectly categorizes some people (those who are muscular for instance) as being overweight despite having a normal or low percentage of body fat and categorizes a greater percentage of people as having a normal BMI but who in reality have a high percent body fat.[4]

An article in the *International Journal of Obesity* sought to address the diagnostic accuracy of BMI in childhood and answer the question of whether children at a high BMI are at greater risk of morbidity. The researchers concluded that a high BMI for age was consistently associated with high specificity (meaning the risk of incorrectly identifying a child as obese was low) and a low-moderate sensitivity (meaning it misses kids who may have a higher percentage body fat but normal BMI).[5] Despite the fact that the BMI measure is imperfect, it can be a useful tool in clinical practice because of its ease of use. However, it is important to be aware of its shortcomings so that its significance is not overly emphasized. It is alarming to see that some schools issue "BMI report cards" despite findings that suggest such BMI reports do not appear to positively impact student weight status and have the potential to cause harm to students (weight stigmatization, teasing, disordered eating, and psychological damage).[6] BMI can be a helpful tool, but it should not trigger a diagnosis or therapeutic plan without thoughtful consideration and exploration.

UNDERWEIGHT

In Chapter 9, we covered many of the feeding issues that can interfere with a child's growth; these principles also apply to children eating a plant-based diet. For any child that is experiencing a lack of appropriate growth or a decline in the expected rate of growth, a work-up should be initiated. It is important to distinguish normal, low but steady growth from poor or inadequate growth. In the case of true failure to thrive, an evaluation, including a thorough history, physical exam, and appropriate testing and referrals are warranted.

In Chapter 1, Health, we detailed how plant-based diets are not only safe but a potentially preferred way of eating for growing children and that children eating a nutritionally adequate and appropriately planned plant-based diet can enjoy normal growth and development. This involves providing sufficient calories and variety of foods. We also mentioned that with young children eating plant-centered diets, care must be taken to ensure that the diet is not too bulky as plant-based foods are generally high in fiber and children can feel full before consuming enough calories. Including some more refined foods (such as grains and oils) can help to ensure that growing children get adequate calories. Additional plant foods that can provide a boost of calories include seeds, nuts, seed/nut butters, avocados, dried fruit, and smoothies made with some of these ingredients. We cannot emphasize enough that our top priority in feeding children must always be to ensure that they grow and develop well. If feeding is not going well or your child is experiencing poor growth, seek out professional support.

WHAT DO WE KNOW ABOUT CHILDHOOD OBESITY?

Over the last three decades, childhood obesity rates have more than doubled and the rate in adolescents has quadrupled. The prevalence of obesity among children in the United States between the ages of two and eighteen is 18.5 percent (13.9 percent in preschool children, 18.4 percent in school-age children, and over 20 percent in adolescents).[7,8] Though the rate of rise seems to be leveling off in the United States over the last few years, the World Health Organization reports that overweight and obesity are linked to more deaths worldwide than underweight and that globally there are more people who are obese than underweight—this occurs in every region except parts of sub-Saharan Africa and Asia.[9]

A large study, following over 50,000 children, published in the *New England Journal of Medicine* found that "among children who were obese at three years of age, the probability of being overweight or obese in adolescence was almost 90 percent and only a minority of young children with obesity returned to a normal weight...Among adolescents who were overweight or obese, the most excessive weight gain had occurred between two and six years of age."[10] Additionally, studies have also reported that an elevated BMI in childhood is associated with a greatly increased risk of being overweight in adulthood.[11,12] In one study, it was reported that close to 70 percent of six- to nine-year-old children with a BMI greater than the 95th percentile were obese as adults, but this number rose to 83 percent for children between the ages of ten and fourteen.[13] These findings emphasize early childhood as a critical age for prevention strategies. It's an age where parents can have an enormous impact in terms of establishing healthy habits such as family meals and a plant-centered diet.

But this is not just a matter of statistics and trends. These figures are connected to real health outcomes for children. If obesity in childhood (and especially during adolescence) puts children at greater risk for obesity in adulthood, it also places them at greater risk for many of the adult diseases and conditions that have been associated with it. A study in the *New England Journal of Medicine* analyzed data to assess the trends in the prevalence of overweight and obesity among children and adults between 1980 and 2015 and quantified the burden of disease related to high BMI. It reported that, "epidemiologic studies have identified high body-mass index as a risk factor for an expanding set of chronic diseases, including cardiovascular disease, diabetes mellitus, chronic kidney disease, many cancers, and an array of musculoskeletal disorders."[14] Additionally, a National Institutes of Health (NIH) expert panel review stated that obesity is a major contributor to chronic disease and it "raises the risk for morbidity from hypertension, dyslipidemia, type 2 diabetes, coronary heart disease, stroke, gallbladder disease, osteoarthritis, sleep apnea and respiratory problems, and some cancers. Obesity is also associated with increased risk in cardiovascular and all-cause mortality. The biomedical, psychosocial, and economic consequences of obesity have substantial implications for the health and well-being of the U.S. population."[15]

Obesity in childhood not only carries greater risk for disease in adulthood but can also have more immediate health consequences.

- In children, obesity is strongly associated with dyslipidemia (abnormal blood lipids, which is a risk factor for cardiovascular disease),[16] and we know from Chapter 1 that early atherosclerotic lesions begin in childhood.
- A study published in *Circulation,* identified that in children between the ages of twelve and eighteen, obesity was the risk factor most strongly associated with a high carotid intima media thickness (a measure of carotid atherosclerotic disease that correlates with a risk of cardiovascular disease), more so than hypertension, smoking, and elevated cholesterol.[17]
- There is a strong link between hypertension and obesity. While only 3 to 5 percent of children in the United States have high blood pressure, this number rises up to 25 percent in children with obesity.[18]
- Overweight and obesity is a key risk factor for the development of type 2 diabetes in youth.[19] Early onset of diabetes in children hastens the complications of diabetes, such as eye, kidney, and vascular damage.
- A high adolescent BMI increases adult diabetes and coronary artery disease risks by nearly threefold and fivefold, respectively.[7]
- Several other pediatric health conditions have been associated with childhood and adolescent obesity including orthopedic problems (slipped capital epiphyses, Blount's disease), intracranial hypertension (pseudotumor cerebri), gall stones, fatty liver disease, menstrual abnormalities, polycystic ovarian syndrome, sleep apnea, and asthma.[20]
- In addition to negative health outcomes, childhood obesity has been associated with a variety of negative psychological consequences including body

dissatisfaction, low self-esteem, disordered eating behaviors, and, in some instances, depression (although the research around the link between childhood obesity and depression is inconsistent). Weight stigmatization, teasing, and bullying all contribute to these negative outcomes. Overweight and obese children not only experience weight-related stigma and teasing from their peers, but can also experience it from parents, educators, and even health care providers. This is exemplified by one study that found that child obesity prevention programs (meant to help children) can actually lead to increased stigmatization towards overweight/obese youths.[21]

THE SNACKWELL EFFECT

In the 1980s and 1990s the *Dietary Guidelines for Americans* urged us all to eat less fat. The food industry promptly rose to the challenge of "helping" us by producing a barrage of low-fat snacks that overtook our grocery and pantry shelves. By complying with the low-fat guidelines (which did not work because Americans actually did not cut their fat consumption), products like Snackwell's actually made the problem of diet-related preventable diseases worse by encouraging us to swap out fat for heavily refined and processed carbohydrates, which was never the intention of the dietary guidelines. In a similar way, we must be cautious to not let our fervor over the childhood obesity epidemic create an even bigger problem. Messaging and programming that encourages families and health care providers to put children on diets have the potential to do the same—no change (or worsening) in obesity with the unintended, but real consequence of childhoods filled with diets, restriction, and a dismantling of self-esteem and self-worth. The intention is good—help our children lead healthy, fulfilling lives—but we must guard against creating an environment where our children are more obese, more unhappy, and unable to feed themselves with care and reliability.

HELPING WITHOUT HARMING

Childhood obesity affects a significant proportion of the population and it is associated with numerous adverse health consequences, both physical and emotional. But it is important to remember that health depends on so much more than a percentile. Weight is not the only determinant of health. Physical activity, stress, relationships, diet quality, and sleep can all influence well-being. Additionally, as is emphasized in a statement by the Academy of Eating Disorders, "weight is not a behavior: A child's weight is not a reliable proxy for health or fitness and focusing on modifying weight may not be as effective as modifying behaviors."[22]

In *Your Child's Weight: Helping Without Harming*, registered dietitian and feeding expert, Ellyn Satter, offers an approach that aims to support children's health and eating without harming. She refrains from using overweight/obesity and instead uses the term "growth acceleration" to define the clinical problem. Growth acceleration, she offers, can be treated by answering the key question: What is undermining this child's ability to grow in a way that is right for him? "Rather than *avoiding overweight*, the emphasis becomes *supporting each child's normal growth*."[23]

In this way prevention (and treatment) programs should target behaviors that promote a healthy lifestyle in a way that is weight neutral. Interventions should focus not only on providing opportunities for appropriate levels of physical activity and healthy eating, but also promote self-esteem, body satisfaction, and respect for body size diversity.[22]

On a daily basis, we are inundated with messages about food, healthy eating, healthy weight, and strategies for weight loss. Increasingly our children are exposed to messages and photoshopped images that can distort ideas of what "normal" looks like. Simultaneously, they see a world of super-sized everything and five-day juice fasts for flat abs. As researcher Dianne Neumark-Sztainer recognizes, "our society is full of pressures that promote obesity but reward thinness." Conflicting advice leaves parents unsure about "how to protect your child from the health hazards of obesity without inadvertently planting the seeds of an unhealthy weight obsession."[24] There has got to be a middle way for parents to help support and guide their children.

Ways That We Might Harm:

- Many teens and their parents misinterpret obesity prevention messages and begin eliminating foods they consider to be "bad" or "unhealthy." Even though most teens who develop an eating disorder (ED) were not previously overweight, it is not unusual for an ED to start with an adolescent "trying to eat healthy." Our messages around food matter.

- In an attempt to lose weight, adolescents who are overweight may engage in disordered eating behaviors. A thoughtful article in the journal *Pediatrics*, "Preventing Obesity and Eating Disorders in Adolescents," addresses this issue by explaining that "initial attempts to lose weight by eating in a healthy manner may progress to severe dietary restriction, skipping of meals, prolonged periods of starvation, or the use of self-induced vomiting, diet pills, or laxatives. Initial attempts to increase physical activity may progress to compulsive and excessive exercise. . . . At first, weight loss is praised and reinforced by family members, friends, and health care providers, but ongoing excessive preoccupation with weight loss can lead to social isolation, irritability, difficulty concentrating, profound fear of gaining the lost weight back, and body image distortion."[7] Dieting has been identified as the most significant predictor of developing an eating disorder.

> Dieting has been identified as the most significant predictor of developing an eating disorder.

- As we saw in Chapter 9, restriction often leads to a pre-occupation and eventual overconsumption of restricted foods. Placing parents in a position of policing instead of guiding or coaching around food is a set-up for cycling of restriction followed by overconsumption.
- Teens who "diet" are at increased risk for weight gain over time. One study found that adolescent dieters had nearly twice the odds for being overweight five years later than non-dieters. The analysis adjusted for baseline BMI so that the association was not due to a difference in BMI at the beginning of the study.[25]
- Weight talk (weight-related comments made to a child about their weight, encouraging a child to diet or lose weight, parents talking about their own weight, discussing other people's weight, and perhaps worst of all, weight teasing) is harmful. Research suggests that "weight talk" may increase risk for both eating disorders and obesity, and one study reported that weight talk, including parental dieting and parental encouragement to diet, predicted the incidence of overweight status five years later in adolescents.[24]
- Media and specifically food marketing targeted at children puts children at risk. Research suggests that not only is screen time a sedentary activity that might take the place of physical activity but that, media with food

advertising directed at children has a specific effect. Food marketers spend nearly two billion dollars annually in child-targeted advertising. Not surprisingly, nearly all (98 percent) of food advertising directed at children is for products that are high in salt, fat, or sugar. An earlier report published by the Institute of Medicine concluded that "food and beverage marketing practices geared to children and youth are out of balance with healthful diets and contribute to an environment that puts their health at risk."[26]

It is understandable why parents worry about their children being overweight. Experts tell us that being overweight puts us at greater risk for chronic diseases such as heart disease and diabetes. The world tells us that being overweight puts our children at risk of being teased, bullied, and stigmatized. But the path to helping our children does not have to include restricting, counting, and shaming. Satter reminds us that "striving for weight loss does harm. It hurts your child, and it hurts you. For your child, getting enough to eat is basic to getting her needs met. For you, giving your child enough to eat is fundamental to nurturing. You don't have to go there. Instead, do the best job of feeding and parenting that you possibly can, and accept your child, just the way she is." And that doing your job "means your child does not have to worry about eating and weight."[23] The last thing parents, teachers, schools, and health care providers want to do is harm. So how is it that we can help?

Ways That We Can Help

It's important enough to repeat once again: weight is not a behavior. We can help our children by modeling healthy lifestyle choices and providing structure, support, and love.

- *Avoid weight talk.* Do not allow weight teasing in your home and refrain from making negative comments about your own weight. These types of comments are so insidious and pervasive that it requires active attention for us to eradicate them from our conversations. For older children, when you observe weight talk, teasing, or stigma, it can be an opportunity to show empathy and invite conversation.

- *Discourage dieting.* A definition of dieting in this context would be "an eating plan that includes rigid rules about what to eat, how much, in what combinations, or at what times, that is usually followed for a specified period, for the purpose of weight loss."[24] As mentioned previously, dieting has not been found to show sustained weight loss, predisposes to future weight gain, and is associated with extreme weight-control behaviors, including eating disorders.

- *Have healthy choices on hand.* Sliced veggies in the fridge, a bright bowl of fruit on the kitchen counter, or overnight oats ready for tomorrow morning's breakfast are simple ways to make the healthy choice the easy choice. If there are foods you are trying to avoid or minimize (for instance sugar-sweetened beverages), it is best not to purchase them in the first place.

- *Plant-centered diets can support a healthy weight for children and adults.* Many epidemiological studies have consistently shown that children and adults following plant-based diets are leaner and have lower BMIs. Some studies have even shown a progressive increase in BMI as meat and animal products were added in the diet.[27] Treatment of obesity in adulthood is difficult, making prevention strategies in childhood that much more critical. While some may argue that a plant-centered diet would fall into the category of "restriction," a well-planned plant-based diet can be abundant, nutritious, and delicious by focusing on all of the foods that are included instead of avoided. If you are just beginning, one way of approaching this is to first add in foods (beans, tofu, plant milks) instead of eliminating foods. As you and your family enjoy more of these foods, it will naturally crowd out the foods you are looking to minimize in the diet. It's not about restricting calories or enjoyment but rather about creating a foundation that supports health.

- *"Calories count but don't count them."*[24] This phrase highlights the tricky situation many parents find themselves in. It's important for older children and teens to have some basic nutrition information, but it can be a slippery slope that can lead to an unhealthy obsession with calorie counting and restriction. When researchers from Project EAT (a study group examining a broad spectrum of weight-related problems among diverse youth from adolescence to adulthood) asked adolescents about this, they found that teens wanted information to make informed decisions but that they also wanted it to be delivered with respect and sensitivity; they did not want to feel badly about themselves or feel guilty about eating "too many" calories. The information you provide will likely vary from child to child depending on what their needs and level of curiosity are and what your concerns may be.

- *Provide structure around meals and snacks.* This goes back to the DOR we discussed in Chapter 9. By avoiding grazing and having structured meals and snacks, you allow your child to come to the table with an appetite and to feel satisfied.

- *Cook more at home.* Multiple studies have found that meals cooked and eaten at home were associated with higher quality diets and better health outcomes. In contrast, meals eaten away from home (full-service restaurants and fast food) were associated with more calories, sodium, and fat.[28] Another study found that less-frequent television and video viewing during family meals and eating more home-cooked family meals were each associated with lower odds of obesity.[29]

- *Prioritize family meals.* We reviewed the vast benefits of family meals in the last chapter. Regular family meals are associated with improved dietary quality and have been found to be protective against disordered eating behaviors in adolescents.

- *Limit screen time as best you can.* This is especially important at the dinner table. Keep televisions in your family room (or common space) and out of children's bedrooms. One study found that teens who had televisions in their bedrooms watched more TV, were less physically active, and had poorer dietary intakes than adolescents who did not have bedroom televisions.[25] It's important to note that many of these behaviors (family meals, home-cooked meals, no screens at meals) cluster together so that a family that tends to implement one of these behaviors is more likely to do the others. This is all good news because it reinforces the same message: family meals, cooked at home, eaten together, and away from screens and devices support health.

- *Encourage joyful movement.* Finding fun ways to stay active (such as running around at the playground, a game of basketball, or riding bikes) makes physical activity enjoyable and sustainable.

- *Model the behavior you want to see.* Whether it's enjoying fruits and vegetables, regular physical activity, prioritizing sleep, or limiting screen time, our actions speak louder than words. Model the behaviors you want to see instead of lecturing or negotiating.
- *Focus less on weight and more on behavior.* If your child comes to you with concerns about his weight, validate his feelings and come up with ideas that might be supportive. Going for a family walk, coming up with fun recipe ideas, and just listening can be helpful.
- *Focus on your child's positive traits*—their kindness, sense of humor, or creativity. Offer unconditional love and support.

There are no easy, one-size-fits-all solutions. Our approach to caring for a child that is under- or overweight might perhaps be the same. In a way, the BMI chart has co-opted our conversations around food and health. Children falling into the "normal" category receive a green light to continue as usual and children falling below or above are often given brief, prescriptive measures with little evidence of their efficacy or benefit and potential to harm. These hasty interventions take the place of more meaningful explorations that might reveal how a child or family might be struggling and answer the question posed by Satter: "What is undermining this child's ability to grow in a way that is right for him?" All families and children deserve the same support and guidance, regardless of BMI. Creating a home environment that sets our children up for success is a great first step.

Eating Disorders and Veg Diets

Eating disorders are the third most common chronic condition in childhood after obesity and asthma. Increasingly, we are seeing eating disorders diagnosed in younger and younger children (as young as five to twelve years of age) as well as in males and minority youth.[7] The American Psychiatric Association recognizes eight distinct eating and feeding disorders—the three most widely recognized of which are anorexia nervosa, bulimia nervosa, and binge eating disorder.[30]

Additionally, an even larger percentage of youth (some estimates put it at close to 15 percent), suffer from disordered eating with similar physical and psychological consequences but do not meet strict diagnostic criteria.[7] Eating disorders are not determined by body weight, gender, or dietary pattern, but rather are mental health disorders. They are characterized by extreme emotions, attitudes, and behaviors toward food, eating, body weight, and shape. There is a complex interplay between genetics, environmental factors, history of dieting, and neuroendocrine abnormalities that are thought to contribute to the development of eating disorders: a combination of genetic predisposition, environmental triggers, and personal experience.[31] Eating disorders have the second highest mortality rate of all mental health disorders, surpassed only by opioid addiction.[32] Eating disorders in children are a serious matter.

We have already talked about the complex interplay between obesity and disordered eating. One area that comes up often is the role that vegetarian and vegan diets may play in the development of eating disorders. Although vegans tend to be significantly leaner than nonvegans, being vegan does not guarantee a healthy body weight, nor does it guarantee a healthy relationship with food. People following a vegan diet tend to have lower rates of overweight and obesity and slightly higher rates of underweight. Like the general population, some vegans struggle with eating disorders. Contrary to popular opinion, however, vegans do not appear to be at increased risk for eating disorders. The research around this topic is a little complicated, but it is worth reviewing and clarifying.

Data suggest that a disproportionate number of those suffering from anorexia nervosa follow a vegetarian diet. Approximately 50 percent of adolescents and young women with anorexia nervosa eat some form of vegetarian diet compared with about 6 to 34 percent of their omnivorous peers.[33] While it may seem logical, based on this information, to conclude that vegetarian diets cause eating disorders, evidence suggests that vegetarian diets are typically adopted after onset and simply mask eating disorders. In other words, vegetarian diets can be used as a means of facilitating calorie restriction and legitimizing the removal of high-fat, high-calorie animal products and processed or fast foods made with animal ingredients such as eggs and dairy.[34, 35] One research team labeled this phenomenon "pseudovegetarianism."[36]

This does not mean that vegetarians don't develop eating disorders or that people with disordered eating can't become committed vegetarians while they are ill. Both are possible; however, true vegetarians—that is, those not motivated by an eating disorder—can typically be distinguished by what their motivation is to follow the diet. A 2012 study of 160 women (93 with a history of eating disorders and 67 healthy controls) examined the motivation for becoming vegetarian in current and former vegetarians. Remarkably, none of the current or former vegetarians in the control group cited weight concerns as a primary motivation for becoming vegetarian, compared with almost one half of those with a history of eating disorders.[39]

A number of studies published between 1997 and 2009 reported a significantly higher incidence of disturbed eating attitudes and behaviors, restrained eating, and disordered eating among vegetarians compared with nonvegetarians.[37, 38, 39, 40, 41] Restrained eating refers to the degree to which individuals control or restrain their eating in order to lose or maintain weight. For lacto-ovo vegetarians, this may mean avoiding or minimizing intake of calorically dense foods such as full-fat dairy products like cheese and sour cream; for vegans, it could mean avoiding avocados, nuts, seeds, and nut and seed butters. In 2012, two published research papers provided valuable insight into the link between vegetarianism and eating disorders. The first reported that vegetarians and fish eaters were not more restrained than omnivores; however, semi-vegetarians (no red meat) and flexitarians (occasional red meat consumption) were significantly more restrained than omnivores or vegetarians.[42] Moreover, the fewer animal products the vegetarians ate (in other words, the closer they came to veganism), the less likely they were to exhibit signs of disordered eating. The authors note that while the semi-vegetarians and flexitarians were motivated by weight concerns, vegetarians (including vegans) and fish eaters were motivated by ethical concerns.

The second research paper carefully separated true vegetarians and vegans from semi-vegetarians and omnivores.[43] Semi-vegetarians were found to be at greater risk for disordered eating than were omnivores or vegetarians. Vegans had the healthiest scores of all dietary groups, and the researchers speculated that vegan diets may actually be protective against eating disorders.[42] This unexpected finding may be, at least in part, explained by the "other-directed" nature of vegan ethics, which tend to focus on issues of compassion for animals, concern for the environment, and human health. This is in contrast to the "inner-directed" nature of eating disorders, which focus on personal body weight and shape. It is unknown whether vegans are at increased risk for orthorexia, a pathological fixation with healthy eating. For people following a vegan diet, orthorexia may involve severe food limitation beyond the elimination of animal products. Some attempt to remove all high-fat foods, not just fats and oils, but highly nutritious foods such as nuts, seeds, and avocados; some call for minimizing carbohydrates, not just added sugars and refined flour products, but wonderfully nourishing carbohydrate-rich foods such as whole grains, starchy vegetables, and legumes; and others claim cooking renders food toxic, so only raw foods should be consumed. It's important to recognize the potential for orthorexia in vegans who adhere to rigid dietary rules. To date, there are no data comparing incidence of binge eating disorder in vegans, vegetarians, and nonvegetarians.

Whether your child is vegetarian or not, eating disorders are a serious matter in children, and parents need to be on the lookout for worrisome signs. We have often been approached by parents (generally following an omnivorous diet) who become concerned when their child wants to adopt a vegetarian or vegan diet. They worry that this could be a red flag for the beginnings of an eating disorder. When a young child becomes interested in dinosaurs, the stars, or state capitals, our first instincts are to ask questions about what piqued their interest. Did they learn about it in school, did they read an interesting book, see something on television, or have a friend that loves it, too? Often, we put our problem-solving (or worse, worry!) hats on before we simply say, "tell me more." If your child comes to you with a desire to stop eating animal foods, try to understand their perspective and motivations. When they sense that you are truly interested, your child will be more likely to share. More often than not, children are genuinely interested in the social, environmental, or health aspects of a vegetarian diet. Some helpful questions to consider include:

- Has your child lost or gained weight recently?
- Does your child seem preoccupied with calories or have other restrictive tendencies around food?
- Has there been a change in your child's mood? Does he seem irritable, sad, or anxious?
- Does your child seem preoccupied by media that focuses on thinness or healthy eating?

- Does your child avoid meals or seem to make excuses around mealtime?
- Does your child avoid social situations that involve food?
- Will your child readily accept vegan alternatives to animal-based foods that he previously enjoyed, such as a vegan cupcake at a birthday party or a veggie burger instead of a hamburger?
- If your child shares that she is moved by the ethical or environmental aspects of a vegan diet, do her choices extend beyond food (recycling, not wearing leather, etc.)?

David was so happy to see Elisa engaged in something that seemed meaningful to her. In an effort to support her, he swapped out the chicken on her dinner plate with some leftover tofu from last night's dinner. He noticed that she did not sprinkle any parmesan over her pasta (usually a favorite of hers) but did take an extra helping of pasta and spinach. She asked her parents if they could try out a new vegan restaurant in town and invite one of her friends from the club to join them on Friday night. They had a double chocolate vegan brownie on the menu that she was dying to try. David felt a bit more at ease as he learned about the initiatives of the environmental club and thought that it might be wonderful for the family to make these changes together.

Our instincts as parents are usually spot on. If you suspect that your child is making a dietary shift in order to conceal disordered eating behaviors, act swiftly and seek out support. Just as with optimizing growth and development, treatment and eating disorder recovery must always prioritize health. If the timing of starting a vegan diet seems suspect or is interfering with treatment and recovery, explore ways in which you might honor her beliefs but ensure that high calorie and "fear" foods (vegan cheeses, milks, meats, baked goods, etc.) are incorporated. If it seems that your child is more of a "pseudovegetarian," consider reverting back to the pre-eating disorder diet. It's important to note that completely discounting a person's ethical beliefs during recovery could be quite traumatizing. Vegan and vegetarian diets do not cause eating disorders, but such diets can certainly be used to mask disordered eating behaviors.

Weight related issues are multifactorial and complex. When it comes to food, weight, and our children, our job as parents is to support their positive growth and development. We can feed our families in a way that is health-promoting, nourishing, and comes from a place of abundance and joy by focusing on parenting and feeding in a way that fosters connection and supports our child's overall health and well-being. In the next and final chapter in this section, we will work to bring all of these concepts together and help guide the way toward a plant leaning diet for your family.

Chapter 12

Raising a Veg Leaning Family

"Everyone can do simple things to make a difference,
and every little bit really does count."

—*Stella McCartney*

Brenda's Story: When Brenda's daughter was four years old, she and her husband decided to go plant-based. They told their daughter that they had decided to not eat animals anymore. They explained that beef was from cows, pork from pigs, and chicken from chickens. Their daughter asked if they had ever eaten horses. She breathed a sigh of relief when they said no, and said, "Thank goodness, I would never want to eat a horse." Then she asked if she could still eat salmon sandwiches. They said, sure, but within a year or so, she came home with a salmon sandwich that had only one bite out of it. Brenda asked why she hadn't eaten her sandwich, and she said, "I don't want to eat salmon anymore. After my first bite, I kept seeing a hook in my mouth—I don't want to do that to any fish." That was that.

A t this point, you may be near the same place I (Reshma) was when I began shifting my diet toward plants. As I learned more about the benefits of maximizing plant foods and minimizing animal-based foods in my own diet, a small panic bubbled inside of me. I knew that this way of eating could optimize health. It seemed to carry so many benefits beyond my own health or the health of my family. Adopting a diet that could also help to preserve our planet and mitigate animal suffering resonated with both my personal and professional values. Yet, this enthusiasm was tempered by a sense of uncertainty and doubt. I had so many questions.

- What if my family wasn't on board?
- How could I manage the change?
- What would I cook every day?
- Would we be able to go to our favorite restaurants?
- What about eating at friends' homes or events?
- What about family holidays and vacations?

Even though I encountered some bumps along the way, the transition was far smoother than I expected. In this chapter, you will learn a stepwise approach to help shift your family's diet towards plants. My experience in changing my own family's diet and working with patients has given me a perspective that will shed some light on how you might make the transition for your own family. The recommendations in this chapter are not meant to be prescriptive but rather supportive. Each family has its own set of values, strengths, and challenges that will determine the level of enthusiasm and pace with which it moves forward. Here is how it happened for us.

Because I grew up in a vegetarian household, I was already equipped with tools to make the transition a little smoother; the idea that families could eat, enjoy, and thrive on a diet centered around plants was not new to me. As a family, we often ate vegetarian meals many times during the week, and I would say that I had pretty typical children when it came to selectivity around foods. I often joked that between my two children, they had perfectly balanced diets. In the beginning, I simply stopped purchasing meat to cook at home. Very quickly, however, I cut out all meat products from my own diet.

For quite a long stretch of time, I ate eggs on occasion, some dairy, and fish only outside of the home. My diet was close to 90 percent plant-based. The last 10 percent happened much more gradually; I substituted when I could but still did not eat solely plant-based outside of our home. Until, one day while eating out at our favorite pizza place in town, I inquired about vegan options. Without batting an eyelash, the server announced, "Of course! We have a vegan pie. It's not on the menu, but it's delicious."

That was the last little bit holding me back. After another month or so of tiptoeing along the edge of the vegan pool, I finally jumped in. It wasn't about being perfect but rather being centered in my values. I would not knowingly eat food that came from animals any longer. The first 90 percent felt relatively easy to me. The last 10 percent took a bit more time and seemed more effortful.

Eating at home was a breeze; managing meals outside of my home took some navigating. It required a shift in expectations (I couldn't simply choose the thing that sounded best to me on the menu) and a hefty dose of creativity (assembling several sides to create a full meal). You may prefer an even more gradual pace or may choose to stop at the 90 percent mark, which is what so many people in the Blue Zones practice. However, you may also choose to jump in headfirst and go completely cold tofu. There is no one, perfect way.

Introducing these changes to my family came with moments of tension until we finally settled into a routine that felt comfortable for all. One of my children ate a mostly plant-based diet before I even contemplated making a change myself. She rarely turned down fruits and vegetables, and anything with bones and skin received a skeptical glare. Half of our family was fully on board. The other half was accommodating but not necessarily invested.

Shortly after I committed to going fully plant-based, I felt an increased sense of urgency to sway the remaining members of my family. Even though I tried to suppress it, at times, I'm sure they felt my disapproving gaze over certain food choices. I know they did not enjoy this side of me, and to be perfectly honest, I didn't particularly enjoy it either. I had to remind myself, after all, that a core aspect of this way of eating was, indeed, compassion.

I did my best to gently persuade them with one of the best tools in my armament: the food. If I insisted on certain changes in the house, the least I could do was to make it as tasty as possible. With a little bit of care but not too much extra fuss or work, I began making fully plant-based meals at home. I actively sought my family's feedback and worked to prepare delicious, nutritious meals we could all enjoy. The single, most effective action I took to shift my family towards plants was to cook good food. You hardly notice what you are missing when the plate in front of you makes your mouth water.

> The single, most effective action I took to shift my family toward plants was to cook good food.

I did my best to prepare and cook real, whole, plant foods for my family. This is not to say that every meal was greeted with joy and excitement. Ours was not and is not a perfect household, nor do we aim to be. Yet, more often than not, day in and day out, it worked. Our new normal became that we ate (mostly) plant based in the home, and everyone made their own choices outside of the home.

It worked quite well until one day while driving home from school my son made a surprising announcement. "I think I'm going to try to be vegetarian for a month." I tried to remain calm and not let my excitement overtake the moment and simply said, "Okay (!)". After the month was up, he decided to continue. When I asked him why, he said, "It actually wasn't that hard, and so I thought, why not?" I loved his answer. That's exactly right, I thought, *why not?* too. Soon after, my husband made a similar change.

While it certainly helps to have your family on board, it is not a prerequisite. Trying to force a change in someone else (especially other adults or older children) is near impossible, not to mention exhausting and unpleasant. It is difficult to insist upon other people making changes in their diet without their full agreement and participation. Having said that, do ask for respect and courtesy. I was fortunate to have a supportive family. In the early stages, they made accommodations in terms of picking restaurants that might work for me, made no objections to not having meat in the house, and willingly subbed in plant-based milks. I felt seen and understood, and that helped immensely.

> Don't worry about being perfect. Focus instead on small changes that seem reasonable, doable, and delicious!

What follows is an approach that can help your family make and maintain the shift toward a plant-based diet. Don't worry about being perfect. Focus instead on small changes that seem reasonable, doable, and delicious! It's much easier and so much more fun when we concentrate on all we are gaining instead of what we are giving up.

PLANT-BASED FROM THE START

If you were fortunate enough to learn about the myriad of benefits of a plant-based diet before having children, consider yourself lucky. This is, by far, the most straightforward situation to manage and navigate. You've hit the plant-based jackpot. As you know from Chapter 7, plant-based diets are appropriate and healthy throughout pregnancy and while breastfeeding. Once baby arrives, you can simply begin the process of feeding. Many families already follow certain dietary practices due to religious or cultural beliefs. In a similar way, your family will have a particular set of (plant-based) traditions and practices around food. Eating a plant-based diet will be the norm for your family. As your child gets older, some explanations about why you eat this way and conversations about how to handle birthday parties and school events may be beneficial. For those families more like my own, some extra steps are required.

ESTABLISH GOALS AND PRIORITIES

It can be helpful to first give some consideration to what you hope to accomplish for your family. Think both in the short and long term. Make a list of your goals. Some points to consider include:

- What is your "why"? If I/we go plant based, I am hoping to gain "x."
- Does your family seem interested? Do they share the same beliefs and goals?
- Have you made changes around food in the past? If so, what worked well and what would you do differently?
- What are the biggest obstacles you foresee?
- Who can you enlist for support?
- Do you have friends or family members that have made similar changes?
- What would be easiest to do? What would be most challenging?

OBSERVE, TAKE NOTES, AND DO A LITTLE EXPERIMENTING

Once you have a better understanding of your goals, supports, and possible challenges, take time to notice the patterns of eating in your family.

- What do typical breakfasts, lunches, dinners, and snacks look like?
- What times of day and days of the week seem to be the most stressful or chaotic?
- Take note of the foods that are front and center in your pantry and refrigerator.
- What meals does everyone (or at least most everyone!) seem to enjoy? Which are the least favorite?
- What routines does your family have around eating? For instance, Friday pizza night or big family dinners on Sundays.

After taking note of your family's routines, preferences, and challenges around food think about simple, barely noticeable changes that you can begin to implement. In our family, since we already ate many vegetarian meals throughout the week, I found it easy to add an extra one or two plant-based dinners. No one noticed the slight adjustment. Freshly baked muffins made with plant-based milks, nuts, seeds, and fruit were generally met with a smile and made for a simple breakfast or snack. This might also be a great time to do a little research and get inspiration from books or blogs for recipes you think your family might enjoy. You will find several resources at the end of the book for your reference.

CAN WE TALK?

After you have spent some time reflecting, noticing, and experimenting, consider how you might talk to the rest of your immediate family. You might approach the adults in the household first. For some families, the adults in the home already agree and such a discussion may not be needed. For others, it may be quite a sensitive issue. Food is an incredibly personal topic. No one wants to feel judged or scolded for what and how they eat. If this is a delicate topic in your family, use a warm, inviting, and nonjudgmental tone.

Begin by asking if they would be open to such a conversation; if so, when might be a convenient time? Let them know about your motivations, what you have already noticed about your family, and some ideas of what you would like to do more of. Ask for feedback and concerns. Take the time to listen and truly understand their perspective. Do your best to find a middle ground that the adults can settle on. In the beginning, it's much more productive to focus on areas of agreement and how to enhance them rather than areas of potential conflict. If you are the one initiating the change, consider offering to do much of the initial work, if possible.

When it comes to discussing the transition with children in the household, age really does matter. For young children, especially under the age of three, not much conversation is required. It's best to keep things simple but also to answer their questions as openly and honestly as possible. Let their questions guide the conversation. Revisit your goals and priorities and use them as the foundation for your answers. You could talk about protecting the environment, compassion for animals, or simply just eating more delicious plants. Be gentle and caring in talking about these issues, especially health. Adopt a nurturing and loving tone so as not to cause anxiety or create bad feelings around food preferences and choices. Framing the changes in a positive light instead of focusing on how "unhealthy" certain foods are and certainly avoiding graphic details about the realities of factory farming will help to build a positive attitude around food. At this age, showing or doing can be much more useful than telling or talking. Making simple ingredient swaps (flax eggs in your baking) or substitutions in family favorites (beans instead of ground meat for taco night) helps you incorporate more plant-based foods without fanfare. Keep it simple, positive, and honest.

For school-age children who may be used to certain routines and traditions around food, a more in-depth conversation may be in order. If there has already been some tension around food in the family, some repair work might be necessary. You could offer, "I know I've been excited about making changes around food in the house, and at times, my enthusiasm may have seemed controlling or unkind. I'm sorry, and I would like to change that." Again, go back to your "why" to lay the foundation and let their questions guide the discussion. Some conversation starters include:

- I've been learning a lot about how our food choices impact our health and our environment. I'm hoping to try some new things at dinner. How would you feel about that?
- Would you like to go to the farmer's market with me this weekend so we can pick out some of your favorite fruits and vegetables?

- Have you heard about something called "Meatless Monday"? It seems like a neat idea, and I thought we could give it a try. What do you think?

Children, by nature, are compassionate beings. They are often quite moved by calls to preserve wildlife or protect our planet. I can remember many a school campaign looking to raise money to save the pandas and tigers or green initiatives meant to reduce waste and promote recycling. These offer opportunities to dig a little deeper and explore how our food choices connect to sustainability and compassion. Books and documentaries can support your efforts. Consider pre-screening books and videos to decide whether or not they feel appropriate for your child. As with most meaningful conversations with children, this is not meant to be a one and done chat. Rather it is a series of ongoing discussions. Be on the lookout for natural opportunities for the topic to present itself and avoid pressuring.

For tweens and teens, the same rules apply, but you may need to exercise a greater degree of patience and acceptance. If your household habits and traditions were centered around animal foods, expecting older to children to immediately change may not only be unreasonable but could also work to undermine your relationship with your child. If your child seems eager or even interested, move forward at a pace that seems comfortable for them. If, however, they are outright resistant, back off and revisit the conversation at a later time with their permission. Acknowledge that you understand they might not be ready to make such changes while, at the same time, make your needs and position clear. In our household, I did not demand that everyone change their diet to exclude animal foods, but I did let them know that I would no longer purchase or cook animal foods. Deliver this information in as neutral a tone as possible without appearing angry or dismissive. After all, you always want to leave the door open.

SEEK INPUT/FEEDBACK AND LISTEN!

If your family seems interested, or even curious, the next step can be to try out a few changes. Let them know you are experimenting and eager for their feedback and input. This can reassure them that how they feel genuinely matters to you. Food is meant to not only nourish our bodies but to connect us to those we love and care about. It can be tempting to want to take complete control over your family's meals when you've been inspired to make changes. For me, it was useful to reflect on times when my eating was not skewed towards plants and the reasons I might have resisted change. Adopting an attitude of inviting instead of imposing may take longer, but I have found that such an approach offers more lasting and meaningful change and helps to preserve a loving connection to your family.

Adopting an attitude of inviting instead of imposing may take longer, but I have found that such an approach offers more lasting and meaningful change and helps to preserve a loving connection to your family.

START WITH WHAT'S ALREADY WORKING AND BUILD IN GRADUAL CHANGE

This is the lowest hanging fruit. Take note of what's already working and do more of it! The reality is that most families already include a variety of abundant plant-based foods in their diets. From there, you can work to build in change gradually. Some simple ideas include:

- Tofu scramble with veggies (on page 336) in place of bacon and eggs for breakfast
- Almond or soy milk in place of cow's milk in your cereal
- Leftovers in a thermos for lunch (such as split pea soup with brown rice on page 352)
- Hummus and veggie pita in the lunch box instead of ham and cheese
- Chickpea salad sandwiches (recipe on page 341) instead of tuna salad
- Bean and veggie burritos instead of beef burritos
- Tofu instead of chicken in your stir-fry

The possibilities are endless. So many meals can easily be made plant-based. The food at home is the simplest place to start. If a gradual approach better serves your family, you can first focus on making changes at home and worry less about what happens outside of your home. I've heard so many parents say that they worry about their child feeling different or left out at play dates and birthday parties (more on that to come), and so they don't think it would work in their household. I encourage such parents to put their energy and focus on the home environment first and to worry less about occasional, outside meals and snacks.

BUT DON'T BE AFRAID TO TAKE LARGER LEAPS

Some families are utterly inspired and decide to make a brisk change. Often, a health scare in a family member or sudden awareness around the horrors of factory farming makes urgent action the most appealing prospect. Even if your family decides to make a dramatic change, it's still best to start with the familiar and easy. Take special care to read through the sections on nutrients and supplements to ensure you cover your nutritional bases. For some people, abruptly increasing fiber consumption can cause gastrointestinal discomfort. It can take the body some time to adjust. If your family consumes a low-fiber diet, consider increasing the fiber more gradually. It can be especially inspiring to have the entire family take the leap together. It makes for easier meal planning and prepping and provides an immediate, robust support system. If your family is entirely on board, don't hesitate to take action.

BUILD IN FLEXIBILITY

When you have family members with different goals and commitments to this way of eating, create a bit of flexibility to maintain a peaceful and joyful environment around food. If your child seems particularly worried or upset about the dietary changes, reassure him that you are responsible for figuring things out and that you will take care of things. Flexibility can mean that instead of focusing on all the foods you aim to remove from the home, first focus on those you want to add: a green salad with diced apple and slivered almonds, a morning smoothie alongside breakfast, hummus and sliced cucumbers or whole grain crackers in the lunch box. Make simple additions from a place of abundance instead of restriction and sacrifice. Once your family gets used to these additions, it can become easier to crowd out some of the foods you aim to limit or eliminate. Perhaps, the best way forward may be to simply lead by example and let go of any expectation of change in others.

TRANSITION FOODS

We often get asked about the role of transition type foods when switching to a plant-based diet. Transition foods are typically thought of as somewhat (from minimally to heavily) processed foods meant to replace animal-based foods such as meat, dairy, eggs, and fish. Examples might include soy milk, plant-based nuggets, vegan cheese, and veggie burgers. Products differ widely in terms of the degree to which they are processed. In general, the less processed a food is, the more wholesome and healthful it tends to be. Think of a short list of ingredients that are easy to pronounce. In some instances, processing can actually be beneficial. For example, many plant-based milks are fortified with vitamins D and B12 and many veggie "meats" provide high quality, absorbable protein as well as added iron and B12. This can help to boost the nutritional quality of the food. In other instances, such as with certain vegan cheeses, the foods contain many additives and chemicals. These transition type foods may serve as occasional foods or become everyday staples in your family's diet. They can be especially useful when families are just beginning to make the shift, when eating out, or when attending functions such as a family barbecue. These foods can also add a degree of convenience during busy weekdays. Most families we know (including our own!) rely on these processed foods to some degree. The degree to which your family enjoys these foods will, of course, be a personal decision. Relying too much on heavily processed vegan foods would not be considered health promoting, but being too strict can create a rigidity around food that can be harmful. There is no absolute right or wrong answer. In general, eat real, whole foods as much as possible and don't worry too much about being perfectly perfect. As you become more comfortable with cooking and eating this way, you will find a natural rhythm and flow that works best for your family.

> In general, eat real, whole foods as much as possible and don't worry too much about being perfectly perfect.

EATING OUT

One of the common obstacles people identify when transitioning to a plant-based diet is eating out at restaurants. Thirty years ago, getting vegan food in a restaurant was hard. Vegan restaurants were few and far between. It's quite a different story today. Increasingly, many larger cities and even small towns feature entirely vegan restaurants or have vegan options on the menu. Additionally, chain restaurants and even fast food restaurants often feature vegan options such as veggie burgers. Ethnic restaurants are also a great option; whether it be

Thai, Ethiopian, or Indian, ethnic foods are delicious and can be very veg-friendly. Though it may seem daunting, eating out is actually quite accessible (and enjoyable!) when following a plant-based diet.

If your family is gradually transitioning or committing to closer to 90 percent plant-based, the choices are actually quite plentiful. Vegetarian offerings can be found at most restaurants. If, however, you eat an entirely plant-based diet and follow a vegan diet, the following simple recommendations can help guide you:

- If you have a say in selecting the restaurant, become familiar with establishments that you know will have something on the menu for you to eat or search online for "vegan restaurants near me." Otherwise, look at the menu online or call ahead to speak to the staff to inquire about vegan options.
- For restaurants that do not have vegan offerings on the menu, you have a couple of choices. The first option is perhaps the most fun and unexpected. Ask the server if the chef would be willing to prepare a vegan meal for you. The worst that could happen is that the restaurant could say no. More often than not, however, chefs are generally willing to make accommodations if they can.
- A slightly easier ask is to look at the menu items to see if an item might easily be made vegan. Perhaps a pasta dish with chicken can be made with extra vegetables instead; pizza, just hold the cheese; oatmeal with soy milk instead of cow's milk, to name a few.
- Yet another option is to browse the menu for sides and see if you can create an entire meal out of them. Roasted potatoes, soup, and side salad or a veggie sandwich, for instance. Consider packing nuts, seeds, or roasted chickpeas in a small container to fortify a salad or side dish.
- The final option is not ideal but can come in handy in a pinch. If there truly are no reasonable options, you can plan on enjoying the company and try to eat before or after the restaurant outing.

In the beginning, eating out can feel challenging for sure. The more you practice, the better skilled you will become at it. Increasingly, plant-based options are becoming available even in smaller towns, airports, and food courts. It can be fun to go out with friends and family for a nice meal, but you may find it more convenient to pack food from home when it's reasonable. Predictable situations, such as work or school, lend themselves perfectly to a packed lunch. As more and more people go plant-based, the demand and supply of plant-based foods will continue to increase such that it will no longer be an obstacle.

PLAY DATES, SOCCER GAMES, AND SLEEPOVERS

Just as with eating out, the degree to which you need to address these specific situations will depend on the extent to which your family eats plant-based. If your family's diet is not fully plant-based you might consider employing flexibility at events such as sleepovers and birthday parties and pack your owns snacks when possible. These days, so many children have food allergies, intolerances, and special diets that parents and coaches are on alert when it comes to food preferences and restrictions. I have found that most parents are relieved to have you bring an appropriate cupcake or meal for your child if they are not able to easily accommodate. Many vegan families keep frozen cupcakes or other vegan treats stored in the freezer and defrost them as needed for just such an occasion. Other parents opt to allow their child to make their own choices at these events, especially if that is what the child prefers or in the case of older children who may be quite vocal about not wanting to feel different. Let your child's preference guide your actions, offering flexibility or a vegan cupcake, whichever seems more fitting. Realize that what happens "sometimes" (birthday parties, sleepovers, etc.) should not deter you from practicing what's important to you most of the time (every meal and snack at home).

HOLIDAYS AND SPECIAL EVENTS

The same principles also hold true for holidays and special events except for one key difference. These types of events often welcome the addition of another dish. Offering to bring a main dish can be a relief for the host and ensures that you will have something to eat. It's also an opportunity for you to share the food you have been enjoying with family and friends. No need to announce it as "your vegan dish." Just place it on the buffet table to be enjoyed. The Ultimate Veggie Lasagna or Kind Shepherd's Pie in Chapter 15 both feed a crowd and are simply delicious. Be prepared to share the recipe.

Letting your host know ahead of time can also be useful. It's best to avoid surprising your host with a last-minute announcement or request. With a little advance notice, many dishes can easily be modified. For instance, cheese on the side for a salad or a store-bought veggie burger to go on the grill.

STANDING FIRM

Another challenge that some families face is a lack of support from well-meaning (and sometimes not-so-well-meaning) friends or family. Ridicule can be presented as "just a joke," but you may experience both direct and indirect pressure for you and your family to "be more flexible." Extended family members may not understand your reasons for change and may even seem to go out of their way to be difficult. While it can be an uncomfortable topic to discuss, often the source of this tension stems from a fear that your new food choices will change the relationship or that you are in some way judging their food choices. This can be especially challenging if you are relying on loved ones for childcare or additional support. An offer of ice cream or a hot dog may be an innocent mistake, but repeated incidents call for action. You can use some of the same strategies from the previous section on having conversations with your immediate family members. Inquire whether they are open to a conversation. If so, when might be a good time? In an honest and kind tone, explain your "why." Take care that your words do not come across as critical. If they sense that you judge them for their food choices, the conversation is likely to go sour quickly. You could arrange visits that are not centered around food or offer to bring food, such as a vegan hot dog or vegan ice cream.

WHEN YOUR HEALTH-CARE PROVIDER
ISN'T ON BOARD

We have been surprised by the number of parents that have shared that one of their biggest obstacles in going plant-based has been a lack of support from their health-care provider or pediatrician. Medical education in nutrition is highly lacking. Only about a quarter of medical schools meet the minimum recommended hours of nutrition education set by the National Academy of Sciences; of that time, very little covers evidence-based nutrition guidelines or how to translate those guidelines into clinical practice. Yet, parents rely on pediatricians to provide dependable dietary advice. If you find yourself clashing with your pediatrician over your decision to go plant-based, the following approach offers some guidance.

- Ask yourself if you feel good about your relationship with your child's pediatrician. Have they been able to offer support and guidance around other issues? Do they seem empathetic and able to answer your questions effectively?
- If you have a good relationship with your pediatrician, consider explaining your "why," and ask about their specific concerns. You can share the Academy of Nutrition and Dietetics Position Statement on Vegetarian Diets (link in Resources) that unequivocally states, "Appropriately planned vegetarian, including vegan, diets are healthful, nutritionally adequate, and may provide health benefits for the prevention and treatment of certain diseases. These diets are appropriate for all stages of the life cycle, including pregnancy, lactation, infancy, childhood, adolescence, older adulthood, and for athletes. Plant-based diets are more environmentally sustainable than diets rich in animal products because they use fewer natural resources and are associated with much less environmental damage."
- The most frequently reported points of contention include dairy and meat. The reason for the concern is our society (including most health professionals) is conditioned to believe that dairy is necessary for calcium and meat is necessary for protein. When we provide information showing that fortified soy milk has as much protein and calcium as cow's milk, and tofu and veggie meats have as much protein as meat, concerns are greatly alleviated. It can also be helpful to share that many children are allergic or intolerant to dairy and require similar substitutions. Chapters 4 and 5 provide detailed information on calcium and protein in plant-based diets.
- Parents can discuss their switch to a plant-based diet with their pediatrician in a way that supports their efforts. It may be that together, you agree on getting some screening laboratory tests and even arrange for a consultation with a registered dietitian knowledgeable about plant-based diets, though neither recommendation is required. Refer to Part II of this book, which covers many of the areas that will likely be of concern.

- If, however, you cannot have a reasonable conversation with your health-care provider, it may be time to find another pediatrician. You should feel comfortable discussing your concerns and experiences without fear of being judged or scolded. Asking friends and family for recommendations is a great place to start. Some organizations maintain a list of plant-based providers (included in the Resources), but often these providers are not local or may not be covered under individual insurance plans. It is not necessary to have a pediatrician that herself is plant-based (although that can certainly be helpful!), but instead seek out a pediatrician who is supportive and well-informed.

RAISING A VEG LEANING CHILD IN A
NON VEG LEANING FAMILY

One last area to discuss is how best to handle the situation when your child is the one initiating change. Many parents ask us for advice when their child comes charging home from school and announces that he has become vegan or vegetarian. Children are often moved by issues around animal cruelty and climate change and want to take action through their food choices. Some parents panic, not knowing what to feed their child (one of the many reasons this book came to be!) and others don't miss a beat as they thumb through vegetarian cookbooks. The first step is to wonder about your child's "why." Be curious. This is the most effective way to gather more information. As we mentioned in the last chapter, "tell me more" is a great way to start the conversation. Interjecting with "why this isn't a good idea" or rushing off to see a dietitian (which not may be a bad idea at some point) is a sure way to halt the conversation. Try to enter their world. Read their books, see their movies, understand their perspective. When they sense you are genuinely interested, your child will be more likely to share. Make sure you take the time to listen.

The next step is to educate yourself about the specifics of following a vegan/ vegetarian diet to ensure that your child meets his nutritional requirements. You will find all the necessary information on nutrients, supplements, and meal planning throughout this book as well as additional resources provided at the end of this book.

Finally, support your child in making the needed changes. Whenever possible and reasonable, work to make it a family affair. Start with meatless Mondays—an entire day of eating where you avoid animal foods. See how your family enjoys it. Notice what seems difficult, what seems easy. Avoid cooking separate meals for everyone in the family. It's time-consuming, exhausting, and can take away from the experience of a shared family meal. Instead, consider keeping much of the same meals your family already enjoys and simply swap out the animal-based foods for plant-based versions for your vegetarian child. Black beans instead of ground meat in tacos, tofu instead of chicken in your stir-fry, pizza piled high with veggies and vegan cheese for Friday night pizza. These simple swaps allow you to feed the family without much extra fuss or work. Involving your child in both the planning and preparation can help to lighten your load and have your child more engaged in the process. If the rest of your family is equally curious and open, perhaps it could be the beginning of a beautiful shift for the whole family.

In the end, we, as parents, are doing the very best we can for ourselves and our families. If you feel overwhelmed, consider revisiting your "why" and adjusting your pace. Look for support, involve your family, and focus on progress over any illusion of perfection. Move forward with love, compassion, and a generous dose of patience.

Part IV

CONNECTION

We've talked about CONSIDERATION, the Health, Home, and Heart of why we should contemplate a plant-centered diet as a way to nourish our families, protect our planet, and serve as a radical act of compassion. We dove deep into CARE, covering the key principles of nutrition to understand how best to implement a plant-centered diet while ensuring nutritional adequacy for our families. We walked through CONFIDENCE, addressing many of the challenges families face around their dinner tables. And now we end with CONNECTION as a way to bring all of these concepts into practice. This section is about finding and giving support as well as providing resources for families. Whether it's time, money, cooking skills, or availability of food, a family's strengths and limitations will determine how the knowledge that we gain and the values that we embrace show up at our dinner tables. Busy work lives often leave little time for shopping and cooking. The best we can do is to work within our constraints and prioritize our resources. A shift in knowledge and values ultimately provides the framework for us to utilize our resources to the best of our ability. We aim to offer strategies for families to begin making the shift at whatever pace is reasonable. We will provide tips for menu planning and shopping as well as simple, accessible (and delicious!) plant-based recipes.

Additionally, resources for further reading, exploration, and recipe ideas are included. Our experience with families has taught us that starting with small changes that are accessible and enjoyable is the easiest and most sustainable way to begin the path forward. The future of food is plants. We provide a path for families to get there.

> The future of food is plants. We provide a path for families to get there.

Chapter 13

Shopping, Planning, and Prepping

"In this food I see clearly the presence of the entire
universe supporting my existence."

—*Thich Nhat Hanh*

Transitioning to a plant-based diet may seem a little daunting, especially if you are a family (like most!) that struggles to get it all done every week —planning, shopping, prepping, cooking, cleaning—only to have the cycle begin again. This chapter will not only provide inspiration for plant-based meals, but also offer strategies to help busy families make mealtimes happen.

PANTRY MAKEOVER

Sometimes a bit of a makeover can be a source of inspiration and help to set you up for success. This could be a project done in stages (one shelf at a time) or a more massive overhaul. Creating an organized pantry space helps to provide meal ideas and displays front and center the foods you are looking to incorporate into your family's diet. Use clear glass containers (such as mason jars) to store dried beans, grains, nuts, seeds, and other pantry essentials. While shelled nuts and seeds are best stored in the refrigerator or freezer to keep them fresh, many will last up to three months in the pantry. Those rich in omega-3 fatty acids, such as walnuts, flax, chia, and hemp seeds, are best kept only in the refrigerator or freezer, as they go rancid more quickly. Label jars for quick identification. This makes them easy to see and ready to use. These are especially handy if you shop from your store's bulk bins (generally cheaper and cuts down on waste). Keep things that will help your meal prep front and center, and keep snacks for children at a level that is accessible to them. Storage baskets are great for onions, potatoes, and packaged snacks. Tiered shelves and dividers for cans, spices, and condiments add extra shelf space when storage is limited. Consider refreshing the pantry every few weeks to keep it organized. Some families keep a dry erase board near the pantry where they can keep a list of items that are running low and need to be restocked.

MENU PLANNING AND SHOPPING

Planning and prepping are the keys to your success for mealtime. Here is a simple technique that you can use to help organize weekly shopping and menu planning:

1. Pick a day during the week when it works best for you to plan and do the bulk of your grocery shopping. Before creating a list, consider asking your crew if they have any "wishes" for the week. This is a great way to get the kids involved and allow them to feel like they have a say. Additionally, it can help to minimize dinnertime complaints when your children know they have had a hand in creating the week's menu.

2. Start by taking a look at your calendar to help you plan for the week. Two soccer practices and a late work meeting might be the perfect night to plan on having leftovers. No commitments on Friday night might make it a great evening to try a new recipe and enjoy a family game night.

3. Let your calendar and family preferences dictate the menu for the week.

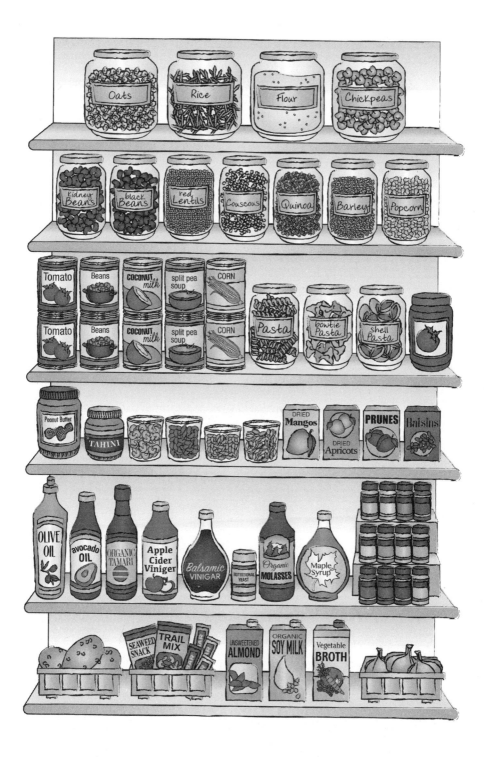

4. Making a quick notecard list can help you create a focused grocery list and be a reminder of what you plan to make for the week. On a notecard, draw a line to separate your menu from your grocery list. Jot down the days of the week and what you plan to make. Let your menu dictate your shopping list. Don't worry if you don't stick to the list precisely. Having a general guide of what the week's menu will be (including room for takeout or dinners out) will ensure that you have meals planned and ready for the week ahead.

5. Plan on making things that won't last long (tender greens, certain produce items) earlier in the week.

6. Leave space for breakfast and lunch ideas.

7. Arrange your list according to the general layout of the grocery store. This way, you can walk through the store and use your list efficiently and avoid forgetting something.

8. Have room for flexibility. If the tomatoes look and smell amazing or the green beans look a little past their prime, consider making adjustments to take advantage of seasonal or sale items.

9. There are many resources that can help with managing menu and grocery planning from apps to worksheets. Find the simplest thing that works for you.

Figure 13.1: Notecard List

Menu & Grocery Planning			MON: _____
Produce	**Grains/Beans**	**Frozen Foods**	TUES: _____
			WED: _____
			THURS: _____
			FRI: _____
Refrigerated (plant milks, tofu, veggie meats)	**Pantry Essentials** (nuts, seeds, nut butters, condiments, snacks)	**Misc.**	SAT: _____
			SUN: _____
			BREAKFASTS: _____
			LUNCHES: _____

SWAPPING IN AND STOCKING UP

If you are a family that is just beginning to make the transition (or really anywhere along in the process) toward a plant-based diet, one of the first steps can be to take stock of your pantry and refrigerator and consider where you might swap in plant-based items. Remember that many of the items your family likely enjoys are already vegan (e.g., peanut butter, ketchup, mustard, etc.). Easy considerations include:

- Vegetable for chicken or beef broth
- Plant-based milks (so many to choose from!) for cow's milk
- Other plant-based dairy alternatives such as cheeses, yogurts, and sour cream
- Tofu, tempeh, or veggie meats in place of meat and eggs
- Plant-based versions of favorite condiments (e.g., dressings, mayonnaise, and dips)

SHOPPING LIST

The following shopping list is a convenient resource that itemizes staples you might want to stock up on. Explore the items you think your family would enjoy. Consider trying a few new things (such as passion fruit, pomelos, jicama, mustard greens, teff, or farro) each time you go to the grocery store. Again, let your menu planning dictate your list. You can add favorite snack items, such as seaweed snacks, and premade foods, such as pizza crust, breads, and frozen bean burritos.

Buy fresh produce as needed and in season. See the recommendations in Chapter 8 for purchasing organic produce. Dry ingredients can be purchased in appropriate amounts and stored in sealed containers in a cool, dry place for several months. Ethnic stores and the ethnic sections of supermarkets and natural foods stores are often good places to find unfamiliar ingredients and great prices on staples such as beans, tahini, spices, and vinegars.

Figure 13.2: Shopping List

VEGETABLES (fresh)

❏ Arugula
❏ Asparagus
❏ Avocados
❏ Beans (green, yellow)
❏ Beet greens
❏ Beets (red, golden)
❏ Bell peppers (green, orange, red, yellow)
❏ Bok choy
❏ Broccoli
❏ Broccolini
❏ Cabbage (Chinese, green, red, Napa)
❏ Carrots
❏ Cauliflower
❏ Celery
❏ Chili (jalapeño)
❏ Chives
❏ Collard greens
❏ Corn (fresh or frozen kernels)
❏ Cucumbers
❏ Garlic
❏ Ginger
❏ Kale
❏ Kohlrabi
❏ Jicama
❏ Lettuce (butterhead, leaf, romaine)
❏ Mushrooms
❏ Mustard greens
❏ Onions
❏ Parsley
❏ Parsnips
❏ Peas
❏ Potatoes
❏ Pumpkin/squash
❏ Radicchio
❏ Radishes
❏ Rutabaga
❏ Spinach
❏ Sprouts (alfalfa, lentil, mung, pea, sunflower)
❏ Sweet potatoes
❏ Tomatoes
❏ Turnips, turnip greens
❏ Winter squash
❏ Yams
❏ Zucchini

FRUITS (fresh)

❏ Apples
❏ Apricots
❏ Bananas
❏ Blueberries
❏ Cherries
❏ Grapefruit
❏ Lemons
❏ Limes
❏ Mangos
❏ Nectarines
❏ Oranges
❏ Papaya
❏ Peaches
❏ Pineapple
❏ Plums
❏ Pomegranate
❏ Raspberries
❏ Strawberries

FRUITS (dried)

❏ Apricots
❏ Blackberries
❏ Blueberries
❏ Cherries
❏ Coconut (unsweetened shredded)
❏ Currants
❏ Dates
❏ Mangoes
❏ Peaches
❏ Pears
❏ Prunes
❏ Raisins

GRAINS AND GRAIN PRODUCTS

❏ Barley
❏ Cornmeal
❏ Flour (buckwheat, oat, spelt, whole wheat)
❏ Kamut
❏ Millet
❏ Oats (groats, old-fashioned rolled, steel cut)
❏ Pasta
❏ Quinoa
❏ Rice (brown, basmati, white, wild rice)
❏ Spelt berries

LEGUMES

❏ Adzuki beans
❏ Black beans
❏ Cannellini beans
❏ Chickpeas (garbanzos)
❏ Great Northern beans
❏ Kidney beans (red, white)
❏ Legume pastas (chickpea, lentil)
❏ Lentils (green, red)
❏ Lima beans
❏ Mung beans
❏ Navy beans
❏ Pink beans
❏ Pinto beans
❏ Red beans
❏ Split peas (green, yellow)
❏ Tempeh
❏ Tofu (medium, firm, extra firm)
❏ Veggie burgers, veggie meats
❏ White beans

NUTS, SEEDS, BUTTERS

- ❑ Almond butter
- ❑ Almonds
- ❑ Brazil nuts
- ❑ Cashews
- ❑ Chia seeds
- ❑ Flaxseeds (whole or ground)
- ❑ Hazelnuts
- ❑ Hemp seeds (shelled)
- ❑ Macadamias
- ❑ Peanut butter
- ❑ Peanuts
- ❑ Pecans
- ❑ Pumpkin seeds
- ❑ Sesame seeds
- ❑ Sunflower seeds
- ❑ Tahini
- ❑ Walnuts

HERBS AND SPICES

- ❑ Allspice (ground)
- ❑ Basil (dried, fresh)
- ❑ Bay leaves
- ❑ Cardamom (ground)
- ❑ Cayenne
- ❑ Celery seeds
- ❑ Chili powder
- ❑ Cilantro
- ❑ Cinnamon (ground)
- ❑ Cloves (ground, whole)
- ❑ Cumin (ground)
- ❑ Curry powder

- ❑ Dill (dried, fresh)
- ❑ Fennel (ground)
- ❑ Garlic powder
- ❑ Ginger (ground)
- ❑ Marjoram
- ❑ Mint
- ❑ Mustard powder
- ❑ Nutmeg
- ❑ Onion powder
- ❑ Oregano
- ❑ Paprika (smoked, sweet)
- ❑ Parsley, dried
- ❑ Pepper (ground black)
- ❑ Poultry seasoning
- ❑ Pumpkin pie spice
- ❑ Red pepper flakes
- ❑ Rosemary
- ❑ Salt
- ❑ Savory
- ❑ Spice blends (berbere, everything bagel, za'atar)
- ❑ Tarragon
- ❑ Thyme (dried)
- ❑ Turmeric (ground)
- ❑ Vanilla extract

NONDAIRY ALTERNATIVES

- ❑ Nondairy milk, unsweetened (almond, cashew, hemp, rice, soy)
- ❑ Nondairy yogurt, unsweetened

MISCELLANEOUS ITEMS

- ❑ Applesauce
- ❑ Arrowroot starch
- ❑ Baking powder
- ❑ Baking soda
- ❑ Bragg Liquid Aminos
- ❑ Cocoa or cacao powder
- ❑ Coconut milk
- ❑ Cornstarch
- ❑ Curry paste
- ❑ Hot sauce
- ❑ Marinara sauce
- ❑ Miso (dark, light)
- ❑ Mustard (Dijon, stone-ground)
- ❑ Nutritional yeast flakes
- ❑ Oil (olive, avocado, sesame)
- ❑ Olives
- ❑ Red peppers, roasted
- ❑ Salsa
- ❑ Sweeteners (coconut sugar, maple syrup, molasses)
- ❑ Tamari
- ❑ Tomato paste
- ❑ Tomatoes (crushed, diced, sun-dried)
- ❑ Vinegar (balsamic, apple cider)
- ❑ Vegetable stock (cubes, powder, liquid)

KITCHEN TOOLS

Setting up your kitchen is a gradual process, but there are certain essentials that make food preparation faster, easier, and more enjoyable. If it is within your means, go for high quality products, as they last longer and perform better. If your budget is tight, look for high quality second-hand equipment. Buy the best knives you can afford—they make a world of difference. You do not need all of these tools in order to prepare delicious plant-based meals. Think about the types of recipes you make (or would like to make), and work on building up your tool set in a way that makes the most sense for you and your family. The following table provides basic supplies, in addition to next level implements, that will enhance your experience as you embark on each new culinary adventure.

Figure 13.3: Tools of the Trade

BASIC EQUIPMENT	NEXT LEVEL EQUIPMENT
baking pans	cast iron skillet
box grater (or hand grater)	citrus squeezer
can opener	Dutch oven (enamelware)
casserole dishes	kitchen scale
colanders (large and small)	mandoline
cutting boards	manual pull-string food processor
garlic press	microplane
glass storage containers (mason jars, lidded containers)	mortar and pestle
knife sharpener	salad spinner
knives (chefs, paring, serrated)	small silicone basting brush
ladle	spiralizer
measuring spoons and cups (dry and liquid)	sprouting lids, sprouting bags, or sprouter
mixing bowls	steamer basket
muffin pans	sushi mats
potato masher	tea kettle
rimmed baking sheets	tofu press
rubber spatulas	vegetable brush
saucepans of various sizes	wok
silicone mats or parchment paper for baking sheets	
skillets of various sizes	
stockpot	

tongs	
vegetable peeler	
whisk	
wooden spoons	
BASIC SMALL APPLIANCES	**NEXT LEVEL SMALL APPLIANCES**
food processor	bread maker
high speed blender	dehydrator
immersion blender	electric mixer (handheld or stand-alone)
	Instant Pot
	rice cooker

WHAT TO COOK

Many people transitioning to a plant-based diet might be concerned that by giving up animal-based foods, they will be signing up for a future of bland, tasteless food and missing out on favorite meals. In reality, moving toward a plant-based diet can actually open you up to a world of new flavors and possibilities. If you are a family that cooks often and has routine and structure that works for you, keep it up! Modify family favorites by swapping out animal-based foods with plant-based foods.

For those families that don't cook often or are not sure where to begin, it may be helpful to start with a bit of structure and routine and expand from there. Most families tend to rotate the same meals (or themes of meals) on a regular basis. This can range from just five to twenty or more recipes and meal ideas. Cookbooks and blogs can be a great source of inspiration, but you shouldn't feel pressured to come up with something new and fancy each night. Here are a few tips to get you started:

- Jot down the types of meals your family enjoys. These are your rotation meals. Some examples include:

  pasta

  tacos/burritos

stir-fry

Buddha bowls/grain bowls

sheet-pan dinners (essentially roast everything on a sheet pan or two
     and create a meal out of it, such as baked tofu with sweet potatoes,
     and roasted broccoli)

burgers and oven fries

soup or stew (one-pot meals mean less clean-up!)

soup and sandwiches

casseroles

- Think about a night when you might have more time to cook. This can be an evening where you try a new recipe. You can make an event out of it by getting the whole family involved. Aim to do this a couple of times a month. This is precisely how to discover new family favorites to put into your regular rotation!

- Consider doubling a recipe for leftovers later in the week or to tuck into the freezer for a later date.

- Hodgepodge nights: toward the end of the week, gather all the bits of leftovers and make a meal out of it, supplementing with a side dish, such as roasted sweet potatoes or fresh bread, if necessary.

- Store-bought staples (veggie burgers, pre-baked pizza crusts, marinara sauce, etc.) can be of enormous help when time is running short.

- Let condiments, sauces, and dips be your friend. A pesto, relish, or the Ginger Miso Sauce in Chapter 15 can transform a simple dish into something special.

- Batch cooking is when you spend a chunk of time (say two to three hours on a Sunday) cooking various components of meals or entire meals ahead of time so you have them on hand for the week. For instance, you might make a batch of grains, lentils, and beans to use throughout the week. Perhaps a stew or casserole made ahead of time can be stored in the fridge. Some families rely on batch cooking and others prefer to cook as they go along. It also does not have to be an all-or-nothing phenomenon. You could make one or two items ahead of time (for instance, the sauce for the Tofu Tikka Masala in Chapter 15) to give yourself a helping hand during the week.

- Repurpose ingredients. If you've got leftover beans, lentils, or grains, they can be thrown in a soup, fill tacos, or be used to create a main dish salad. Leftover rice can be transformed into a rice casserole, stir-fried rice, a Buddha bowl, or rice pudding. Leftover steamed vegetables can be turned into a cream soup, tossed onto a salad, thrown into a pasta sauce, or added to scrambled tofu.
- Prep breakfasts and lunches on the weekend. A batch of steel cut oats, overnight oats, tofu scramble, or muffins are great to have on hand for weekday breakfasts. For lunches, try spiral pasta salad, curried chickpea salad for sandwiches, or split pea soup to put in a thermos.

NO RECIPE MEALS

Recipes are a fun way to explore and find foods your family may enjoy. But day in and day out, we all need quick and easy meals to keep our families fed and out the door. Here are some simple "no recipe" meal ideas that come together quickly:

Table 13.1: Almost Instant Meals

BREAKFAST	LUNCH	DINNER	DESSERTS/ SNACKS
Sprouted toast with nut butter, sliced fruit	Hummus and veggie wrap, orange	Lentil or chickpea pasta with marinara sauce, salad	Bean dip (hummus or white bean), veggies
Avocado toast sprinkled with hemp seeds, fresh berries	Peanut butter and jelly sandwich, carrot and celery sticks, apple	Bean and vegan cheese quesadillas, guacamole, coleslaw	Steamed edamame in the pods with lime and sea salt
Smoothie with frozen fruit, greens, soy milk, nut butter	Canned bean or pea soup, whole grain roll, kale chips, pear	Baked potato with black beans, salsa, steamed broccoli	Fruit, crackers and nut cheese or peanut butter
Plant-based yogurt with granola and berries	English muffin veggie "pizzas," grapes	Tacos with seasoned veggie crumbles, guacamole, green salad	Dried fruit, nuts, dark chocolate
Veggie sausage, toast with fruit	Seasoned tofu sandwich, sugar snap peas, cherries	Pasta with chickpeas and roasted veggies	Fruit plate, non-dairy yogurt dip

Bagel with vegan cream cheese and tomato slices, fresh grapefruit	Frozen bean burrito, broccoli florets, dressing, banana	Store-bought pizza crust with sauce, veggies, veggie sausage, vegan cheese	Seasoned seaweed
Ready-to-eat cereal, walnuts, blueberries, soy milk	Store-bought veggie burger with bun, sliced cucumbers, apple	Rice and beans, sautéed kale	Apples slices with nut butter

PLANT-BASED ON A BUDGET

Some people assume that plant-based foods are simply too expensive to fit within their family budget. While some ingredients such as nuts, seeds, fresh or organic produce, and specialty or convenience items, such as nut cheeses, dairy-free yogurts, and veggie burgers, can certainly be more expensive, the basics of plant-based eating don't have to break the bank. Beans and grains are very inexpensive staples; many of the poorest populations in the world can't afford animal products and, so, are largely plant-based. Basic whole foods can be very affordable.

Money-saving tips:

- Menu planning and grocery shopping can help to cut down on food waste.
- Use all the leftovers! Either for lunches, a second dinner, or hodgepodge dinner nights.
- Dried beans and grains bought in bulk are generally less expensive than canned or ready to eat.
- Frozen vegetables are great to have on hand and are often less expensive than fresh.
- Seasonal fruits and vegetables can be less expensive (plus, produce tastes best when in season!).
- If you have the storage space, buying in bulk can help save money.

We hope the tips and tools provided in this chapter will help to create a road map for your plant-based journey. Remember, look for progress over perfection, go at a pace that seems doable and sustainable, and don't forget to have fun along the way.

Chapter 14

Sample Menus

"Even in this high-tech age, the low-tech plant continues
to be the key to nutrition and health."

—*Jack Weatherford*

From infancy through adolescence, this chapter provides sample menus to help parents understand how they might create balanced nutritional offerings for their family. Remember that any given meal or even day of eating is not the marker of adequate nutrition, but instead that the overall day-in and day-out food choices create a foundation for good health. They need not be followed in any precise way, but rather offer an idea of what you might consider offering.

> Remember that any given meal or even day of eating is not the marker of adequate nutrition, but instead that the overall day-in and day-out food choices create a foundation for good health.

Instead of being a daily burden, menu planning and preparation can become a fascinating and rewarding shared process. Plant-based foods offer an array of tantalizing aromas, flavors, and textures. Including children in food preparation is a wonderful opportunity to not only establish good nutrition habits for life but also a way to connect. We don't need to create exotic meals that are complicated to prepare. In fact, most youngsters will reject a fancy casserole and instead go for finger foods that they can easily identify—raw veggies, fruit, chunks of tofu, and toast or crackers with a spread.

317

We offer a sampling of menu ideas to provide inspiration and guidance. Feel free to let your family's preferences and your creativity do the rest.

The menus are divided into age categories as follows:

- Infants (six to twelve months)
- Toddlers (one to three years)
- Children (four to twelve years)
- Adolescents (thirteen to eighteen years)
- Competitive Adolescent Athletes

Each menu is an example of the types of foods you might offer. Feel free to make swaps as you see fit—if it's not peach season, serve a pear or apple instead. You can vary menu items to suit your family's preferences and the foods available in your pantry. For each menu, time for food prep varies. On days where more food prep time is needed at dinnertime, other meals and snacks may be simple, so the menu doesn't get too overwhelming. You'll notice that menus do not list serving sizes as they will vary depending on age, gender, activity level, health, and metabolism. Remember that once food is on the table, it's up to your child how much they eat. Most children need at least one or two snacks a day.

Table 14.1: Menus for Infants

TIME	6 TO 8 MONTHS	9 TO 12 MONTHS
Early morning	Breast milk *or* formula Vitamin D drops for breastfed babies	Breast milk *or* formula Vitamin D drops for breastfed babies
Breakfast	Iron-fortified infant cereal with thinned* nut or seed butter; breast milk *or* formula; mango cubes	Iron-fortified infant cereal with thinned* nut or seed butter; breast milk *or* formula; strawberries
Snack	Breast milk *or* formula	*Baby Biscuits* (page 380) Kiwi
Lunch	Steamed broccoli and yam cubes Soft-cooked black beans Avocado slices Ripe honeydew Breast milk *or* formula	Steamed green beans Soft-cooked kidney beans and millet Avocado slices Orange sections Breast milk *or* formula

*Thin nut or seed butter with breastmilk, formula, or water. Mix 1 part nut or seed butter with 2 to 3 parts liquid. Use it as a sauce or stir into cereal.

Snack	Breast milk *or* formula	Hummus Whole wheat pita bread Lightly steamed carrot sticks
Dinner	Steamed tofu cubes, carrots, and peas Thinned* nut or seed butter Cooked quinoa Applesauce Breast milk *or* formula	Chickpea pasta Marinara sauce Steamed, chopped baby kale Watermelon cubes Breast milk *or* formula
Snack	Breast milk *or* formula	Breast milk *or* formula Toast with thinly spread nut or seed butter and banana slices

Table 14.2: Menus for Toddlers (1 to 3 years)

MEAL	MENU #1	MENU #2	MENU # 3

Breakfast	*Banana Walnut*
	  Pancakes (page 339)
	Nut butter
	Fruit Compote
	  (page 340)
	Fortified soy *or* pea milk
		Oatmeal with iron-
		  fortified infant cereal
		Hemp hearts
		Sliced strawberries
		Fortified soy *or* pea milk
			Nut butter and banana
			  wrap with sunflower and
			  chia seeds
			Fresh orange sections
			Fortified soy *or* pea milk

Snack	*Toddler Cookies*
	  (page 381)
	Cantaloupe cubes
		Clever Crackers (page
		  382) with nut butter
		and banana slices
			Cashew *or* soy yogurt with
			  raspberries

Lunch	*Split Pea Soup*
	  (page 352)
	Whole grain roll
	Carrot Raisin
	  Salad (page 342)
	Mango slices
		Whole grain toast with
		  avocado and seasoned
		  tofu slices
		Snap peas
		Peach slices
			Whole wheat English
			  muffin pizza
			Raw broccoli, carrots,
			  peppers, and *Dilly*
			  Dip (page 358)
			Watermelon cubes

Snack	Cherry tomatoes, pita
	  bread, and hummus
		Smart Start Smoothie
		  Ice Pops (page 334)
			Chia pudding with
			  blueberries

Dinner	Chickpea spaghetti
	Marinara sauce
	Steamed broccoli
	Grapes (cut in half)
	Fortified soy *or* pea milk
		Tofu Stir-Fry (page 364)
		Brown rice
		Apple Crisp (page 389)
		Cashew Pear
		  Cream (page 390)
		Fortified soy *or* pea milk
			The Ultimate Veggie
			  Lasagna (page 374)
			Green salad
			Lemon tahini dressing
			Nice Cream (page 391)
			Fortified soy *or* pea milk

Note: If toddler is breastfeeding, breast milk can replace soy or pea milk.

Table 14.3: Menus for Children (4 to 12 years)

MEAL	MENU #1	MENU #2	MENU # 3
Breakfast	Whole grain toaster waffles Nut butter *Mixed Berry Compote* (page 340) Tangerine Fortified soy *or* pea milk	*Essential Overnight Oats* (page 333) Sliced strawberries Fortified soy *or* pea milk	*Pumpkin Muffins* (page 337) Non-dairy yogurt, berries, and walnuts Fortified soy *or* pea milk
Snack	Watermelon Seasoned seaweed	Pear Almonds	Mango slices Cashews
Lunch	*Black Bean, Corn, and Salsa Soup* (page 354) Crackers Nut cheese Watermelon slices *Chickpea Chocolate Chip Cookies* (page 385)	Macaroni and *Velvety Cheeze Sauce* (page 361) with peas Diced apples with *Cashew Pear Cream* (page 390), cinnamon and walnuts	Whole grain bun with veggie patty, lettuce, tomato, pickles Carrot and celery sticks Fruit and nut bar
Snack	Granola with cashew yogurt and banana slices	*Clever Crackers* (page 382) with nut butter and banana slices	Crackers and *Snickerdoodle Hummus* (page 383)
Dinner	Baked stuffed sweet potato (stuff with canned black beans, corn, salsa and guacamole) Steamed broccoli *Velvety Cheeze Sauce* (page 361) Grapes Fortified soy *or* pea milk	*Taco Night* (page 368) *Nice Cream* (page 391) Fortified soy *or* pea milk	*Tofu Tikka Masala* (page 363) Steamed broccoli Basmati rice *Peanut Butter Brownies* (page 387) Fortified soy *or* pea milk
Snack	Popcorn Apple slices	Toasted whole grain bagel Nut cheese	Cold cereal Fortified soy *or* pea milk

Table 14.4: Menus for Adolescents (13 to 18 years)

MEAL	MENU #1	MENU #2	MENU # 3
Breakfast	*Golden Scrambled Tofu and Veggies* (page 336) Whole grain toast Fortified soy *or* pea milk	*Smart Start Smoothie Bowl* (page 334)	Cold cereal Sliced bananas Walnuts Fortified soy *or* pea milk
Lunch	Sandwich–whole grain bread, seasoned tofu slices, lettuce, tomato Carrot sticks Granola bar Orange	*Curried Chickpea Salad Spread* (page 341) in a whole wheat pita Cherry tomatoes Fresh peach Dark chocolate almonds	Whole grain bagel with cashew cheese and veggie deli slices Sliced cucumber and *Dilly Dip* (page 358) *Crispy Seedy Cookies* (page 384)
Snack	Banana Mixed nuts	Cantaloupe slices Roasted chickpeas	Apple Pumpkin seeds
Dinner	*Lemony Chickpea Pasta with Mushrooms and Broccoli* (page 372) Whole grain garlic bread Fruit salad with *Cashew Pear Cream* (page 390) Fortified soy *or* pea milk	*Burger Night* (page 366) Veggie tray (carrot and celery sticks, broccoli and cauliflower florets, cherry tomatoes), Ranch dip *Nice Cream* (page 391) with blueberries and nuts	*Crispy Tofu Fingers* (page 362) Roasted potato wedges Green salad (use ready-to-eat greens, cherry tomatoes, and cucumber slices), dressing Watermelon Fortified soy *or* pea milk
Snack	Baked taco chips Salsa	Cold cereal Blueberries Fortified soy *or* pea milk	Cashew yogurt parfait with berries and granola

Table 14.5: Menus for Competitive Adolescent Athletes

MEAL	MENU #1	MENU #2	MENU # 3
Breakfast	*Essential Overnight Oats* (page 333) Fortified soy *or* pea milk Berries Toast with nut butter and jam	*Banana Walnut Pancakes* (page 339) Nut butter *Fruit Compote* (see page 340) Fortified soy *or* pea milk	*Smart Start Smoothie Bowl* (page 334) *Cranberry Orange Almond Muffins* (page 338)
Snack	Trail mix Apple	Energy bar Orange	Nut mix Cherries
Lunch	Sandwich–seasoned tofu, tomatoes, lettuce, pickles Power bar Apple with nut butter	Veggie wrap with *White Bean, Garlic, and Lemon Spread* (page 360), grated carrots, lettuce, sprouts *Chickpea Chocolate Chip Cookies* (page 385) Orange	*Rainbow Spiral Noodle Salad* (page 347) Whole grain roll Nut butter *Molasses Tahini Energy Balls* (page 386)
Snack	English muffin with nut butter and jam	*Berry Bliss Smoothie* (page 335)	Cold cereal, sliced strawberries, fortified soy *or* pea milk
Dinner	*Peanut Dragon Bowl* (page 370) *Apple Crisp* (page 389) with *Cashew Pear Cream* (page 390) Fortified soy *or* pea milk	*Kind Shepherd's Pie* (page 376) Steamed broccoli *Velvety Cheeze Sauce* (page 361) *Oatmeal Bars* (page 388) Fortified soy *or* pea milk	Frozen burritos Green salad (use ready-to-eat greens, cherry tomatoes, and cucumber slices), dressing Watermelon Fortified soy *or* pea milk
Snack	*Chocolate Peanut Butter Smoothie* (page 335)	Toasted bagel with nut cream cheese, avocado, and tomato slices	Nondairy yogurt parfait (yogurt, berries, granola)

Chapter 15

Recipes

"It's easy to be convincing when the food is delicious.
It doesn't feel like a sacrifice—it feels like a step up."

—Tal Ronnen

Our final chapter provides simple, delicious, plant-based recipes for the whole family. From weaning to adolescence, we fully endorse the idea that "kid food" should be real food. While it's important to make meals that are enjoyable and accessible to kids, having children participate in family meals where everyone eats the same meal is a great habit to get into. Introducing kids to a variety of flavors, textures, and ingredients is key to having them accept new foods. If you are just beginning to do more cooking at home, recipes can be an invaluable resource. They provide precise amounts and instructions that can take some of the fear out of cooking. As you begin to gain more confidence in the kitchen, you'll be able to easily modify recipes or even prepare meals based on what you have on hand. Anywhere along the process, we encourage you to substitute, experiment, and explore.

Before we dive into the recipes, there are a few practical points to consider.

ADDED SALT, OIL, AND SUGAR

There is a spectrum of eating styles within the whole-food, plant-based world. At one end of the spectrum are those who eat mostly whole foods, but include moderate amounts of added salt, oil, and sugar for flavor and to allow greater flexibility with food purchases and when eating out. At the other end are those who completely avoid added salt, oil, and sugar, otherwise known as an "SOS-free" whole-food, plant-based diet. Those who choose an SOS-free diet often do so to prevent or manage chronic diseases such as heart disease or type 2 diabetes. Significantly reducing or removing salt, oil, and sugar, while maximizing intake of high fiber, whole plant foods, can be an effective strategy for treating chronic disease. However, as we reviewed in Part III, being overly restrictive with foods, especially for children, has potential harms. Additionally, it is important to keep in mind that the vast majority of added salt, sugar, and oil comes from processed foods and meals eaten outside of the home. Working on increasing the amount of meals cooked and eaten at home is the best way to increase the nutritional value of the food your family eats and enjoys. Of course, it makes good sense to be judicious with the use of added salt, oil, and sugar, and to incorporate whole food alternatives, when possible and practical.

Nourish recipes are designed to be family friendly, and some of the recipes that follow do include small amounts of added salt, oil, and sugar. For those who are looking to cut back on or omit these additions, nearly all of the recipes are easily adjusted. Following are some simple ways to modify recipes to reduce or remove added salt, oil, and sugar. Feel free to make other substitutions or alterations that suit your taste or dietary needs.

No Oil Cooking

- **Sautéing**—use broth, water, or wine in place of oil. Alternatively, if you are looking to brown onions or mushrooms, you can dry sauté until browned and then deglaze with broth, water, or wine.
- **Baking**—swap out oil with nut or seed butter, applesauce, prune or pumpkin puree, or bananas. You may need to adjust the sweetness (if using applesauce, bananas, or prune puree, cut back a little on the

sweetener) or add a little plant-based milk to thin out if using a nut butter.
- **Salad dressings**—use nut butters, avocado, or tahini for thick, creamy oil replacements.

Sweet Sugar Substitutes
- Substitute sugar or syrup with dried fruits and dried fruit purees such as date paste (page 384). They work especially well in baking, in main dishes, and in salad dressings.
- Use fresh fruit to sweeten some baked goods, granola, and salad dressings.
- Generally, avoid artificial sweeteners for your family. If you want a low-calorie sweetener, stevia or monk fruit are reasonable options.

Slashing Salt
- Add a splash of lemon, lime, or vinegar to brighten the flavor of food, which reduces the need for salt.
- Sprinkle on a variety of fresh or dried herbs and spices to give your dish a flavor boost.
- Increase the garlic, onions, shallots, and green onions called for in the recipe.
- Include a little nutritional yeast in your sauces, dressings, or popcorn.

SALT, OIL, AND SUGAR — YOUR BEST BETS

When a recipe calls for salt, oil, or sugar, there are many options for each. Generally, purchase the least processed, highest quality products you can manage. Of course, since you are using less salt, oil, and sugar, selecting a higher quality product is often more doable.

- *Salt.* Good old-fashioned iodized salt is a reasonable option if you are relying on salt for iodine. It's the least expensive salt, dissolves quickly, and works well in most cooking and baking. Kosher salt is coarser and flakier than table salt, so it is less dense (note that one teaspoon of kosher salt equals about one-half to two-thirds of a teaspoon of table salt). Chefs tend to prefer kosher salt as it is more "pinchable" and has better texture and flavor than table salt. Other varieties such as sea salt, Celtic sea salt, black salt *(kala namak)*, Himalayan pink salt, and *fleur de sel,* while more costly, can be fun to experiment with. Feel free to explore while also ensuring an adequate source of iodine. When trying a new variety of salt, season judiciously as it is easy to add more but nearly impossible to reduce added salt.

- *Oil.* Vegetable oils vary tremendously in their processing, flavor, nutrition, and suitability for various cooking applications. More heavily refined oils have fewer phytochemicals and less flavor. However, they tend to have higher smoke points so are more suitable for higher temperature cooking than less refined oils. The best oils for cooking (oils with a high smoke point) are refined avocado, olive, or high-oleic sunflower oils. For salads, opt for omega-3-rich oils, less refined avocado, or extra-virgin olive oils. Omega-3-rich oils such as flax or hemp seed oil are intensely flavored oils and are best cut with other oils in salad. Toasted nut and seed oils add deep flavor to dishes and work beautifully in salads or to finish a dish. Both omega-3-rich oils and toasted nut and seed oils do not withstand heat.

- *Sugar.* Go for less refined, more nutritious options. For example, maple syrup, blackstrap molasses, date sugar, and coconut sugar are choices that provide some nutrition. Of all the natural sugars, blackstrap molasses provides the most impressive supply of iron, calcium, and other minerals.

COOKING BEANS AND GRAINS

Cooking Legumes

It's both practical and economical to cook legumes in quantity so you'll have different types on hand whenever you want them. You can freeze individual or meal-sized portions of cooked legumes in labeled containers for as long as six months.

One option is to invest in a slow cooker, pressure cooker, or multi-use programmable Instant Pot, and follow instructions that accompany it for cooking legumes. If you prefer to cook your beans on your stove top, here are our recommendations.

Spread your legumes on a tray, so you can easily see any small rocks, twigs, or other debris that might have come through the mechanical cleaning process. Rinse the legumes well to remove dirt, and place in a cooking pot. Soaking is generally recommended prior to cooking to improve digestibility and reduce cooking time. While soaking is not necessary for lentils and split peas, some people do find it helpful. To soak, add enough water to cover the beans, split peas, or lentils, plus an extra two or three inches of water on top. Soak for six hours or overnight. If you want to speed up the soaking process, cover the legumes with water as you did to soak, bring to a boil for one minute, cover, then remove from the heat and let sit for one hour.

Once the legumes have been soaked (or to cook lentils and split peas), drain, rinse, and place in a pot with a heavy, tight-fitting lid. Add the amount of water indicated in the cooking chart, bring to a boil, then lower the heat and simmer for the time indicated. During cooking, skim off any foam that rises to the top, as this can also cause flatulence.

If you'd like to flavor the legumes while they cook, add herbs and spices (including salt) at the beginning of the cooking process. Add acidic ingredients (such as vinegar, tomatoes, or lemon juice) near the end of the cooking time, when the beans are just tender. If these ingredients are added sooner, they can make the beans tough and slow the cooking process. Beans are done when you can soften them on the roof of your mouth with your tongue. At this stage, they're the most digestible. The following chart provides specific guidelines for cooking different types of beans on a stove top.

Table 15.1: Cooking Legumes

For 1 cup dry beans, peas, or lentils

LEGUME	PRESOAK?	COOKING WATER	COOKING TIME FOR SOAKED BEANS*	APPROXIMATE YIELD
adzuki, black, black-eyed peas, cannellini	yes	4 cups	45 minutes to 1 hour	2½ cups
Great Northern, kidney, lima, navy, pink, pinto, red (small)	yes	3 cups	1½ to 2 hours	2 to 2½ cups
chickpeas, red (large)	yes	4 cups	2 to 3 hours	2½ cups

lentils, brown, green, or black	optional	3 cups	Presoak: 15 to 20 minutes No presoak: 30 to 40 minutes	2¼ cups
red lentils	no	3 cups	15 to 20 minutes	2¼ cups
split peas, green or yellow	optional	3 cups	Presoak: 30 to 45 minutes No presoak: 1 to 1½ hours	2¼ cups

*Beans that have been stored for several months may take longer to cook.

Cooking Grains

Just as with legumes, having cooked grains on hand makes it easy to add to soups, salads, and meals throughout the week. You can freeze individual or meal-sized portions of cooked grains in labeled containers for as long as six months.

Cook whole grains in a heavy-bottomed pot with a tight-fitting lid to retain moisture. Bring the amount of water recommended in the cooking chart to a boil, add the grain, return to a boil, then lower the heat, cover, and simmer. Many whole grains will fluff up if you turn off the heat and leave them covered for a few minutes after all the water has been absorbed; this will also help the grains separate and not stick together as much when stored. If your cooked grains have stuck to the bottom of the pot, turn off the heat, add a very small amount of liquid, cover the pan, and let it sit a few minutes. The grain will loosen, easing serving and cleanup. Recommendations for specific grains are given in the cooking chart.

For those that are looking to reduce the potential arsenic content of rice, rather than using the traditional preparation method, use six to ten parts water to one part rice. Cook for the usual amount of time and drain excess water before serving.

Table 15.2: Cooking Grains

Based on 1 cup dry grain

GRAIN	COOKING WATER	COOKING TIME	APPROXIMATE YIELD
barley, hulled, whole-grain, pot, or Scotch	3½ cups	1 hour	3½ cups
buckwheat groats	2 cups	20 minutes	3 cups
Kamut	3 cups	45 to 60 minutes (30 to 40 if soaked 6 hours or overnight)	3 cups
oats, steel cut	4 cups	20 minutes	4 cups
rice, brown, brown basmati, long grain, short grain	2 cups	35 to 40 minutes (let stand covered 5 to 10 minutes)	3½ cups
spelt	3 cups	45 to 60 minutes	2½ cups
wild rice	3 cups	40 to 45 minutes (let stand covered 10 minutes)	3½ to 4 cups

RECIPE INDEX

Breakfast

Creamy Steel Cut Oats   *332*

Essential Overnight Oats   *333*

Smart Start Smoothie Bowl   *334*

5 Quick Smoothies   *335*

Golden Scrambled Tofu and Veggies   *336*

Pumpkin Muffins   *337*

Cranberry Orange Almond Muffins   *338*

Banana Walnut Pancakes   *339*

Fruit Compotes   *340*

Salads

Curried Chickpea Salad Spread   *341*

Carrot Raisin Salad   *342*

Mango, Avocado, and Black Bean Salad   *343*

Build Your Own Full-Meal Salad   *344*

Not Your Everyday Kale Salad   *346*

Rainbow Spiral Noodle Salad   *347*

Lentil, Wheat Berry, and Roasted Veggie Salad   *348*

Soups

Better Broth Base   *349*

Rustic Lentil Soup   *350*

Curried Red Lentil Soup   *351*

Split Pea Soup   *352*

Creamy Broccoli Soup   *353*

Black Bean, Corn, and Salsa Soup   *354*

Roasted Pepper and Tomato Soup   *355*

Dips, Dressings, and Spreads

Lemon Tahini Dressing   *356*

Ginger Miso Sauce   *357*

Dilly Dip   *358*

Spinach Artichoke Dip   *359*

White Bean, Garlic, and Lemon Spread   *360*

Velvety Cheeze Sauce   *361*

Mains

Crispy Tofu Fingers   *362*

Tofu Tikka Masala   *363*

Tofu Stir-Fry   *364*

Burger Night   *366*

Taco Night   *368*

Peanut Dragon Bowl   *370*

Lemony Chickpea Pasta with Mushrooms and Broccoli   *372*

The Ultimate Veggie Lasagna   *374*

Kind Shepherd's Pie   *376*

Snacks and Sweets

Roasted Chickpeas   *378*

Edamame with Lime and Sea Salt   *379*

Baby Biscuits   *380*

Toddler Cookies   *381*

Clever Crackers   *382*

Snickerdoodle Hummus   *383*

Crispy Seedy Cookies   *384*

Chickpea Chocolate Chip Cookies   *385*

Molasses Tahini Energy Balls   *386*

Peanut Butter Brownies   *387*

Oatmeal Bars   *388*

Apple Crisp   *389*

Cashew Pear Cream   *390*

Nice Cream   *391*

Creamy Steel Cut Oats

Hot cereal is a welcome treat, especially during the cold days of winter. This one is soaked overnight to speed cooking time in the morning. If you forget to soak, cook oats in water/milk mixture for about 25 minutes. Quinoa could be used in place of the oats, if desired. Leftovers can be covered and refrigerated for up to 5 days. Heat before serving or eat cold with toppings.

5 cups boiling water

2 cups steel cut oats

2 cups fortified nondairy milk

¼–½ teaspoon salt

1. Before going to bed, bring water to a boil in a medium to large pot.

2. Add the oats to the pot. Stir, cover, and let sit overnight.

3. In the morning, add the milk and salt and simmer on low heat for about 15 minutes or until cereal is soft and creamy.

4. Add your choice of toppings: chia, flax, or hemp seeds; walnuts, raisins, spices (e.g., cinnamon, cloves, nutmeg), berries, compote, chopped fruit, and non-dairy milk.

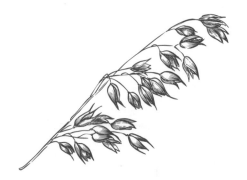

Essential Overnight Oats

This overnight oats recipe provides a base for so many oatmeal varieties. The hemp and chia seeds add nice texture and a boost of omega-3 fatty acids. Use the basic recipe and let your creativity flow. Getting the kids involved allows them to customize to their taste and makes it a fun experience. Make several jars at a time to have breakfast ready for days. You may want to halve the recipe for younger children. A perfect breakfast on the go!

½ cup rolled oats

½ teaspoon ground cinnamon

1 teaspoon hemp seeds

1 teaspoon chia seeds

1 cup plant-based milk (we recommend soy *or* pea for younger children and milk of choice for older kids)

1 teaspoon maple syrup, optional

SUGGESTED TOPPINGS

Peanut butter and banana: swirl in a tablespoon of peanut butter and top with sliced banana

Peanut butter and jelly: swirl in a tablespoon of peanut butter and top with fruit compote (page 340)

Blueberry almond: swirl in a tablespoon of almond butter and top with fresh blueberries and toasted almonds

Raspberry coconut: top with fresh raspberries and shredded coconut

The possibilities are endless!

1. Place the oats, cinnamon, and seeds in a mason jar. Stir to combine.

2. Add the plant-based milk and optional maple syrup if desired. Mix. Close with a lid and store in the fridge overnight.

3. In the morning, add your toppings of choice.

Smart Start Smoothie Bowl

MAKES 2 TO 3 SMOOTHIE BOWLS

Smoothie bowls make breakfast fun. Frozen peas are an unexpected ingredient that add fiber, protein, and a gorgeous bright green color. Hemp seeds provide additional protein and an omega-3 boost. Frozen ingredients are the key to thick, rich-tasting smoothie bowls—make sure all other ingredients are very cold. To turn the smoothie bowl into a smoothie, increase the milk to 2 to 2½ cups (depending on how thick you like it). A high-powered blender is ideal for smoothies, but if you don't have one a regular blender will usually do the trick. If you have extra, use to make ice pops.

SMOOTHIE BOWL

1½ cups unsweetened fortified soy milk *or* other non-dairy milk

3 cups greens (e.g., kale, power greens, spinach)

4 tablespoons hemp seeds

½ small *or* medium ripe avocado

¾ cup frozen peas

2 frozen sliced bananas

1 cup frozen pineapple *or* mango chunks

TOPPINGS

Seeds (e.g., chia, ground flax, pumpkin, sunflower)

Nuts, chopped *or* whole (e.g., almonds, cashews, pecans, walnuts)

Shredded coconut, unsweetened

Granola

Fresh berries

Chopped fruit (e.g., kiwi, peaches, nectarines, pineapple)

1. Put ingredients in the order listed (it's best to put in the liquids first, then fresh ingredients and finally the frozen ingredients) into a high-speed blender and blend on low speed, increasing speed slowly. Blend until smooth and creamy.

2. Divide into 2 or 3 bowls. Let each person decorate their bowl with the toppings provided.

5 Quick Smoothies

MAKES 1 TO 2 SERVINGS

Almost anything goes in smoothies. Experiment with a variety of fruits and vegetables. Soy milk is suggested in these smoothies to boost protein, but any milk can be used. You can also replace some of the milk with yogurt. To make smoothies, blend ingredients until smooth (preferably using a high speed blender). To make blending easier, add liquid ingredients first and frozen ingredients last.

1. CHOCOLATE PEANUT BUTTER SMOOTHIE

1½ cups soy milk, 3 tablespoons peanut butter, 3 tablespoons hemp seeds, 2 tablespoons cocoa powder, and 2 frozen bananas (add 2 to 3 soft dates *or* a tablespoon of maple syrup if you like it sweeter).

2. BERRY BLISS SMOOTHIE

1 cup soy milk, ½ cup yogurt (e.g., cashew, almond, coconut), 1 cup frozen berries (e.g., blueberries, raspberries, blackberries), and 1 frozen banana.

3. TROPICAL GLOW SMOOTHIE

1½ cups soy milk, 1 tablespoon lemon *or* lime juice, ¼ cup hemp seeds, 1 cup frozen mango, 1 frozen banana, and ½ cup frozen pineapple.

4. CITRUS KALE SMOOTHIE

1 cup soy milk, 1 fresh orange, 2 cups washed and trimmed kale leaves, ¼ cup almonds *or* cashews, and 1 frozen banana.

5. PUMPKIN PIE SMOOTHIE

1 cup soy milk, ½ cup pumpkin puree (or cooked butternut squash), 1 teaspoon pumpkin pie spice (or a mix of cinnamon, ginger, and nutmeg), 2 tablespoons cashew *or* almond butter, and 1 frozen banana.

Golden Scrambled Tofu and Veggies

MAKES 2 TO 4 SERVINGS

Scrambled tofu is a delicious protein-packed breakfast. One of the great nutritional benefits of tofu over eggs is the calcium. Compare brands to find the biggest calcium kick for your buck. Get creative with the vegetables and seasonings. Add a few tablespoons of versatile Velvety Cheeze Sauce (page 361) for a special treat! Serve with whole grain toast, sweet or white potatoes, and a sunny smile.

16 ounces medium firm tofu *or* firm tofu

1 tablespoon avocado *or* olive oil *or* 2 tablespoons vegetable stock

½ cup diced onion

2 cloves garlic, minced

1 cup diced mushrooms

½ cup diced red peppers

¼ to ½ teaspoon turmeric

½ teaspoon salt

2 cups coarsely chopped spinach *or* other leafy greens

2 tablespoons diced fresh herbs *or* 2 teaspoons dried herbs (e.g., basil, oregano, parsley)

2 tablespoons nutritional yeast

Freshly ground pepper to taste

1. Drain tofu and pat dry.

2. Place oil or stock in a nonstick pan over medium-high heat; add onions, garlic, mushrooms, and red peppers and sauté for 3 to 5 minutes.

3. Mash tofu into chunks in a bowl. Add mashed tofu, turmeric, and salt, and sauté for about 5 minutes or until the consistency resembles scrambled eggs.

4. Add greens and herbs and cook just until greens are wilted (about 1 minute for spinach, and 2 to 3 minutes for heavier greens).

5. Sprinkle on nutritional yeast and fresh ground pepper and give it a quick stir to distribute evenly.

> CHEF'S TIP: Using tamari or liquid aminos in place of salt provides many recipes with a wonderful burst of flavor. In this recipe, replace the salt with 1 tablespoon of tamari. Another option is to replace salt with black salt (kala namak) for an "egg-like" flavor.

Pumpkin Muffins

Pumpkin muffins are a fall favorite, brimming with warming spices that make them irresistible. There is nothing like pumpkin muffins fresh from the oven to celebrate autumn. This wonderfully healthy version features almond butter, spelt flour, and maple syrup. They are perfect for breakfast, in a lunch box, or as an after-school snack.

2 cups spelt flour

2 teaspoons baking powder

½ teaspoon baking soda

2 teaspoons pumpkin pie spice mix

¼ teaspoon salt

½ cup maple syrup

⅓ cup unsweetened plant-based milk

⅓ cup smooth almond butter

1 teaspoon vanilla extract

15-ounce can 100% pumpkin puree

1 cup chocolate chips (substitute raisins if you prefer!)

1. Preheat oven to 375° F and line a 12-muffin tin with parchment liners.

2. In a medium-sized bowl, combine flour, baking powder, baking soda, pumpkin pie spice, and salt.

3. In a small bowl, combine the maple syrup, plant-based milk, almond butter, and vanilla. Mix in the pumpkin puree.

4. Add the wet mixture to the dry mixture and mix until just combined, being careful not to overmix. Gently stir in the chocolate chips or raisins.

5. Fill the muffin tins ¾ full with an ice cream scoop or spoon. Sprinkle a few more chocolate chips on top if you like.

6. Bake for 22–28 minutes or until fluffy and a toothpick inserted into the center comes out clean.

7. Allow to cool in the pan for 5 minutes, then transfer to a wire rack to cool completely. Store in an airtight container. These muffins also freeze well if you happen to not eat them all first.

CHEF'S TIP: Pumpkin Pie spice is not just for pumpkin pie. It is perfect for muffins, pancakes, crumbles, cookies, so well worth keeping on hand. If you don't have pumpkin pie spice, make your own by combining 1 teaspoon of cinnamon, and ¼ teaspoon each of nutmeg, ginger, allpice, and cloves.

Cranberry Orange Almond Muffins

MAKES 12 MUFFINS

These muffins are bursting with flavor from the citrus and cranberry. They also look bright and festive and are perfect to share.

1½ cups spelt flour

½ cup almond meal

2 teaspoons baking powder

½ teaspoon baking soda

½ teaspoon salt

⅓ cup maple syrup

Zest from 1 orange (about 1 tablespoon)

¾ cup freshly squeezed orange juice

½ cup unsweetened apple sauce

1 teaspoon pure vanilla extract

¼ teaspoon almond extract

1½ cups fresh *or* frozen cranberries

½ cup sliced almonds

1. Preheat oven to 375° F. Line a 12-muffin tin with parchment liners.

2. In a medium bowl, combine the flour, almond meal, baking powder, baking soda, and salt.

3. In a separate bowl, mix to combine the wet ingredients (maple syrup through almond extract).

4. Add the wet ingredients to the dry and mix to combine. Gently fold in the cranberries.

5. Fill the muffin tins ¾ full with an ice cream scoop or spoon and top with sliced almonds.

6. Bake for 20–25 minutes, until lightly browned on top and a toothpick or knife inserted through the center comes out clean. When cool enough to handle, transfer to cooling racks to cool completely.

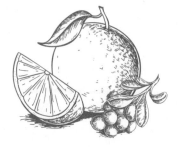

Banana Walnut Pancakes

These pancakes are denser and heartier than traditional white flour pancakes. They are gluten-free if you select gluten-free oats. They rise best when the batter is spread thinly on the pan. Make sure the pan is hot enough that drops of water dance when a few are dropped on the surface. Serve with peanut butter (or other nut or seed butter), sliced bananas, and maple syrup or fruit compote.

1½ cups rolled oats

3 tablespoons ground flaxseeds

1½ teaspoons baking powder

1 teaspoon cinnamon

⅛ teaspoon nutmeg

½ teaspoon salt

2 ripe bananas (about 1 cup mashed)

1½ cups fortified nondairy milk

½ teaspoon vanilla

⅓ cup coarsely chopped walnuts

Cooking spray *or* oil

1. In a blender, pulse the oats, flaxseeds, baking powder, cinnamon, nutmeg, and salt to a flour-like consistency.

2. Put the bananas, nondairy milk, and vanilla in the blender with the oat mix and pulse until the batter is smooth. Add the walnuts and pulse until just mixed into the batter. (You want the walnuts to remain in chunks.)

3. Place a large nonstick skillet on medium heat.

4. Spray or lightly coat the hot pan with oil so the pancakes do not stick. Make 3 small pancakes, using about ¼ cup of the batter per pancake. Spread the batter with a spatula so the pancakes are not too thick. Cook about 2–3 minutes or until pancakes are browned. Flip and cook about 2 minutes on the other side.

Fruit Compotes

Fruit compotes are great to have on hand. They take minutes to make and add a special touch to oatmeal, pancakes, or waffles. The recipes are more of a suggestion than a set of precise instructions. Spices and additional flavorings make it seem fancy, but the preparation is so easy that it almost feels like cheating. All of these compotes can be stored in a glass container and will keep for several days.

MIXED BERRY COMPOTE

12-ounce bag mixed
  frozen berries

½ teaspoon ground cinnamon

In a small pan add frozen berries and a hefty sprinkle of cinnamon. Mix to combine and warm gently until berries are softened and sauce forms.

ITALIAN PRUNE PLUM COMPOTE

4 cups Italian prune plums,
  quartered

2 tablespoons water

1. Place the prune plums and water in a large saucepan.
2. Over the lowest heat possible, stew until plums are covered in their own juice, stir occasionally. Cooking can take an hour or more. If the plums start to stick, add a bit more water.
3. Remove from heat, pour into jars, cover, and let cool.
4. For slight variations consider adding a pinch of ground cloves or 1 tablespoon of orange zest and replacing the water with orange juice.

RASPBERRY VANILLA COMPOTE

12-ounce bag frozen raspberries

1 teaspoon vanilla extract

1 teaspoon maple syrup, optional

In a small pan, warm the berries. When they have softened and created a sauce, remove from heat and stir in the vanilla and optional maple syrup.

BLUEBERRY AND GREEN APPLE COMPOTE

1 medium-sized Granny Smith
  apple, diced into small pieces

Zest of one lemon, preferably Meyer

12-ounce bag frozen blueberries

1 to 2 teaspoons fresh lemon juice

1 teaspoon vanilla extract

1. Place the diced apple, lemon zest, and blueberries in medium-sized pot. Squeeze in just a bit of lemon juice.
2. Over medium heat, bring the mixture to a boil and gently simmer until it is well combined and the fruit has softened.
3. Remove the pot from the heat, stir in the vanilla, and let it sit to come to room temperature.

Curried Chickpea Salad Spread

This is a plant-based version of a "tuna-less" or "egg-less" salad. The recipe is so forgiving that it really does lend itself to your creativity or simply to what you have on hand. Serve over toasted bread and with homemade tomato soup and call it dinner.

15-ounce can chickpeas, rinsed and drained

2 teaspoons olive oil, divided (optional)

1 teaspoon curry powder

Salt and pepper

¼ to ½ cup hummus

1 to 2 teaspoons Dijon mustard

1 cup finely diced crunchy things (celery *or* watermelon radish work well)

¼ cup finely diced red onion

1 tablespoon capers

1. Preheat oven to 375° F. Line a rimmed baking sheet with parchment paper.

2. Lightly pat the chickpeas dry and place on the baking sheet. Drizzle with 1 teaspoon of optional olive oil. Sprinkle on the curry powder, ¼ teaspoon of salt, and freshly ground black pepper. Gently mix to coat the chickpeas.

3. Bake the chickpeas in a single layer on the baking sheet for about 15 minutes. The chickpeas should be beginning to brown but not be crispy. They should still be soft and mashable.

4. Place the chickpeas in a glass bowl. Add ¼ cup of hummus and the mustard. Fold to combine and then with a potato masher or hefty fork, mash the chickpeas until they are the consistency of really lumpy mashed potatoes. A few whole chickpeas here and there are perfectly fine—they can be charming. You can add a little olive oil here or a little extra hummus if the mixture seems too dry.

5. Add the crunchy things, red onion, and capers. Fold in to combine. Season with salt and pepper to taste.

6. Pile onto toasted sourdough bread or serve with your favorite crackers.

7. The spread can be stored in an airtight container for several days. The flavor is even better the next day.

Carrot Raisin Salad

This carrot raisin salad is dressed with a delicious peanut sauce. The combination is a hit with kids and adults alike.

3 tablespoons natural peanut butter

3 tablespoons lemon *or* lime juice *or* apple cider vinegar

1 tablespoon water (*or* more if peanut butter is very thick)

1 teaspoon sesame oil

2 teaspoons tamari

1 tablespoon freshly grated ginger

Pinch crushed red pepper flakes

2 cups grated carrots, packed

½ cup chopped cilantro *or* parsley

⅓ cup raisins

3 tablespoons chopped peanuts

1. In a small bowl, stir together peanut butter, lemon or lime juice or apple cider vinegar, water, sesame oil, tamari, ginger, and red pepper flakes to make the peanut dressing.

2. In a medium-sized bowl toss carrots, cilantro or parsley, and raisins.

3. Add the peanut dressing and toss together.

4. Top with chopped peanuts. Serve immediately or refrigerate.

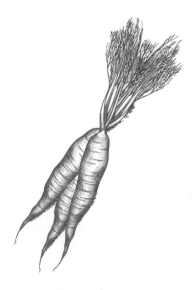

Mango, Avocado, and Black Bean Salad

This salad is like sunshine on the table—it's festive and fabulous. It can also be served as a salsa with pita chips (cut veggies and fruits smaller if using this way). If you prefer to omit the oil, add an extra tablespoon of lime juice.

DRESSING

3 tablespoons fresh lime juice

1 tablespoon olive *or* avocado oil

½ teaspoon chili powder *or* cumin

¼ teaspoon salt

¼ teaspoon black pepper

SALAD

1 cup frozen corn kernels, thawed

14-ounce can black beans, drained and rinsed

1 large orange pepper, chopped

½ to 1 small jalapeño *or* chipotle pepper, seeded and minced (optional)

2 green onions, diced (*or* ½ small red onion, chopped)

½ cup cilantro, finely chopped

2 medium-sized mangoes *or* 3 Ataulfo mangoes, peeled and chopped

1 medium avocado, chopped

1 large tomato, chopped

1. In a jar, combine the lime juice, oil, chili powder or cumin, salt, and pepper.

2. In a large bowl, place the corn, black beans, peppers, onion, and cilantro. Stir to combine.

3. Gently fold in the mangoes, avocado, and tomato.

4. Pour the dressing over the salad and toss very gently.

5. Serve immediately or refrigerate for a few hours before serving. Salad will keep in the refrigerator for about 2 days.

Build Your Own Full-Meal Salad

MAKES 1 OR MORE LARGE SERVING

This full-meal salad is fun for the whole family as each individual can build their own plate. The trick to transforming a salad into a full meal is to add a starch for satiety, a plant-based, protein-rich option, and a higher fat topping for essential fats and to enhance absorption of nutrients. The serving sizes are for adults or adolescents, so adjust for smaller children. Serve as a salad bar in many separate little bowls allowing each person to build their own. Alternatively, make a full-meal salad in a large bowl to use for a few days. Add items that discolor, such as avocados, just before serving.

Build Your Own Full-Meal Salad Selection Chart

Category	Suggested Amount per Person (adjust as needed)	Suggested Choices	Notes
Leafy Greens	4 cups per person	Any greens: arugula, kale (sliced matchstick thin), lettuce, radicchio, spinach, watercress, wild greens	When selecting greens, go for intense color—darker greens are generally more nutrient-dense. Include some leafy greens with red or purple tones when possible.
Veggies	1 or more cups per person	Pick vegetables to cover every color of the rainbow. Aim for 5 color families when you can. Examples include: Green: asparagus, broccoli, broccolini, celery, cucumber, snow peas, sugar-snap peas, zucchini Yellow-orange: carrots, peppers, grape tomatoes, golden cauliflower florets, sweet potato cubes, yellow. Pink-red: beets, cherry tomatoes, red onion, red peppers, radish, watermelon radish Purple-blue: purple cabbage, purple carrots, purple cauliflower, purple peppers White-beige: cauliflower, jicama, kohlrabi, salad turnips, sweet onion	Be creative in your selection and your preparation of each choice. Grate, spiral, shred, chop diagonally, or cut in fancy shapes. Engage children! See if they can find an item from each color group. Get them searching when you're at the market or at home.

Sprouts* **and Microgreens**	½ cup per person	Alfalfa sprouts, broccoli sprouts, lentil sprouts, microgreens, radish sprouts, sunflower sprouts, pea shoots	Sprouts and microgreens add a huge phytochemical punch to a salad. Consider growing your own microgreens or sprouts. Kids love to watch plants grow, especially when they grow as quickly as sprouts!
Fruits	½ cup per person	Apples, berries, grapefruit, grapes, kiwi, mangoes, oranges, peaches, pears, pomegranate seeds, and starfruit all make great choices.	If you are short on a color in your veggie selection, fill in with fruit such as blueberries in the purple/blue group.
Plant Protein	½–1 cup per person	Cooked or canned chickpeas, beans, or lentils; scoop of hummus or bean spread; smoked or flavored tofu cubes, tempeh strips, or veggie meat. Tofu, tempeh, or veggie meat can be hot or cold; both work well on salads.	Purchase ready-to-eat flavored tofu or prepare it yourself. Cube firm or extra-firm tofu, and coat with tamari and seasonings (e.g., turmeric, black pepper, and herbs), then place on a cookie sheet lined with a silicone mat and bake at 350° F for 20 minutes or until crispy.
Superb Starches	½–1 cup per person	Starchy vegetable: Steamed or baked and cubed potatoes, squash, or sweet potatoes; corn. Whole grains: cooked barley, kamut, or spelt berries, quinoa, or wild rice.	Starchy vegetables or grains add fiber, texture, and calories, making the meal more satisfying.
Healthy Fats	2–4 tablespoons per person	Great options include seeds such as chia, hemp, pumpkin, sesame, or sunflower seeds; nuts such as almonds, hazelnuts, pecans, pine nuts, or walnuts; avocado cubes or slices, peanuts, and sliced olives.	Choose at least 1 healthy whole-food fat option. Try to include an omega-3-rich choice such as chia seeds.
Herbs	¼–½ cup per person	Basil, chives, cilantro, dill, or parsley all work well.	Fresh herbs add a boost of flavor and unique phytochemicals.
Dressing	3–4 tablespoons per person	Homemade dressings (see pages 356–358) or a high-quality store-bought dressing.	When you make dressing from scratch, make enough to last a week—use nuts and seeds as a base to boost nutritional value.

Sprouts are not recommended during pregnancy due to the potential for food poisoning.

1. Wash and prep all produce (greens, vegetables, fruit), placing each in individual bowls.
2. Let everyone layer and assemble their bowl as desired, topping with microgreens, nuts, seeds, avocados, olives, herbs, and dressing.
3. Alternatively, you could assemble one large salad for everyone to enjoy.

Not Your Everyday Kale Salad

MAKES 8 TO 10 SERVINGS

This salad is essentially one specific version of the full-meal salad. It may seem like quite a bit of work with many ingredients, but it's actually easy to prep. It's flavorful and satisfying, and because the kale holds up well, it is a perfect pick for potlucks!

1 cup quinoa

1¾ cups water *or* vegetable broth

2 15-ounce cans chickpeas, rinsed, drained, and dried

Olive oil

1 teaspoon curry powder

2 apples, diced (Granny Smith works well)

Squeeze of lemon juice

1 large bunch kale (*or* 2 small), stems removed and shredded into thin ribbons

2 to 3 limes, zested and juiced (about 4 to 6 table-spoons of lime juice)

½ cup red onion, minced

3 ribs celery, diced

½ cup golden raisins

½ cup chopped mint

½ cup chopped cilantro

½ cup toasted almonds (pumpkin seeds, toasted cashews, *or* sunflower seeds would also be delicious)

Salt and pepper

1. Preheat the oven to 375° F.

2. Prepare the quinoa. In a dry skillet or pot, lightly toast the quinoa for 2 to 3 minutes over medium heat. When you begin to smell a nutty aroma, add 1¾ cups water (or broth) and a ¼ teaspoon of salt. Bring to a boil and then reduce to simmer and cover until the quinoa is cooked through (about 15 minutes). Let sit covered for 5 minutes and then fluff with a fork. Set aside.

3. Rinse, drain, and gently pat dry the chickpeas. Place the chickpeas on a parchment-lined baking sheet. Drizzle with about a teaspoon or so of olive oil. Sprinkle the curry powder, about ½ teaspoon of salt, and freshly ground black pepper over the chickpeas, and gently toss to combine. Roast at 375° F for 15 to 20 minutes. You want the chickpeas to have a little bite but not be overly crunchy. Set aside to cool.

4. While the quinoa and chickpeas are cooking, prepare the rest of your ingredients. Toss the diced apples with a squeeze of fresh lemon juice to prevent them from browning.

5. In a large bowl, gently massage the kale with a drizzle of olive oil (about 1 teaspoon) and two tablespoons of lime juice. Season with ¼ teaspoon of salt.

6. Next, fold in the quinoa and curry roasted chickpeas. Add the onion, celery, golden raisins, apples, lime zest, and herbs. Mix to combine.

7. Taste and add additional lime juice, salt, and pepper to taste. Top with toasted almonds. Watch it disappear!

Rainbow Spiral Noodle Salad

This salad is perfect for a picnic, a potluck, or a lunch box. It's pretty enough to serve to guests. Add additional vegetables, such as steamed asparagus, broccoli, cauliflower, or sliced Brussels sprouts, if desired. Other great additions are fresh or dried oregano, sundried tomatoes, and diced artichoke hearts. Double the vinaigrette, so you have extra to add if it gets dry (the pasta tends to absorb liquids).

RAINBOW SPIRAL NOODLE SALAD

1 pound whole grain (or regular) rotini noodles

4 cups spinach or thinly sliced kale or other greens

14-ounce can kidney beans, rinsed and drained

14-ounce can garbanzo beans or cannellini beans, rinsed and drained

3 cups cherry tomatoes

1 cup fresh parsley, chopped

½ cup fresh basil, chopped

4 green onions, finely chopped

2 peppers, 1 orange and 1 yellow, diced

¾ cup kalamata olives, sliced

2 plant-based Italian sausages, boiled for 10 minutes, and cut in half lengthwise, then sliced (optional)

1. Boil pasta in a large pot of salted water according to package directions. Add the spinach to the pot just before draining, to wilt. Drain and rinse in cold water immediately. Do not overcook.

2. In a large bowl, put the pasta and spinach, beans, tomatoes, parsley, basil, green onions, peppers, olives, and sausage, if using.

3. Toss gently with balsamic vinaigrette or your favorite dressing. Refrigerate and serve cold.

BALSAMIC VINAIGRETTE DRESSING

½ cup balsamic vinegar

¼ cup extra virgin olive oil

¼ cup water

2 tablespoons tamari

1 tablespoon Dijon mustard

1 tablespoon maple syrup

2 cloves garlic, peeled

1 tablespoon nutritional yeast

Fresh ground black pepper

Place all ingredients in a blender and blend until smooth.

Lentil, Wheat Berry, and Roasted Veggie Salad

MAKES 8 TO 10 SERVINGS

This recipe is great for potlucks or to have on hand for lunches during the week. Note, this is not a one-pot meal, but it is a one-bowl meal. That's to say the ingredients need to be cooked separately so that the dish is a salad and not a stew. There are lots of options for variations so make note of the (*).

1 cup wheat
   berries*

1 cup black lentils**

1 small *or* ½ a
   large purple
   cabbage,
   shredded***

1 tablespoon olive
   oil, divided

Salt and pepper

1 medium onion,
   finely diced

½ cup frozen green
   peas, thawed

½ cup golden
   raisins

Juice of ½ a lemon
   or 1 tablespoon
   red wine vinegar

Chopped fresh
   cilantro

½ cup toasted
   pumpkin seeds

1. Preheat the oven to 375°F.

2. Put the wheat berries and lentils into two separate pots. Cover with 2 inches of water. Bring to a boil and then lower the heat to simmer. Cook separately until just tender and cooked through. About 10 to 15 minutes for the lentils and 20 to 30 minutes for the wheat berries. You may need to add additional water. Be careful not to overcook the lentils. You want them cooked through but nowhere close to mushy. Drain both separately and set aside.

3. Meanwhile, place the shredded cabbage on a baking sheet and toss with a drizzle of olive oil (about 1 teaspoon), ½ teaspoon of salt, and freshly ground black pepper. Roast the cabbage for about 20 to 25 minutes until slightly browned.

4. Drizzle an additional 2 teaspoons of olive oil into a large pan. Sauté the onion until golden brown.

5. Add the cooked wheat berries and lentils followed by the peas and raisins. Season with salt and pepper to taste, and place the mixture into a large mixing bowl. Fold in the roasted cabbage.

6. Finish with a hefty squeeze of lemon juice or vinegar and chopped cilantro.

7. Right before serving, garnish with toasted pumpkin seeds.

You could also substitute Kamut, spelt, barley, quinoa, farro, or another hearty grain, but the wheat berry does have a nice bite!

**Again, you could substitute with another bean or lentil that is not mushy. Avoid using red, brown, or green lentils—you will end up with a mushy mess.*

***You get the idea! Substitute whatever veggies you prefer or have on hand (a combination of roasted eggplant, zucchini, mushrooms, and red pepper would work very well!).*

Better Broth Base

MAKES ABOUT 2¼ CUPS BROTH BASE

(enough to make about 36 cups of broth)

Many vegetable broth cubes or powders are based on palm oil or other hard fats and sugar. This one is based on B vitamin-rich nutritional yeast and seasonings. Use in place of broth in soups and stews. Feel free to adjust the herbs and spices to suit your palate. Store in an airtight glass jar for up to a year.

1 cup nutritional yeast flakes

½ cup dried onion flakes
    (*or* 3 tablespoons onion powder)

2 tablespoons dried garlic flakes
    (*or* 1 tablespoon garlic powder)

1 tablespoon iodized salt

1 teaspoon black pepper

½ teaspoon turmeric

1 teaspoon paprika

1 teaspoon celery seed

1 teaspoon thyme

1 tablespoon oregano

1 tablespoon parsley flakes

1. Mix well. Seal in airtight container.

2. Stir 1 tablespoon of broth base into 1 cup of hot water to make 1 cup of broth.

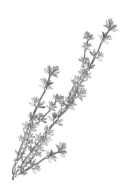

Rustic Lentil Soup

This classic soup pairs perfectly with crusty bread. The French lentils hold their shape better than regular brown lentils, giving the soup a nice texture. If you cannot find them, brown lentils will also work but they will just be a little softer/mushier and take less time to cook.

1 tablespoon olive oil

Medium-sized yellow onion, finely chopped

2 carrots, diced

3 ribs of celery, diced

2 garlic cloves, minced

1 teaspoon dried thyme

¾ teaspoon salt

Freshly ground black pepper

1 cup of French or green lentils

14.5-ounce can petite diced tomatoes

6 cups low-sodium vegetable broth (or 4 cups broth and 2 cups water)

3 to 4 cups chopped greens (such as Swiss chard, spinach, or kale)

Juice of half a lemon (about 2 to 3 teaspoons)

Chopped fresh parsley

1. Warm the olive oil in a medium-sized pot or Dutch oven.

2. Sauté the onions until golden brown. Next add the carrots and celery and continue to sauté until the vegetables are tender.

3. Add the garlic, thyme, salt, and black pepper (to taste), along with the lentils, tomatoes, and broth.

4. Bring to a boil and then lower to a simmer. Cook until the lentils are tender and cooked through (about 20 to 25 minutes for the French, a little less for brown lentils).

5. Stir in the greens and allow them to wilt down.

6. Finish with a squeeze of lemon, additional salt and pepper to taste, and fresh parsley.

Curried Red Lentil Soup

MAKES 4 TO 6 SERVINGS

This soup is a variation on our simple, more traditional lentil soup. It's great for an easy weeknight dinner because red lentils cook quickly. You can serve it over steamed brown rice or toasted naan alongside a salad. Leftovers are great in the lunch box.

1 tablespoon olive oil

1 teaspoon whole cumin seeds

Medium yellow onion, chopped

1-inch piece fresh ginger, minced

2 garlic cloves, minced

1 teaspoon ground cumin

1 teaspoon garam masala

½ teaspoon ground turmeric

¼ to ½ teaspoon ground red chili
    or red pepper flakes

1 teaspoon salt

Freshly ground black pepper to taste

1 tablespoon tomato paste

1 cup red lentils

6 cups low-sodium vegetable broth
    (*or* 4 cups broth and 2 cups water)

4 cups spinach *or* greens of choice

1 to 2 teaspoons fresh lemon juice

Chopped cilantro for garnish

1. In a medium-sized pot, warm the olive oil. Add the whole cumin seeds and warm for about a minute or two until you hear a sizzling sound (they should be fragrant but not burn).

2. Add the onion and sauté until golden brown. Add the minced ginger and garlic and sauté for about a minute until fragrant.

3. Add the ground cumin, garam masala, turmeric, ground red chili, salt, and black pepper. Next, add the tomato paste and mix together well, being careful not to let the spices burn (only cook for about a minute or so).

4. Add the lentils and vegetable broth to the pot. Bring to a boil and then lower the heat to simmer until lentils are almost cooked through, about 20 minutes.

5. Stir in the greens and cook until just wilted (spinach will only take a minute or two, heartier greens like kale will take a few minutes longer) and the lentils are soft and cooked through.

6. Finish with a fresh squeeze of lemon juice and chopped cilantro to garnish.

Split Pea Soup

This soup is made of simple ingredients and is adaptable to the stove top or Instant Pot.* You could also add one or two diced potatoes to the soup to give it a little more heft. It is a welcome treat in a thermos for lunch. Serve with crusty bread or steaming rice and a simple salad.

16 ounces (about 2 cups) dried, green split peas

1 tablespoon olive oil

Medium onion, chopped

2 ribs celery, diced

2 medium carrots, diced

2 cloves garlic, minced

1 teaspoon salt

1 teaspoon dried thyme

8 cups low-sodium vegetable broth

Chopped parsley *or* scallions

Hot sauce (optional)

1. Soak the split peas overnight or in the morning if you plan to make for the evening. This cuts down on the cooking time significantly.

2. Warm the olive oil in a medium- to large-sized pot. Sauté the onions, celery, carrots, and garlic until soft and translucent (5 to 10 minutes).

3. Add the rinsed and drained split peas, salt, and dried thyme.

4. Pour in the vegetable broth. Bring to a boil, then lower the heat to simmer. Cook for 30 to 40 minutes until the peas are mushy/tender. Add more water to thin out, if needed, and finish with salt and pepper to taste.

5. Garnish with chopped parsley or scallions and an optional drizzle of hot sauce.

CHEF'S TIP: To save time, use an electric pressure cooker such as an Instant Pot. No need to soak split peas ahead of time. Place the electric pressure cooker on sauté mode. Prepare vegetables as above. Add the split peas, salt, thyme, and broth. Pressure cook on manual for 15 minutes and allow the pressure to release naturally.

Creamy Broccoli Soup

MAKES 6 SERVINGS

You may wonder how a cream soup could be made without cream. It is actually very simple--we make or our "cream" by blending cashews. The flavor is fabulous, and the cashews make the soup lower in saturated fat and higher in trace minerals than soups made with cream.

4 cups vegetable broth

1 large white *or* yellow onion, chopped

3 cloves garlic, minced

2 medium-sized potatoes, chopped

1 bunch broccoli (about 6 cups chopped)

¼ cup fresh chopped basil (*or* 1 heaping tablespoon dried basil)

2 cups unsweetened fortified nondairy milk (almond, coconut, soy, etc.)

1 cup raw cashew pieces, rinsed

3 tablespoons light *or* white miso

Salt and pepper to taste

Lemon wedges

1. Place broth, onions, garlic, and potatoes in a large saucepan. Bring to a boil and simmer for about 30 minutes.

2. Chop broccoli and set aside 2 cups of small florets. Add the rest of the broccoli and the basil to the soup. Cook for 5 minutes or until the broccoli is tender crisp.

3. Blend milk, cashews, and miso until smooth and creamy. Add to soup, and heat until warmed through

4. Blend the soup in batches or use an immersion blender to puree until smooth. Add the reserved florets to the creamy soup and cook until the florets are tender crisp.

5. Serve hot with lemon wedges.

Black Bean, Corn, and Salsa Soup

MAKES 8 SERVINGS

This soup is satisfying and flavorful. Make it more fun for the family by providing a variety of toppings. Serve with a green salad and taco chips, guacamole, and salsa, or your favorite crusty bread.

SOUP

1 onion, chopped

1 tablespoon oil *or* 3 tablespoons vegetable broth

4 cups vegetable broth

2 cloves garlic, minced

1 teaspoon chili powder

1 teaspoon ground cumin

1 green pepper, chopped

1 14-ounce can crushed tomatoes

1 cup salsa (mild, medium, *or* hot)

2 14-ounce cans black beans, rinsed and drained

2 cups whole kernel corn

Salt and pepper to taste

OPTIONAL TOPPINGS

Lime wedges (for squeezing on the hot soup just before eating)

Fresh cilantro, chopped

Avocado cubes

Sliced green onions

Sliced black olives

Hot sauce

Plant-based sour cream

Baked tortilla chips

1. In a large saucepan, sauté onion in oil or broth for about 10 minutes until onion is softened. If using vegetable broth, add one tablespoon at a time as needed to prevent sticking.

2. Stir in garlic, chili powder, and cumin. Cook for another minute.

3. Add 4 cups vegetable broth, green peppers, crushed tomatoes, and salsa. Stir together and cook over medium heat until the broth comes to a boil. Lower heat and simmer for 15–20 minutes.

4. Add the beans and corn. Simmer for another 15–20 minutes.

5. Dish into individual bowls. Put out small bowls of additional toppings so each person can add the flavors they enjoy.

Roasted Pepper and Tomato Soup

MAKES 4 TO 6 SERVINGS

Homemade tomato soup is a breeze to make. The addition of roasted red pepper adds a sweet flavor. You could also use jarred peppers but roasting at home is so simple and the flavor is fantastic.

1 large *or* 2 small red bell peppers

1 tablespoon olive oil

Medium onion, diced

Pinch red pepper flakes (optional)

½ teaspoon salt

4 garlic cloves, sliced

1 teaspoon dried thyme *or* basil

28-ounce can whole peeled tomatoes (San Marzano preferred for extra flavor and sweetness)

2 cups low-sodium vegetable stock

1. Preheat the oven to 400° F. Line a rimmed baking sheet with foil and place the peppers on the baking sheet. Roast in the oven for 20 to 30 minutes, flipping the peppers halfway through. The skin of the peppers should look charred and the flesh should be soft and cooked through. Once the peppers are nicely charred, allow them to cool enough so that you can handle them without burning yourself. Gently peel away the charred skin from the pepper and pull out the stem along with the seeds. Slice the roasted peppers and set them aside.

2. While the peppers are roasting, in a medium-sized pot, warm the olive oil over medium heat. Add the diced onions and sauté until they begin to brown just slightly. Add the optional pinch of red pepper flakes, salt, garlic, and thyme. Cook them for another minute or two.

3. Next, add the roasted peppers, tomatoes, and vegetable stock. Bring to a boil, and then lower the heat to a simmer and cook for 20 to 30 minutes to allow the flavors to meld.

4. Use an immersion blender to puree until smooth. If you do not have an immersion blender, carefully and in batches, transfer the soup to a blender and puree until smooth.

5. Season with salt and pepper to taste.

Lemon Tahini Dressing

MAKES 2⅓ CUPS

Tahini is sesame seed butter, and it's a staple in Mediterranean cuisine. It can be used to flavor sauces and soups or to make salad dressings creamy. If available get Mediterranean tahini as it is thinner and less bitter than other tahini. This dressing is wonderful on salads, dinner bowls, steamed vegetables, or baked potatoes. It thickens up a lot when refrigerated. If too thick, it can be thinned with a little water.

¾ cup water

⅔ cup tahini

½ cup fresh lemon juice

2 tablespoons tamari

4 cloves garlic, peeled and coarsely chopped

1 tablespoon maple syrup *or* 1 Medjool date (optional)

Pinch cayenne (optional)

Put the water, tahini, lemon juice, tamari, garlic, optional maple syrup or date, and optional cayenne in a blender and process until smooth, about 30 seconds. Stored in a sealed container in the refrigerator. The dressing will keep for 2 weeks.

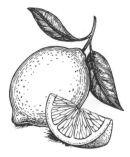

Ginger Miso Sauce

MAKES ROUGHLY HALF A CUP

Another wonderful way to use tahini is in this ginger miso sauce that can transform dinner into something special. It keeps in the fridge for several days and adds a punch of flavor to leftovers. Great over baked tofu, on a salad, or over roasted veggies (especially Japanese sweet potatoes!).

1 tablespoon minced ginger

2 tablespoons yellow miso paste

2 tablespoons tahini

1 tablespoon maple syrup

1 tablespoon rice wine vinegar

4 tablespoons warm water

If you have a small blender attachment or mini food processor, add all of the ingredients and blend until smooth and creamy. If you don't have one of these implements, simply place the ingredients in a mason jar with a lid and shake until combined. The texture won't be quite as creamy, but it will remain delicious. Store in a glass container for up to one week.

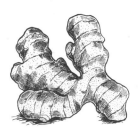

Dilly Dip

This dill dip is reminiscent of traditional vegetable dips. It is a hit with the kids, and is a snap to pull together. If you prefer, use a clove of fresh garlic (or two) instead of the garlic powder. Using the fortified non-dairy milk gives a nutrition boost. Vary the seasonings to suit your taste.

1 ½ cups raw cashew pieces

¾ cup unsweetened fortified non-dairy milk *or* water

3 tablespoons apple cider vinegar *or* lemon juice

¾ teaspoon salt

½ teaspoon garlic powder

1 teaspoon onion powder

3 tablespoons fresh chopped dill

1 tablespoon fresh chopped chives

1. Soak the raw cashews in hot water for 15 to 30 minutes.

2. Drain and rinse cashews. Place in blender, along with nondairy milk, vinegar or lemon juice, salt, garlic powder, and onion powder. Blend until very smooth, scraping down sides, if needed.

3. Transfer into a bowl and fold in the dill and chives. Store in the refrigerator for up to a week. Serve with vegetables as a dip, or with salads, as a dressing. If using as a dressing, you can thin with a little extra unsweetened non-dairy milk or water.

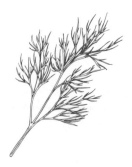

Spinach Artichoke Dip

Spinach artichoke dip is always a crowd favorite. This healthy, plant-based version is a welcome addition to any party or potluck, or a wonderful treat for the family. Leftovers are delicious, and can be enjoyed cold with bread, crackers, pita chips, or veggies. Feel free to vary the heat from red pepper flakes, fresh hot peppers, or hot sauce to suit your palate.

1 sweet onion, diced

5 cloves garlic, minced

1 red pepper, diced

3 tablespoons white wine *or* 1 tablespoon avocado *or* olive oil

1¼ cups raw cashew pieces, soaked 4 to 6 hours *or* overnight (or do a quick 30-minute soak using boiling water), drained and rinsed

1¼ cups unsweetened plain cashew milk (not vanilla) *or* other nondairy milk

2 to 3 tablespoons fresh squeezed lemon juice (juice of about 1 lemon)

1 tablespoon white *or* light miso

⅓ cup nutritional yeast

¾ teaspoon salt

14-ounce can artichoke hearts (packed in water), drained and chopped

10-ounce package chopped frozen spinach, thawed and squeezed dry

¼ teaspoon red pepper flakes, ½ to 1 jalapeno pepper, diced, *or* hot sauce to taste

¼ teaspoon paprika

3 tablespoons vegan parm (optional)

1. Preheat oven to 375° F.

2. In a medium saucepan, sauté onions, garlic, and red pepper in white wine or oil for about 5 to 7 minutes or until onions are tender.

3. In a high-powered blender, put the cashews, cashew milk, lemon juice, miso, nutritional yeast, and salt. Blend until very smooth and creamy.

4. In a medium-sized bowl, stir together cashew mixture, cooked vegetables, spinach, artichokes, and red pepper flakes.

5. Transfer mixture to an oven-safe casserole or pie dish. Sprinkle with paprika and vegan parmesan.

6. Bake for 25 to 30 minutes or until browned on top. Serve immediately with sourdough bread, sliced baguette, or pita chips.

White Bean, Garlic, and Lemon Spread

MAKES 4 SERVINGS (ABOUT 1½ CUPS)

This creamy spread is simple yet bursting with flavor. It's great over a sliced baguette, as a spread on sandwiches, or even alongside sliced veggies as a dip.

15-ounce can cannellini beans, rinsed and drained

1 to 2 cloves garlic, sliced*

1 tablespoon tahini

1 tablespoon olive oil

Juice of ½ lemon (or more)

1 cup loosely packed parsley

½ teaspoon salt

¼ teaspoon freshly ground black pepper

1. Put all of the ingredients (setting aside a few sprigs of parsley) into a food processor and pulse until roughly smooth (no big chunks of beans but not into a complete paste).

2. Season with additional salt, pepper, and lemon juice to taste.

3. Garnish with remaining chopped parsley. Store in a glass container for up to 3 to 4 days.

CHEF'S TIP: Garlic adds a nice punch of flavor to many dishes, but you may want to go lightly for younger kids as the flavor can be too strong for budding palates.

Velvety Cheeze Sauce

MAKES ABOUT 2½ TO 3 CUPS

This versatile "cheese" sauce is simply the best! It is fabulous on steamed vegetables, burgers, loaves, or sandwiches and it makes a fine filling for celery sticks or a dip for veggies. Stir it into soups or stews just before serving to impart a creamy texture and cheesy taste. It also makes a wonderful macaroni and cheese. For each cup of cooked, drained macaroni, add about 3 tablespoons of sauce and heat. Soaking the cashews prior to blending helps improve mineral availability and makes it even creamier, but if you have a high-powered blender, it is not critical. Use jarred roasted red peppers if you like—they are inexpensive and handy. Raw peppers can also be used if you prefer. Water works well, but fortified non-dairy milk adds a substantial nutrition boost.

2 cups unsweetened fortified nondairy milk *or* water

¾ cup raw cashews, rinsed well *or* soaked for 4 to 6 hours, drained, and rinsed

1 to 2 roasted red bell peppers, seeded and coarsely chopped

3 tablespoons cornstarch

¼ cup nutritional yeast flakes

2 tablespoons lemon juice

½ teaspoon garlic powder

1 teaspoon onion powder

1 teaspoon salt

1. Put all ingredients in a high-powered blender and process until very smooth and creamy.

2. Pour mixture into a medium saucepan and bring to a boil over medium heat, stirring constantly. Immediately decrease the heat to medium low and cook, stirring or whisking frequently, until thickened, for about 5 minutes. Blend again for an extra silky sauce, if desired. Serve hot on vegetables or on anything needing cheese sauce.

CHEF'S TIP: Substitute cashews with sunflower seeds for an economical, nut-free version. Sunflower seeds can replace cashews in other recipes as well, such as the dilly dip or cashew pear cream.

Crispy Tofu Fingers

This tofu can be used as a main dish for a dinner meal, as a sandwich filling, or as a snack. Kids love it! You only need to press tofu if it is packed in water.

1 package (14- to 16-ounce) firm *or* extra-firm tofu, pressed *or* patted dry

3 tablespoons tamari *or* soy sauce

½ cup nutritional yeast

¾ teaspoon Spike seasoning *or* other favorite seasoning mix (for less sodium, use salt-free Spike)

1 tablespoon avocado oil

1. Preheat oven to 375° F.
2. Slice the tofu into ¼" to ⅓" pieces. Each piece will be about 4 x 1.5 inches. You can be creative with shapes, cutting diagonally if you prefer.
3. Pour the tamari into a bowl.
4. On a plate, mix the nutritional yeast and seasoning.
5. Dip each piece of tofu into the tamari, then into the nutritional yeast mixture coating both sides.
6. Place the tofu on an oiled cookie sheet or on a silicone mat on a cookie sheet (oil is optional if using a mat). Be sure that the pieces of tofu are not touching one another. Bake at 375° F for about 30 minutes or until golden brown, flipping once during baking. Alternatively, cook the tofu in a small amount of oil in a hot non-stick skillet about 5 minutes per side or until golden brown.

> CHEF'S TIP: To press, place tofu between 2 plates with a couple of cans on top for weight. Allow to drain for an hour or more. For tofu not packed in water, simply pat dry using paper towel or clean cloth.

Tofu Tikka Masala

This is a take on a restaurant-style Indian dish. It's a bit lighter but still full of flavor. It's best served with rice or naan and perhaps some roasted cauliflower.

2 14-ounce packages of organic sprouted tofu, cut into half-inch cubes

1 tablespoon olive oil

3 whole cloves

1 dried bay leaf

1 stick whole cinnamon

1 large yellow onion, diced

3 cloves garlic, minced

1 tablespoon fresh ginger, minced

4 ripe tomatoes, roughly chopped

2 tablespoons tomato paste

2 teaspoons ground cumin

½ to 1 teaspoon ground red chili powder, depending on level of spice desired

½ teaspoon ground turmeric

¾ teaspoon garam masala

1 teaspoon salt

½ cup coconut, plain almond, *or* soy milk

1 cup frozen peas

Chopped fresh cilantro for garnish

1. On a baking sheet lined with parchment paper, bake the tofu at 375° F for about 15 minutes. The tofu should firm up and just start to brown. Set the tofu aside.

2. Warm the olive oil in a medium-sized pot or Dutch oven. Add the cloves, bay leaf, and cinnamon. Cook for just about a minute, until fragrant.

3. Add the onions and sauté until beginning to brown. Next, add the garlic and ginger and sauté for a minute, being careful not burn the garlic and ginger.

4. Add the tomatoes and sauté until they are cooked down a bit (about 5 minutes). Mix in the tomato paste followed by the remaining spices, including the salt, and cook until fragrant and the spices have been incorporated into the mixture (2 to 3 minutes).

5. This next step is optional, but recommended to create a smooth and creamy sauce. Carefully fish out the cloves, cinnamon, and bay leaf. Add 1 cup of water and use an immersion blender or transfer the sauce to a regular blender. Puree the mixture until smooth and return to the pot. Bring the sauce to a simmer and stir in the coconut milk.

6. Add the baked tofu and frozen peas. Cook on medium-low heat for 10 to 15 minutes to allow the flavors to meld.

7. Season with additional salt and pepper to taste. Garnish with cilantro.

CHEF'S TIP: Sprouted tofu can be used in place of regular tofu in almost any recipe. It is higher in protein and thought to be more easily digested than regular tofu. Its texture tends to be quite firm, so pressing isn't necessary. In this recipe, if you select regular tofu, press it between plates or paper towels for about a half hour before baking.

Tofu Stir-Fry

MAKES 4 SERVINGS

A family favorite! This recipe does have several steps so might be easier to prep on a night when you have a little extra time. If your family likes things on the milder side, decrease (or omit) the chili sauce. Consider doubling the recipe if you've got older kids or are aiming for leftovers. Feel free to add extra veggies (mushrooms, snap peas) along with the red bell pepper. This recipe works best if you have a wok, but a large pan/skillet also works.

15-ounce package extra-firm tofu

1 medium head broccoli, cut into small florets

½ cup low sodium vegetable broth

¼ cup soy *or* tamari sauce

1 tablespoon maple syrup

1 to 2 teaspoons garlic chili sauce

2 teaspoons cornstarch *or* arrowroot powder

2 teaspoons high heat cooking oil
(such as avocado)

½ small yellow onion, sliced

1 cup Thai basil (do not sub with regular basil; if you can't find, just skip it; if you can find, definitely add it!)

2 garlic cloves, minced

1 tablespoon fresh ginger, minced

1 red bell pepper, sliced

ACCOMPANIMENTS

Steamed rice *or* wide rice noodles

Toasted sesame seeds *or* crushed peanuts

Sliced scallions

1. Preheat the oven 375° F and line a rimmed baking sheet with parchment paper. This first step involves prepping the tofu. It may seem like extra work, but these extra couple of steps give the tofu a great texture and are well worth the effort. You will press and then bake the tofu before adding it to the stir-fry. Begin by wrapping the tofu in a kitchen towel or paper towels. Place the wrapped tofu on a plate and a cutting board on top of the tofu. Weigh down the tofu by placing a heavy item (canned beans, pot) on top of the cutting board. Feel free to use a tofu press if you have one. Allow the tofu to be pressed (20 to 30 minutes) to remove some of the moisture while you prep your remaining ingredients.

2. Cut the pressed tofu into roughly ¾-inch cubes and lay them in a single layer on the baking sheet. Bake for 15 to 20 minutes. You want the tofu slightly browned on the outside but still soft inside. Set the baked tofu aside.

3. While the tofu bakes, you can prep the rest of your ingredients, beginning by blanching your broccoli florets in a pot of boiling water for 3 to 5 minutes (the broccoli should be soft but still have a little bite to it). Rinse and set aside.

4. Make the sauce. In a glass measuring cup, combine the broth, tamari, maple syrup, and chili garlic sauce. In small bowl gently stir the cornstarch in a teaspoon or two of water to make a slurry. Add the slurry to the sauce and stir to combine. (Adding the cornstarch directly to the sauce without making the slurry can create clumps.)

5. The next few steps will move quickly so make sure all of your ingredients are prepped and ready to go. Warm your wok on medium-high heat. Warm the oil. Next add the sliced onions and sauté until golden brown. If you have Thai basil leaves, add them now. Next add the garlic and ginger and sauté for only a minute. Next add the peppers (and any additional veggies such as mushrooms or snap peas) and sauté for another couple of minutes.

6. Create a well in the middle by shifting the vegetables to the sides. Add your baked tofu and sauté for another couple of minutes. Next, add the broccoli. Mix to combine it all.

7. Give your sauce a quick stir before pouring it all over the stir-fry. Gently mix to combine. Simmer for 5 minutes, which will allow the flavors to combine and the sauce to thicken.

8. Serve over steamed rice or wide rice noodles and garnish with optional toasted sesame seeds or crushed peanuts and sliced scallions.

Burger Night

Burger night is a favorite among people of all ages. A delicious burger has certain prerequisites—a fresh whole grain bun (homemade or from a good bakery–grilled or toasted if you like), a firm and flavorful patty, and all the right fixings. To save time, you can purchase ready-made burger patties. There are a wide variety of tasty options from a traditional meat-like veggie patty, to whole food variations such as black bean and quinoa burgers. Serve burgers with a salad or veggies and dip. To make the meal extra special, add in a tray of baked potato wedges.

BEET BURGERS

1 large *or* 2 medium onions, coarsely chopped (about 2 cups)

6 cloves garlic, cut into quarters

1 tablespoon oil *or* 2 tablespoons broth

⅔ cup rolled oats

1 cup walnuts, pecans, *or* sunflower seeds

1 large *or* 2 medium beets, peeled and cut into chunks (about 2 cups shredded)

1 cup cooked brown, black, *or* red rice

2 cups cooked brown lentils

¼ cup ground flaxseed

2 tablespoons tamari *or* liquid aminos

1 teaspoon smoked paprika

2 tablespoons seasoning blend (store-bought *or* homemade— see on following page)

Salt and pepper to taste

1. Sauté the onions and garlic in oil or broth in a skillet on medium heat. Cover and cook for about 10 minutes, stirring occasionally, until soft. Let cool.

2. Pulse the oats, walnuts, pecans, or sunflower seeds to a course texture using a food processor. Transfer mixture to a large bowl.

3. Shred the beets in the food processor. Add to the bowl with the walnuts and oats.

4. Pulse the rice, lentils, and onion mixture until somewhat chunky.

5. Transfer to the large bowl with oats, walnuts, and beets.

6. Add the flaxseed, tamari, paprika, seasoning mix, salt, and pepper. Stir the dough until all the ingredients are evenly distributed.

7. Preheat the oven to 375° F.

8. Divide the dough into 12 patties. Start with a ball and flatten it out. Place on a lightly sprayed nonstick baking sheet or a silicone mat on a cookie sheet. Bake for 50 to 60 minutes, flipping burgers about halfway through baking. Serve on a whole grain bun with all the fixings.

SEASONING BLEND

MAKES ABOUT 1 CUP

2 tablespoons dried basil

2 tablespoons dried oregano

2 tablespoons onion powder *or* minced onion

1 tablespoon garlic powder *or* granules

1 tablespoon smoked paprika *or* regular paprika

1 teaspoon black pepper

1 teaspoon salt

1 teaspoon cayenne pepper

Place all ingredients in a glass jar. Shake well.

Stick with traditional burger toppings, or let your imagination run wild. Beyond the usual ketchup, mustard, relish, and mayo, consider the following:

THE FIXINGS

Avocado slices

BBQ sauce

Caramelized onions *or* thinly sliced sweet *or* purple raw onions

Velvety Cheeze Sauce (page 361)

Nut cheese

Lettuce

Salsa

Sautéed sliced mushrooms

Sliced dill pickles

Sliced tomatoes

Sprouts

Veggie bacon

Taco Night

MAKES 4 TO 6 SERVINGS

Taco night is a family favorite in many households. Once you make the filling, you can stuff it into hard taco shells, flour tortillas for a burrito, or use it as the base for a taco salad. You can use your favorite store-bought taco seasoning to save time or make the one included at the end of this recipe. Baking the tofu into crumbles gives the filling a nice texture. For an easy weeknight swap, you could also use ground veggie crumbles in place of the baked tofu crumbles.

14-ounce package extra-firm tofu

2 to 3 teaspoons olive oil

Medium onion, chopped

Green bell pepper, chopped

15-ounce can dark red kidney beans, rinsed and drained

15-ounce can black beans, rinsed and drained

Corn taco shells, flour tortillas, or corn tortilla chips

1 package store-bought taco seasoning or the following homemade recipe:

1. Preheat the oven to 375° F. Line a rimmed baking sheet with parchment paper.

2. If you are making the homemade taco seasoning, combine the spices in a small bowl and set aside.

3. Wrap the tofu with a kitchen towel or paper towels. Place the wrapped tofu on a plate and a cutting board on top of the tofu. Weigh down the tofu by placing a heavy item (canned beans, pot) on top of the cutting board. Feel free to use a tofu press if you have one. Allow the tofu to be pressed to remove some of the moisture while you prep your remaining ingredients.

4. Once the tofu has been pressed for 20 to 30 minutes, break it up into crumbles on the baking sheet. Bake for 20 to 25 minutes until beginning to brown.

5. While the tofu crumbles bake, warm the olive oil in a medium-sized pot. Add the onions and pepper and sauté until tender and beginning to brown.

6. Add the baked tofu crumbles, beans, and store-bought or homemade taco seasoning. Mix to combine.

7. Add ½ to ¾ cup of water to deglaze the bottom of the pot. Mix to combine and simmer for 5 to 10 minutes.

8. Use the taco filling in whatever way you like. Allow everyone at the table to add their own toppings.

TACO SEASONING MIX

2 tablespoons chili powder

1 tablespoon ground cumin

1 teaspoon smoked paprika

1 teaspoon garlic powder

1 teaspoon onion powder

½ teaspoon dried oregano

½ teaspoon salt

Freshly ground black pepper to taste

ACCOMPANIMENTS

Shredded romaine lettuce

Sliced black olives

Sliced scallions

Salsa

Plant-based shredded Cheddar

Peanut Dragon Bowl

MAKES 4 SERVINGS

This recipe is fun, filling, and flavorful. It is also versatile, as it can be prepared with a wide range of vegetables and toppings. If you end up with too much sauce, use leftovers as a dip for lettuce wraps or as a dressing for a full-meal salad.

SPICY PEANUT SAUCE

1 cup natural crunchy peanut butter

1 cup water

3 tablespoons tamari, soy sauce, *or* coconut aminos

3 cloves garlic, minced

1 tablespoon fresh grated ginger

1 tablespoon hot chili sauce (adjust to your taste)

½ can (200 ml) coconut milk (*or* other unsweetened, non-dairy milk)

2 teaspoons sesame oil

2 tablespoons lemon juice

BOWLS

10 cups washed and chopped vegetables of your choice (e.g., asparagus slices, small beet cubes, broccoli florets, Brussels sprout slices, cauliflower florets, carrot strips, green beans, chopped kale *or* other greens, thin purple onion slices, pepper slivers, snow peas, squash cubes, sweet potato cubes)

4 cups hot, cooked barley, farro, quinoa, *or* rice

3 cups hot, cooked beans (e.g., shelled edamame, garbanzo, cannellini) *or* veggie protein of your choice (e.g., tofu, tempeh, veggie chicken)

1. *Prepare sauce.* Put peanut butter and water in a medium saucepan. Heat on a low temperature stirring until smooth and creamy. Add tamari, garlic, ginger, hot sauce, coconut milk, and sesame oil. Cook on low heat for 15 to 20 minutes, stirring occasionally. Remove from heat. Stir in lemon juice.

2. *Prepare optional toppings.* Place toppings into small bowls so each person can top their own bowl with the favorites.

3. *Steam vegetables.* In a large saucepan, steam vegetables in a steamer basket. Put the longer cooking vegetables in the steamer first (squash, beets, sweet potatoes). Steam for about 15 minutes. Add in all other vegetables except greens. Cook another 7 to 8 minutes. Add greens and cook another 2 to 3 minutes or just until they are wilted.

4. *Assemble bowls.* To assemble the meal, place cooked grains into 4 bowls (use ½ cup for smaller bowls and 1 cup for larger bowls). Top each bowl with 2½ cups steamed vegetables. Add ¾ cup beans or other plant protein to each bowl. Sprinkle on optional toppings, as desired. Drizzle each bowl with dressing to taste.

OPTIONAL TOPPINGS

½ cup unsalted peanuts

2 tablespoons roasted black sesame seeds

½ cup green onions, chopped

½ cup parsley *or* cilantro

1 cup sprouts (your choice)

1 avocado, chopped

Lemon *or* lime wedges

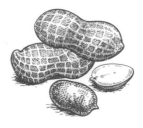

Lemony Chickpea Pasta with Mushrooms and Broccoli

MAKES 3 TO 4 SERVINGS

This pasta dish comes together for a quick weeknight meal. You can double the recipe to have extra for lunch boxes. The chickpea pasta has a nice hearty flavor. When using citrus in a recipe, try to remember to use the zest as well. It adds amazing flavor and puts all of your lemon to good use.

8-ounce package chickpea pasta (shells, elbow, *or* rotini work well)

2 teaspoons olive oil

Pinch red pepper flakes, optional

Medium onion, diced

2 to 3 garlic cloves, minced

Half pound sliced mushrooms

2 to 3 cups spinach

1 large head broccoli, cut into small florets

Zest of a lemon

Juice from ½ lemon

Salt

Pepper

OPTIONAL:

Chopped fresh parsley,

Vegan parm (see recipe next page)

1. Bring a large pot of salted water to boil for the pasta. Add the pasta.

2. While the pasta is cooking, heat a large skillet or pan (make sure it is large because your pasta will also go in this pan). Warm the olive oil. Add a pinch of optional red pepper flakes and the onions. Sauté until golden brown.

3. Next, add the garlic and sauté for another minute or so.

4. Add the sliced mushrooms and ½ teaspoon of salt to the onions. Sauté the mushrooms until they are caramelized and soft, adding a bit of water if they are sticking to the pan. Lastly, add the spinach and cook until wilted.

5. When your pasta is almost cooked through, add the broccoli florets directly into the pot with the pasta and cook for an additional 3–5 minutes until both the pasta and broccoli are cooked through.

6. Drain and toss the pasta/broccoli mixture into the pan with the mushrooms. Mix to combine. Add the lemon zest and finish with a squeeze of lemon juice and salt and pepper to taste.

7. Garnish with fresh parsley and optional vegan parm.

CHEF'S TIP: The stems of broccoli are quite delicious! Trim away the woody part of the stalk as well as the tough outer edges using a knife or vegetable peeler. The middle part has a mild flavor and can be sliced up and used in whatever recipe you are making.

BONUS VEGAN PARM

This cashew-free vegan parm comes together in sixty seconds or less!

- ¾ cup almond meal
- ¼ cup nutritional yeast
- 1 teaspoon onion granules
- 1 teaspoon garlic granules
- ½ teaspoon salt

Mix to combine in a mason jar. Great over pastas, soups, salads, and popcorn.

The Ultimate Veggie Lasagna

Lasagna is a perennial family favorite. It's a wonderful way to feed a crowd, and is always a hit at a potluck. This one is entirely plant-based, veggie-rich, dairy-free, and yummy! Lasagna is always a bit of a project, so to speed the process, prepare the tofu ricotta ahead of time. You could also cook the lentils and prepare the veggies in advance. You can skip a step and select no-boil noodles, but you'll need to add an extra cup of tomato sauce. Use the extra sauce to cover the top of the lasagna so the noodles on top will cook. Add hot sauce or hot peppers to the sauce if you want to spice it up.

1 recipe tofu ricotta (on right)

1 bunch fresh spinach (about 4 cups, chopped) *or* 1 10–12 ounce package frozen spinach

2 cups mushrooms, sliced

1 onion, diced

4 cloves garlic, minced

1 pepper (any color), thinly sliced

1 zucchini, cut in half lengthwise and thinly sliced

1 tablespoon olive oil *or* 3 tablespoons vegetable broth, water, *or* wine

1 tablespoon Italian seasoning (*or* a mix of basil, oregano, and thyme)

½ teaspoon salt

¼ teaspoon pepper

12 lasagna noodles (whole wheat, spinach, brown rice, *or* your choice)

4½ cups marinara sauce

1½ cups cooked red *or* small brown lentils *or* 1 package burger crumbles

1 cup plant-based shredded mozzarella *or* Vegan Parm (see page 373)

2 tomatoes, sliced

2 tablespoons fresh basil *or* 2 teaspoons dried basil

TOFU RICOTTA

1 cup cashews

½ cup water

3 tablespoons fresh lemon juice *or* 2 tablespoons apple cider vinegar

4 cloves garlic, minced

¾ teaspoon salt

¼ cup nutritional yeast

1 package (12–16-ounce) firm tofu, pressed

1. *Prepare the tofu ricotta.* Soak the cashews in enough water to cover them completely. Let sit 4–6 hours or overnight. For a quick soak method, soak in boiling water for 30 minutes. Drain cashews and rinse well. In a food processor, combine soaked cashews, water, lemon juice, garlic, salt, and nutritional yeast. Blend until fairly smooth. Crumble the tofu into the processor and pulse until distributed through the cashew mixture, but not smooth (you want it to look and feel like ricotta cheese).

2. *Prepare the vegetables.* Thaw spinach if using frozen and squeeze out excess moisture. If using fresh, wash and coarsely chop. In a large hot pan, dry sauté the mushrooms over medium heat for 5 to 10 minutes. Do not stir. Add onions, garlic, peppers, zucchini, and broth, wine or oil, and cook covered another 5 to 10 minutes or until vegetables are tender. Add spinach and cook just until wilted (about a minute). Drain any excess liquid. Turn off the heat. Stir in Italian seasoning, salt, and pepper.

3. *Cook the noodles (unless using no-boil noodles).* Prepare noodles as directed on the package. Drain with cold water to prevent noodles from sticking to one another.

4. *Prepare sauce.* Stir lentils or burger crumbles into marinara sauce.

5. Preheat oven to 350° F.

6. Assemble the lasagna in a 9 x 13-inch casserole dish:

   a. Spread 1½ cups sauce on the bottom of the casserole dish.

   b. Top with 4 cooked lasagna noodles, 3 lengthwise and 1 sideways, to fill the gap (cut a little off to make it fit).

   c. Spread half the ricotta on the noodles, then top with half the vegetables.

   d. repeat the layering with sauce, noodles, ricotta, and vegetables, ending with a final layer of noodles.

   e. Place sliced tomatoes attractively on top.

   f. Cover with foil and cook for 25 to 30 minutes. Remove foil, and sprinkle with vegan mozzarella cheese. If you are not using the mozzarella, sprinkle with vegan cheese and herbs.

   g. Bake uncovered for another 30 to 35 minutes or until golden brown. If the cheese and top don't brown well, broil for 2 to 3 minutes or until it browns nicely. Let stand 10 minutes to set, slice, and serve with a green salad.

Kind Shepherd's Pie

MAKES ABOUT 8 HEARTY SERVINGS

This classic comfort food is composed of a rich, savory base, a veggie center, and a smooth topping of mashed potato. If you prefer, substitute sweet potatoes for some or all of the potatoes. You can also replace up to half of the potatoes with parsnips and/ or cauliflower. If you have any Velvety Cheeze Sauce on hand (page 361), you can add a thin layer on top before baking. French lentils or small brown lentils are preferred in the base layer, but regular lentils can be substituted, if need be.

BASE LAYER

3 cups mushrooms, sliced

¼ teaspoon salt

1 large onion, diced

4 cloves garlic, minced

1 tablespoon avocado *or* olive oil *or* 2 tablespoons vegetable broth

3 cups cooked lentils (see page 327 for cooking instructions)

¾ cup walnuts, finely chopped

1 tablespoon optional vegetarian Worcestershire sauce

4 tablespoons tamari *or* liquid aminos

1 teaspoon marjoram

1 teaspoon rosemary

1 teaspoon sage

1 teaspoon thyme

3 tablespoons cornstarch

1½ cups unsweetened, nondairy milk

Freshly ground pepper, to taste

MIDDLE LAYER

5 cups mixed vegetables (carrots, cauliflower, corn, green beans, peas, peppers, etc.), chopped into small pieces

2 tablespoons all purpose, whole wheat, *or* gluten-free flour

¼ cup unsweetened soy milk *or* other non-dairy milk

½ teaspoon salt

Pepper to taste

TOP LAYER

½ cup unsweetened soy milk, *or* other unsweetened non-dairy beverage

¼ cup cashews, soaked *or* rinsed well (optional addition)

4 to 6 large potatoes (about 2 ½ to 3 pounds/ 1.1 to 1.4 kg), washed, peeled, cut in halves *or* quarters, and boiled

¾–1 teaspoon salt

White *or* black pepper, to taste

Rosemary, thyme, *or* paprika as optional garnish

1. Prepare the base layer. Begin by dry sautéing the mushrooms. Heat a large saucepan over medium heat, add mushrooms and a dash of salt. Let cook for 5 to 10 minutes until the mushrooms begin to caramelize—do not stir. Add onion, garlic, oil, or broth, and cook another 5 to 7 minutes. Add cooked lentils, walnuts, optional Worcestershire sauce, tamari, marjoram, rosemary, sage, and thyme. Cook on low heat for 10 to 15 minutes. Whisk together cornstarch and non-dairy milk. Add to lentil mixture and stir until the gravy thickens. Add pepper to taste.

2. Prepare the middle layer. If using frozen vegetables, thaw in a bowl, and toss with flour, milk, salt, and pepper. If using fresh or a combination of fresh and frozen, steam the fresh vegetables for about 5 minutes before tossing. They should be very tender crisp as they will cook more fully in the oven.

3. Prepare the top layer. If you're making cashew cream, blend milk and cashews until a thick cream is formed. Drain cooked potatoes and mash with nondairy milk or cashew cream, salt, and pepper.

4. Preheat oven to 375° F.

5. Assemble the pie. Use a large casserole dish (or two smaller casserole dishes). Begin by spreading the base layer evenly in the dish. Add the vegetable layer evenly on top. Spread the mashed potato layer evenly over the vegetables. Score potatoes with a fork and sprinkle with rosemary, thyme, and/or paprika, if desired. Bake uncovered for 50 to 60 minutes or until heated through and nicely browned on the top. Serve hot.

Roasted Chickpeas

These chickpeas are great tossed in a salad, on top of a cream soup, or to enjoy as a snack. They travel well in a small container, and make the perfect addition to restaurant meals that may be lacking protein (e.g., veggie stir fries, salads, soups)

15-ounce can chickpeas

1 teaspoon olive oil

½ teaspoon salt

¼ teaspoon freshly ground black pepper

Optional: 1 teaspoon curry powder, cumin powder, *or* smoked paprika

1. Preheat oven to 400° F. Line a baking sheet with parchment paper.

2. Rinse and drain the chickpeas. If you have a few extra minutes, allow the chickpeas to dry in a single layer on a dish towel. Removing the moisture creates a crispier texture.

3. Lay the chickpeas on the lined baking sheet. Drizzle with olive oil, salt, pepper, and your choice of spice. Gently mix to coat.

4. Bake in a single layer at 400° F. For softer chickpeas, bake for 15 to 20 minutes (great for the curried chickpea salad on page 341) or on top of salads. For a crispier texture bake for an additional 5 to 10 minutes.

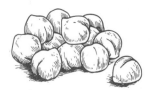

Edamame with Lime and Sea Salt

MAKES 3 TO 4 SERVINGS

Seasoning the outside of the edamame gives them a boost of flavor as you can eat them by squeezing the edamame directly into your mouth. Consider saving this snack for older children as the pods can be difficult for younger children and can pose a choking risk. Perfect for after-school snack, the lunch box, or as a dinner side.

10-ounce frozen package edamame in the pod

Juice of ½ lime

½ teaspoon kosher *or* flaked sea salt*

Toasted sesame seeds

1. Bring a medium-sized pot of salted water to boil.

2. Add the frozen edamame (no need to defrost).

3. Cook for about 5 minutes. You can test one for doneness. You want them fully cooked through but not mushy.

4. Drain the edamame and place into a bowl.

5. Squeeze the lime juice over the edamame. Sprinkle with salt and toss to combine.

6. Garnish with toasted sesame seeds.

Please note that Kosher salt is not iodized, so if using as your primary salt, be sure to include a source of iodine.

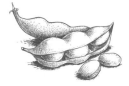

Baby Biscuits

MAKES ABOUT 30 TO 36 BISCUITS

If you look at the ingredient list of traditional teething biscuits, the first 3 ingredients are generally white flour (listed as enriched wheat flour), sugar, and oil. In contrast, these biscuits are nutrition gems with fresh banana as the only sweetener. Peanut butter, fortified infant cereal, oats, and hemp seeds are the other key ingredients. In place of hemp seeds you could also use chia seeds or ground flaxseed.

1 very ripe medium-sized banana

½ cup smooth peanut butter

1 teaspoon vanilla

½ cup iron-fortified infant oatmeal

½ cup instant oatmeal or ground rolled oats

2 tablespoons hemp seeds

½ teaspoon baking powder

½ teaspoon cinnamon (optional)

1. Preheat oven to 200° F.
2. In a medium bowl, mash the banana, and stir in the peanut butter and vanilla.
3. In a small bowl combine the dry ingredients—infant oatmeal, instant oats, hemp seeds, baking powder, and cinnamon. Stir to combine.
4. Add dry ingredients to banana mixture.
5. Line a cookie sheet with a silicone mat or parchment paper, or spray lightly.
6. Roll the dough to about ¼-inch thick or less. Sprinkle a little infant oatmeal on a board or on your counter surface to keep the dough from sticking.
7. Using a cookie cutter, cut out shapes and use a spatula to lift cookies onto the cookie sheet.
8. Bake for about 45 minutes or until nicely browned. Remove from oven and let sit for about a day to get crispy. Store in an airtight container in the freezer to retain crispiness. Serve right out of the freezer.

Toddler Cookies

MAKES 30 COOKIES

These cookies pack a powerful nutrition punch and are great for toddlers. The key ingredients are black beans, nut butter, and iron-fortified infant cereal–amazing!

15-ounce can black beans
(drained and rinsed)

½ cup nut butter

2 tablespoons maple syrup

1 teaspoon vanilla

½ cup fortified baby oatmeal

2 tablespoons ground flax

1 teaspoon baking powder

1 teaspoon cinnamon

½ cup raisins (optional)

1. Preheat oven to 325° F.

2. In a food processor, process the beans until smooth.

3. Add nut butter, maple syrup, and vanilla, and process until well combined.

4. In a small bowl, combine infant oatmeal, ground flax, baking powder, and cinnamon. Add to processor and pulse until dough is smooth.

5. Remove dough and stir in raisins.

6. Line 2 cookie sheets with silicone mats or parchment paper, or spray lightly. Roll dough into 1-inch balls and press down to flatten.

7. Bake for 12 to 15 minutes or until lightly browned.

VARIATIONS

1. Add 2 tablespoons cocoa powder and 1 extra tablespoon maple syrup.

2. Replace raisins with semi-sweet chocolate chips or dark chocolate chunks.

Clever Crackers

MAKES ABOUT 48 SMALL CRACKERS

These crackers are tasty, nutritious, and fun to make with your little ones. Feel free to use whatever seeds you have on hand—mix and match. You can also vary the flour by using ½ cup whole wheat flour, and ¼ cup of almond, coconut, buckwheat, or other flour.

4 tablespoons cold avocado oil

½ cup fortified baby oatmeal

¾ cup whole wheat flour

1 teaspoon baking powder

½ teaspoon salt

2 tablespoons hemp seeds

2 tablespoons sesame seeds

2 tablespoons ground flaxseed

½ cup ice cold water

1. Put avocado oil in the freezer for at least an hour until very cold.

2. Put baby oatmeal, flour, baking powder, salt, hemp, sesame, and flaxseeds in a medium-sized bowl. Stir to combine.

3. Remove oil from freezer. Stir oil and water together in a measuring cup or small bowl.

4. Pour the wet ingredients into the dry ingredients and stir just until a dough is formed.

5. Roll as thin as possible (thinner is crispier). Cut into squares or use a smaller cookie cutter for fun shapes.

6. Place on a sprayed baking sheet or on a baking sheet lined with a silicone mat.

7. Preheat oven to 375° F. Bake for about 15 minutes or until nicely browned (watch closely as they finish quickly).

Snickerdoodle Hummus

MAKES ABOUT 1½ CUPS

If you've never tried a sweet hummus, you don't know what you're missing. It's great with sliced apples, crackers, pretzels, or even straight off a spoon. Full of protein, fiber, and, of course, deliciousness. Use ¼ cup of maple syrup if you prefer a less sweet version.

15-ounce can chickpeas, rinsed and drained

½ cup almond butter

¼ to ½ cup maple syrup, depending on desired level of sweetness

1 teaspoon ground cinnamon

¼ teaspoon sea salt

1. Place chickpeas, almond butter, maple syrup, cinnamon and sea salt in a food processor and process until smooth and creamy.

VARIATIONS

1. *Peanut Butter Hummus:* replace almond butter with peanut butter and cinnamon with 1 teaspoon vanilla extract.

2. *Chocolate Hummus:* using either almond or peanut butter, replace the cinnamon with ¼ cup cocoa powder.

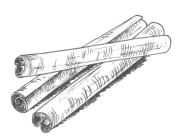

Crispy Seedy Cookies

MAKES ABOUT 45 COOKIES

These crispy cookies are flour free and gluten free (when gluten-free oats are selected). Also rich in essential fatty acids, they are simply delicious!

1 cup nut *or* seed butter

2 tablespoons oil

½ cup maple syrup

¾ teaspoon salt

1 teaspoon vanilla

⅓ cup ground flaxseed

⅓ cup chia seeds

½ cup sunflower seeds

½ cup finely chopped walnuts

1 cup rolled oats

1. Preheat oven to 325° F.

2. In a medium to large bowl, stir together nut butter, oil, maple syrup, salt, and vanilla.

3. Add flaxseed, chia seeds, sunflower seeds, walnuts, and rolled oats. Stir until well mixed.

4. Drop by heaping teaspoons onto sprayed cookie sheet or silicone mats on cookie sheets. Flatten with a fork dipped in water (re-dip for each cookie). Cookies should be as flat as possible to make them crispy.

5. Bake for about 20 minutes or until golden brown. Cooking time varies and is generally longer if using silicone mats. Watch carefully, so as not to burn the bottoms.

6. Remove from oven, cool, and store in an airtight container. To help maintain crispiness, leave out only what you will use within a day or two. Freeze the rest—they are great right out of the freezer!

VARIATION

To make these cookies oil free and sugar free, replace the maple syrup with one cup of date paste and omit the oil.

BONUS DATE PASTE

1½ cups dates, packed

1 cup boiling water

½ teaspoon vanilla

1. Place dates in a large glass measuring cup, then cover with boiling water and let sit for 15 minutes.

2. Pour into a blender. Add vanilla and blend until smooth.

Chickpea Chocolate Chip Cookies

This isn't your typical chocolate chip cookie. It's much denser and heartier. It's incredibly satisfying and delicious. The flaked sea salt is an optional addition. A little goes a long way and it adds a special touch.

15-ounce can chickpeas, drained and rinsed

½ cup maple syrup

½ cup creamy peanut butter (or other nut butter)

1 teaspoon vanilla extract

1 cup rolled oats

½ cup walnuts, chopped

½ cup almond flour

¼ cup chia seeds

¼ cup hemp seeds

1 to 2 cups chocolate chips *or* raisins (depending on how chocolatey you want them!)

flaked sea salt, optional

1. Preheat the oven to 375° F.

2. In a food processor, puree the chickpeas with the maple syrup, peanut butter, and vanilla until smooth.

3. Empty the puree into a medium-sized mixing bowl. Without bothering to clean out the food processor, pulse the oats until they are coarse (somewhere between whole oats and oat flour). If you have larger walnuts, pulse them a few times with the oats.

4. Add the oats and remaining ingredients to the bowl. Mix until combined.

5. Using a mini ice cream scooper, place the dough on a parchment lined baking sheet, making roughly 20 to 24 smaller cookies.

6. Gently press down to flatten. Sprinkle each cookie with the tiniest pinch of salt.

7. Bake for 10 to 15 minutes until cooked through and slightly golden. If you prefer a softer cookie, take them out on the earlier side. Leaving them in for too long will dry out the cookie.

Molasses Tahini Energy Balls

MAKES ABOUT 32 TO 36 BALLS

These protein-rich energy balls are high in calcium, iron, and omega-3 fatty acids. Add a tablespoon of fresh grated ginger for a flavor boost, if desired. If you prefer, roll in hemp seeds, coconut, or a mix of seeds.

1 cup walnuts

½ cup sunflower *or* pumpkin seeds (or a combination)

1 cup dates, tightly packed (soak in hot water for 15–30 minutes to soften, if hard)

¼ cup tahini

¼ cup almond butter (*or* other nut butter)

¼ cup organic blackstrap molasses

1 teaspoon pure vanilla extract *or* ½ teaspoon of vanilla powder

¼ cup hemp seeds

¼ cup chia seeds

¼ teaspoon salt

4 to 5 tablespoons sesame seeds (raw *or* roasted)

1. In a food processor, coarsely chop walnuts and sunflower/pumpkin seeds. Pour into a bowl.

2. Process dates, tahini, almond butter, blackstrap molasses, and vanilla in the food processor until it forms a smooth dough.

3. Add hemp seeds, chia seeds, and walnut mixture to the dough and pulse just until nuts and seeds are distributed through the dough—don't over-process.

4. With a spatula, put the dough into a bowl. If it is sticky, place in the fridge for an hour or more for easier handling.

5. Form into 1-inch balls. Roll in sesame seeds. Refrigerate or freeze.

Peanut Butter Brownies

MAKES 16 BARS

These brownies can be made peanut-free by substituting another nut butter or sunflower butter for the peanut butter in both recipes. If you would rather not ice the brownies, you can drizzle with melted chocolate after baking.

2 cups dates, packed

1 cup water

½ cup peanut butter

1 teaspoon vanilla

¼ cup avocado oil*

2 tablespoons ground flaxseed

½ cup whole wheat flour (*or* other flour)

6 tablespoons cocoa powder

2 teaspoons baking powder

½ teaspoon salt

1 cup walnuts, chopped (optional)

1. Preheat oven to 350° F.

2. In a medium saucepan, bring dates and water to a boil, then simmer on low heat until dates are soft. Mash well.

3. In a large bowl, stir together peanut butter, vanilla, avocado oil, flaxseed, and dates.

4. In a small bowl, combine whole wheat flour, cocoa powder, baking powder, and salt.

5. Stir flour mixture into wet ingredients. Add walnuts and stir just until blended.

6. Spread into a sprayed 8 x 8 baking pan. Bake for 30–40 minutes until a cake tester comes out clean. Cool before icing.

7. Store in an airtight container for up to 4 days. They freeze beautifully.

If you prefer not to use oil, substitute an equal amount of apple sauce for the oil. This does affect texture and richness, but it works!

CHOCOLATE/PEANUT BUTTER FROSTING

2 cups soft dates (if dates are hard, soak in hot water for 15 minutes and drain, *or* steam until soft)

½ cup non-dairy milk (e.g., almond, cashew, *or* coconut)

¼ cup cocoa powder

½ cup peanut butter

1 teaspoon vanilla

1. Blend all ingredients in a food processor until smooth.

2. Use to frost brownies. You need only about ½ to ⅔ the recipe for the brownies. With leftover frosting, use as a filling for Medjool dates (remove pits and stuff with frosting and a Brazil nut or 2 to 3 hazelnuts or almonds). The dates freeze beautifully and make a lovely dessert or lunch box treat.

Oatmeal Bars

MAKES 16 SQUARES

These bars are great for an afternoon pick-me-up, a quick breakfast on the go, or even a sweet treat for dessert. Be adventurous and play around with the dried fruit, nuts, and/or seeds, and additional seasonings.

2 cups old-fashioned oats

½ cup walnuts

¼ cup ground flaxseed

½ teaspoon cinnamon

¼ teaspoon salt

2 ripe bananas (about ¾ cup)

½ cup raisins

¼ to ½ cup dark chocolate chips (optional)

1 tablespoon sesame seeds

¼ cup dried, unsweetened coconut

1. Preheat the oven to 350° F and line a 9-inch square baking pan with parchment paper, allowing for an overhang of paper on the sides.

2. Pulse the oats a few times in a food processor and empty into a bowl.

3. Pulse the walnuts (especially if they are large chunks or walnut halves) in the food processor a few times to create small pieces and empty into a bowl with the oats.

4. Add the ground flaxseed, cinnamon, and salt, and mix through.

5. Place the bananas in the food processor (no need to clean out in between) and pulse until the bananas are roughly pureed, being careful not to over-process (a few chunks are okay, but you don't want any big pieces).

6. Add the bananas to the oat mixture and mix in. Add the raisins and optional chocolate chips.

7. Press the mixture into the lined baking pan. You can use the bottom of a small bowl or measuring cup to smooth the filling into the pan. Sprinkle the sesame seeds and coconut on top. Gently press into the dough.

8. Bake at 350° F for 15 to 20 minutes until cooked through.

9. Allow to cool in the pan for 5 to 10 minutes, and then lift out gently using the parchment overhang. Cool for another 10 minutes or so. Slice into squares and enjoy!

Apple Crisp

This simple, wholesome apple crisp is a great addition to any family dinner. Once the chopping is done, this dessert pulls together in just a few minutes. If you like, top each serving with vanilla "Nice Cream" (page 391) or Cashew Pear Cream (page 390).

FILLING

8 apples, washed, cored, and thinly sliced (no need to peel)

1 tablespoon lemon juice

2 tablespoons maple syrup

1 teaspoon ground cinnamon

½ teaspoon fresh grated nutmeg (optional)

1 teaspoon vanilla

1 tablespoon cornstarch

Pinch of salt

TOPPING

3 tablespoons maple syrup

3 tablespoons cashew *or* almond butter

2 tablespoons nondairy milk

1 teaspoon vanilla extract

1 cup old-fashioned rolled oats

¼ cup whole wheat flour, almond, *or* other flour

⅓ cup chopped walnuts *or* pecans

1 teaspoon cinnamon

Pinch of salt

1. Preheat the oven to 350° F.

2. For the filling, in a large bowl, toss apples with lemon juice, maple syrup, cinnamon, nutmeg, vanilla, cornstarch, and salt.

3. For the topping, in a medium bowl, stir together maple syrup, nut butter, non-dairy milk, and vanilla. Add in oats, flour, walnuts, cinnamon, and salt. Stir until nicely combined.

4. Spray or oil a large deep casserole dish. Put the apple mixture in the dish and flatten. Sprinkle the topping evenly over the apple mixture and press down with a spatula or moistened hands to flatten.

5. Bake for about 40 minutes or until golden brown. Serve hot with milk or Nice Cream (see page 391).

VARIATION

Peach or berry crisp. Follow instructions but swap out the apples with an equal amount of peaches or berries, and replace the cornstarch with ¼ cup flour. Coat berries or peaches with flour and proceed with recipe.

Cashew Pear Cream

MAKES 3½ CUPS

This cream is an excellent topping for pancakes, waffles, or breakfast bowls, or with desserts such as puddings, fruit salads, baked fruit, fruit crisps, or parfaits. To make a thicker cream that is suitable as a whipping cream substitute on pumpkin pie or other desserts, use 1¾ cups cashews, and for a thinner cream sauce, use 1 to 1¼ cups cashews. If you have a high-powered blender, you can just rinse the cashews before blending, although soaking is preferred. The recipe can be cut in half using a 14-ounce jar of pears if you want a smaller batch.

1 28-ounce jar *or* can pears in water *or* juice

1½ cups raw cashews

1 teaspoon vanilla

1. Place the cashews in a bowl and cover with at least an inch of water. Soak for 2 to 3 hours. Drain and rinse the cashews.

2. Put pears with juice, cashews, and vanilla in a blender, and blend on high speed for 1 to 2 minutes until very creamy and smooth.

3. Store in a glass jar in the refrigerator for 5 to 7 days.

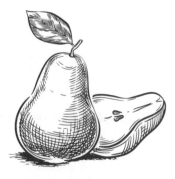

Nice Cream

This simple nondairy dessert is reminiscent of soft-serve ice cream. It's high in potassium and protective phytochemicals and is a superb sweet treat without added sugar.

2 large *or* 3 regular bananas, peeled, cut into chunks and frozen solid (freeze on a cookie sheet in a single layer then transfer into a freezer bag).

2 cups frozen berries, cherries, diced mango, *or* pineapple chunks

¼ cup fortified unsweetened soy milk *or* other nondairy milk

SUGGESTED TOPPINGS

Berries

Fruit sauce

Nuts (e.g., chopped almonds, hazelnuts, peanuts, pecans, *or* walnuts)

Seeds (e.g., chia seeds, roasted sunflower, *or* pumpkin seeds)

Chocolate chips *or* chunks

Granola

Shredded coconut

Put all the ingredients in a food processor and process until smooth. Serve immediately with your choice of toppings.

VARIATIONS

1. *Vanilla Nice Cream.* Double the bananas and eliminate the other fruit. Add ½ teaspoon vanilla extract or ¼ teaspoon vanilla powder.

2. *Chocolate Nice Cream.* Make vanilla Nice Cream and add 2 tablespoons cocoa powder. You may want to add 1 or 2 tablespoons of maple syrup to increase sweetness.

CHEF'S TIP: A high-powered blender with a tamper can be used instead of the food processor. Increase milk to ⅓ cup. Alternatively, Nice Cream can be made without any milk using a Champion or Green Star juicer or a Yonana machine (less expensive option).

Resources

"The single greatest lesson the garden teaches is that
our relationship to the planet need not be zero-sum, and that as long
as the sun still shines and people still can plan and plant,
think and do, we can, if we bother to try, find ways to provide
for ourselves without diminishing the world."

—*Michael Pollan*

Website, books, cookbooks, and other resources are provided for continued exploration. The list is not exhaustive but rather provides a sampling of resources that you might find useful. We have most likely missed many wonderful resources, so do continue to explore and share what you have found to be particularly helpful. While we don't endorse any specific program or service, we hope you find these resources valuable.

WEBSITES

Authors' Websites

nourishthebook.com
reshmashahmd.com
brendadavisrd.com

Nutrition

drfuhrman.com
ewg.org/foodnews/dirty-dozen.php
fdc.nal.usda.gov
foodrevolution.org
health.gov/our-work/food-nutrition/2015
    -2020-dietary-guidelines/guidelines
healthychildren.org
lpi.oregonstate.edu/mic
nal.usda.gov/fnic/dietary-reference-intakes
nutritionfacts.org
ods.od.nih.gov/factsheets/list-all
pcrm.org
plantbaseddietitian.com
plantbaseddocs.com
theveganrd.com
veganhealth.org
vegetariannutrition.net
vndpg.org
vrg.org

Getting Started with a Plant-Based, Vegan Lifestyle

byanygreensnecessary.com
colleenpatrickgoudreau.com
farmsanctuary.org
happycow.net
humanesociety.org
mercyforanimals.org/files/VSG.pdf
nomeatathlete.com
onegreenplanet.org/
pcrm.org/good-nutrition/plant-based-diets/
    vegan-starter-kit
peta.org/living/food/free-vegan-starter-kit
plantricianproject.org/quickstartguide
plantstrong.com

Cooking Blogs

acouplecooks.com
deliciouslyella.com
emilieeats.com
frommybowl.com
minimalistbaker.com
ohsheglows.com
pickuplimes.com
plantbasedartist.com
plantbasedonabudget.com
rainbowplantlife.com
simpleveganista.com
sweetpotatosoul.com
sweetsimplevegan.com
thefirstmess.com
thefullhelping.com
thevegan8.com
veganricha.com

BOOKS

Cookbooks

Artisan Vegan Cheese by Miyoko Schinner
Eat to Live Quick and Easy Cookbook by Joel
    Fuhrman
Frugal Vegan by Katie Koteen and Kate Kasbee
I Can Cook Vegan by Isa Chandra Moskowitz
Master Plants Cookbook by Margarita Restrepo
    and Michele Lastella
Plant Powered Families by Dreena Burton
Plant-based on a Budget by Toni Okamoto
Plant-Powered for Life by Sharon Palmer
Power Plates by Gena Hamshaw
Simple Green Meal by Jen Hanscard
Sweet Potato Soul by Jeanne Claiborne
The 22 Day Revolution Cookbook by Morco Borges
The Blue Zones Kitchen by Dan Buettner
The College Vegan Cookbook by Heather Nicholds
The Conscious Cook by Tal Ronnen
The How Not to Die Cookbook by Michael Greger
The Kick Diabetes Cookbook by Brenda Davis and
    Vesanto Melina

The No Meat Athlete Cookbook by Matt Frazier
and Stephanie Romine

The Plantpower Way by Rich Roll and Julie Piatt

The Ultimate Vegan Cookbook by Emily von Euw,
Kathy Hester, Linda and Alex Meyer, Marie
Reginato, Celine Steen, and Amber St Peter

The Vegan Instant Pot Cookbook by Nisha Vora

The Vegetarian Flavor Bible by Karen Page

The Whole Foods Cookbook by John Mackey

Vegan 100 by Gaz Oakley

Vegan Meal Prep by JL Fields

Vegan Richa's Everyday Kitchen by Richa Hingle

Vegan Under Pressure by Jill Nussinow

Veganomicon by Isa Chandra Moskowitz

Vegetable Kingdom by Bryant Terry

Nutrition/Plant-Based Books

31-Day Food Revolution by Ocean Robbins

Becoming Vegan: Comprehensive and Express
Editions by Brenda Davis and Vesanto Melina

Disease-Proof Your Child by Joel Fuhrman

How Not to Die by Michael Greger

How to Eat by Mark Bittman and David Katz

The Alzheimer's Solution by Ayesha Sherzai and
Dean Sherzai

The Book of Veganish by Kathy Freston

The Engine 2 Diet by Rip Esselstyn

The Idiot's Guide to Plant-Based Nutrition by
Julieanna Hever

The Mindful Vegan by Lani Muelrath

The Plant-Powered Diet by Sharon Palmer

The Whole Foods Diet by John Mackey

Vegan for Life by Jack Norris and Virginia
Messina

Whole by T. Colin Campbell

Your Complete Vegan Pregnancy by Reed Mangels

Environment

Comfortably Unaware by Richard Oppenlander

Eat for the Planet by Nil Zacharias and Gene Stone

Food Is the Solution by Matthew Prescott

Kiss the Ground by Josh Tickell

The Uninhabitable Earth by David Wallace-Wells

We Are the Weather by Jonathan Safran Foer

Ethics

A Plea for the Animals by Matthieu Ricard

Animalkind by Ingrid Newkirk and Gene Stone

Dominion by Matthew Scully

Eating Animals by Jonathan Safran Foer

Empty Cages by Tom Regan

How to Create a Vegan World by Tobias Leenaert

The Ethics of What We Eat by Peter Singer and
Jim Mason

The Face on Your Plate by Jeffrey Moussaieff
Masson

Why We Love Dogs, Eat Pigs, and Wear Cows
by Melanie Joy

Feeding

Helping Your Child with Extreme Picky Eating
by Katja Rowell and Jenny McGlothlin

Secrets of Feeding a Healthy Family by Ellyn Satter

Your Child's Weight: Helping Without Harming
by Ellyn Satter

References

Introduction

1. http://www.worldwatch.org/peak-meat-production-strains-land-and-water-resources-1

Chapter 1: Health

1. Satija A, Bhupathiraju SN, Spiegelman D, et al. Healthful and Unhealthful Plant-Based Diets and the Risk of Coronary Heart Disease in U.S. Adults. *J Am Coll Cardiol.* 2017;70(4):411–422.

2. Messina V, Mangels AR. Considerations in Planning Vegan Diets: Children. *Journal of the American Dietetic Association.* 2001;101: 661–669.

3. Jacobs C and Dwyer JT. Vegetarian Children: Appropriate and Inappropriate Diets. *American Journal of Clinical Nutrition.* 1988; 48; 811–818.

4. O'Connell JM, Deibly MJ et al. Growth of Vegetarian Children: The Farm Study. *Pediatrics.* 1989; 84 (3): 475–481.

5. https://www.cdc.gov/nccdphp/dnpao/growthcharts/who/breastfeeding/index.htm

6. Sander TA. Growth and Development of British Vegan Children. *American Journal of Clinical Nutrition.* 1988; 48: 822–825.

7. Sabaté, J. Attained Height of Lacto-Ovo Vegetarian Children and Adolescents. *European Journal of Clinical Nutrition.* 1991; 45: 51–58.

8. Nathan I, Hackett AF, Kirby S. A Longitudinal Study of the Growth of Matched Pairs of Vegetarian and Omnivorous Children, Aged 7–11 Years, in the Northwest of England. *European Journal of Clinical Nutrition.* 1997; 51: 20–25.

9. Sanders TA, Manning J. The Growth and Development of Vegan Children. *Journal of Human Nutrition and Dietetics.* 1992; 5: 11–21.

10. Yen CE, Yen CH, Huang MC, Cheng CH, Huang YC. Dietary intake and nutritional status of vegetarian and omnivorous preschool children and their parents in Taiwan. *Nutr Res.* 2008;28(7):430–436.

11. Leung SSF, Lee RHY, Sung RYT, et al. Growth and nutrition of Chinese vegetarian children in Hong Kong. *J Paediatr Child Health.* 2001;37(3):247–253.

12. Weder S, Hoffmann M, Becker K, Alexy U, Keller M. Energy, macronutrient intake, and anthropometrics of vegetarian, vegan, and omnivorous children (1–3 years) in Germany (VeChi diet study). *Nutrients.* 2019;11(4):1–18.

13. Richter M, Boeing H, Grünewald-funk D, et al. Vegan Diet. *Ernahrungs Umschau.* 2016;63(05):92–102.

14. Baroni L, Goggi S, Battaglino R, et al. Vegan nutrition for mothers and children: Practical tools for healthcare providers. *Nutrients.* 2019;11(1):1–16.

15. Melina V, Craig W, Levin S. Position of the Academy of Nutrition and Dietetics: Vegetarian Diets. *J Acad Nutr Diet.* 2016;116(12):1970–1980.

16. Renda M, Fischer P. Vegetarian Diets in Children and Adolescents. *Pediatr Rev*. 2009;30(1):e1–e8.

17. Amit M, Cummings C, Grueger B, et al. Vegetarian diets in children and adolescents. *Paediatr Child Health (Oxford)*. 2010;15(5):303–314.

18. https://www.bda.uk.com/resource/british-dietetic-association-confirms-well-planned-vegan-diets-can-support-healthy-living-in-people-of-all-ages.html

19. https://www.eatforhealth.gov.au/sites/default/files/content/n55_australian_dietary_guidelines.pdf

20. Agnoli C, Baroni L, Bertini I, et al. Position paper on vegetarian diets from the working group of the Italian Society of Human Nutrition. *Nutr Metab Cardiovasc Dis*. 2017;27(12):1037–1052.

21. Position of the Academy of Nutrition and Dietetics: Vegetarian Diets. *J Acad Nutr Diet*. 2016;116:1970–1980.

22. Murray CJL, Mokdad AH, Ballestros K, et al. The state of US health, 1990–2016: Burden of diseases, injuries, and risk factors among US states. *JAMA*. 2018;319(14):1444–1472.

23. Banfield EC, Liu Y, Davis JS, Chang S, Frazier-Wood A. Poor adherence to U.S. dietary guidelines for children and adolescents in the NHANES population. *J Acad Nutr Diet*. 2016;428(4):709–719.

24. Krebs-Smith SM, Guenther PM, Subar AF, Kirkpatrick SI, Dodd KW. Americans Do Not Meet Federal Dietary Recommendations. *J Nutr*. 2010;140(10):1832–1838.

25. Fulgoni VL, Keast DR, Bailey RL, Dwyer J. Foods, Fortificants, and Supplements: Where Do Americans Get Their Nutrients? *J Nutr*. 2011;141(10):1847–1854.

26. Clarys P, Deliens T, Huybrechts I, et al. Comparison of nutritional quality of the vegan, vegetarian, semi-vegetarian, pesco-vegetarian and omnivorous diet. *Nutrients*. 2014;6(3):1318–1332.

27. Katz DL, Meller S. Can We Say What Diet Is Best for Health? *Annu Rev Public Health*. 2014;35(1):83–103.

28. Buettner D, Skemp S. Blue Zones: Lessons From the World's Longest Lived. *Am J Lifestyle Med*. 2016;10(5):318–321.

29. Orlich MJ, Chiu THT, Dhillon PK, et al. Vegetarian Epidemiology: Review and Discussion of Findings from Geographically Diverse Cohorts. *Adv Nutr*. 2019;10:S284–S295.

30. Le LT, Sabaté J. Beyond meatless, the health effects of vegan diets: findings from the Adventist cohorts. *Nutrients*. 2014;6(6):2131–2147.

31. Spencer EA, Appleby PN, Davey GK, Key TJ. Diet and body mass index in 38 000 EPIC-Oxford meat-eaters, fish-eaters, vegetarians and vegans. *Int J Obes*. 2003;27(6):728–734.

32. Orlich MJ, Fraser GE. Vegetarian diets in the Adventist Health Study 2: a review of initial published findings. *Am J Clin Nutr*. 2014;100(suppl_1):353S–358S.

33. Craig WJ. Health effects of vegan diets. *Am J Clin Nutr*. 2009;89(5):1627S–1633S.

34. Satija A, Hu FB. Plant-based diets and cardiovascular health. *Trends Cardiovasc Med*. 2018;28(7):437–441.

35. Crowe FL, Appleby PN, Travis RC, Key TJ. Risk of hospitalization or death from ischemic heart disease among British vegetarians and nonvegetarians: Results from the EPIC-Oxford cohort study1–3. *Am J Clin Nutr*. 2013;97(3):597–603.

36. Chiu THT, Chang HR, Wang LY, Chang CC, Lin MN, Lin CL. Vegetarian diet and incidence of total, ischemic, and hemorrhagic stroke in 2 cohorts in Taiwan. *Neurology*. 2020;94(11):e1112–e1121.

37. Tong TYN, Appleby PN, Bradbury KE, et al. Risks of ischaemic heart disease and stroke in meat eaters, fish eaters, and vegetarians over 18 years of follow-up: Results from the prospective EPIC-Oxford study. *BMJ*. 2019;366.

38. Appleby PN, Key TJ. The long-term health of vegetarians and vegans. *Proc Nutr Soc*. 2016;75(3):287–293.

39. Song M, Fung TT, Hu FB, et al. Association of animal and plant protein intake with all-cause and cause-specific mortality. *JAMA Intern Med*. 2016;176(10):1453–1463.

40. Ornish D, Brown SE, Billings JH, et al. Can lifestyle changes reverse coronary heart disease? *Lancet*. 1990;336(8708):129–133.

41. Esselstyn CB. Updating a 12-year experience with arrest and reversal therapy for coronary heart disease (an overdue requiem for palliative cardiology). *Am J Cardiol*. 1999;84(3):339–341.

42. Chiu THT, Pan WH, Lin MN, Lin CL. Vegetarian diet, change in dietary patterns, and diabetes risk: A prospective study. *Nutr Diabetes*. 2018;8(1).

43. Papier K, Appleby PN, Fensom GK, et al. Vegetarian diets and risk of hospitalisation or death with diabetes in British adults: results from the EPIC-Oxford study. *Nutr Diabetes.* 2019;9(1).

44. Satija A, Bhupathiraju SN, Rimm EB, et al. Plant-Based Dietary Patterns and Incidence of Type 2 Diabetes in US Men and Women: Results from Three Prospective Cohort Studies. *PLoS Med.* 2016;13(6):1–18.

45. Tonstad S, Stewart K, Oda K, Batech M, Herring RP, Fraser GE. Vegetarian diets and incidence of diabetes in the Adventist Health Study-2. *Nutr Metab Cardiovasc Dis.* 2013;23(4):292–299.

46. Rizzo NS, Sabaté J, Jaceldo-Siegl K, Fraser GE. Vegetarian dietary patterns are associated with a lower risk of metabolic syndrome: The Adventist Health Study 2. *Diabetes Care.* 2011;34(5):1225–1227.

47. Barnard, ND et al. A low-fat vegan diet and a conventional diabetes diet in the treatment of type 2 diabetes: a randomized, controlled, 74-wk clinical trial. *Am J Clin Nutr.* 2009;89(5):1588S–1596S.

48. Orlich MJ, Fraser GE. Vegetarian diets in the Adventist Health Study 2: a review of initial published findings. *Am J Clin Nutr.* 2014;100(suppl_1):353S–358S.

49. Craig WJ. Health effects of vegan diets. *Am J Clin Nutr.* 2009;89(5):1627S–1633S.

50. Key TJ, Appleby PN, Spencer EA, et al. Cancer incidence in British vegetarians. *Br J Cancer.* 2009;101(1):192–197.

51. Key TJ, Appleby PN, Crowe FL, Bradbury KE, Schmidt JA, Travis RC. Cancer in British vegetarians: Updated analyses of 4998 incident cancers in a cohort of 32,491 meat eaters, 8612 fish eaters, 18,298 vegetarians, and 2246 vegans. *Am J Clin Nutr.* 2014;100(SUPPL. 1):378–385.

52. Tantamango-Bartley Y, Jaceldo-Siegl K, Fan J, Fraser G. Vegetarian diets and the incidence of cancer in a low-risk population. *Cancer Epidemiol Biomarkers Prev.* 2013;22(2):286–294.

53. Dinu M, Abbate R, Gensini GF, Casini A, Sofi F. Vegetarian, vegan diets and multiple health outcomes: A systematic review with meta-analysis of observational studies. *Crit Rev Food Sci Nutr.* 2017;57(17):3640–3649.

54. Bouvard V, Loomis D, Guyton KZ, et al. Carcinogenicity of consumption of red and processed meat. *Lancet Oncol.* 2015;16(December):1599–1600.

55. Kushi LH, Doyle C, McCullough M, et al. American Cancer Society guidelines on nutrition and physical activity for cancer prevention. *CA Cancer J Clin.* 2012;62(1):30–67.

56. Tomova A, Bukovsky I, Rembert E, et al. The effects of vegetarian and vegan diets on gut microbiota. *Front Nutr.* 2019;6 (April).

57. Crowe FL, Appleby PN, Allen NE, Key TJ. Diet and risk of diverticular disease in Oxford cohort of European Prospective Investigation into Cancer and Nutrition (EPIC): Prospective study of British vegetarians and non-vegetarians. *BMJ.* 2011;343(7817):1–15.

58. Appleby PN, Allen NE, Key TJ. Diet, vegetarianism, and cataract risk. *Am J Clin Nutr.* 2011;93(5):1128–1135.

59. Chen YC, Chang CC, Chiu THT, Lin MN, Lin CL. The risk of urinary tract infection in vegetarians and non-vegetarians: a prospective study. *Sci Rep.* 2020;10(1):1–9.

60. Chiu T, Lin M-N, Pan W-H, Chen Y-C, Lin C-L. Vegetarian diet, food substitution, and nonalcoholic fatty liver. *Tzu Chi Med J.* 2018;30(2):102.

61. Huang T, Yang B, Zheng J, Li G, Wahlqvist ML, Li D. Cardiovascular disease mortality and cancer incidence in vegetarians: A meta-analysis and systematic review. *Ann Nutr Metab.* 2012;60(4):233–240.

62. Key TJ, Fraser GE, Thorogood M, et al. Mortality in vegetarians and nonvegetarians: Detailed findings from a collaborative analysis of 5 prospective studies. In: *American Journal of Clinical Nutrition.* Vol 70.; 1999:516–524.

63. Ornish D, Scherwitz LW, Billings JH, et al. Intensive lifestyle changes for reversal of coronary heart disease. *J Am Med Assoc.* 1998;280(23):2001–2007.

64. Kahleova H, Levin S, Barnard N. Cardio-metabolic benefits of plant-based diets. *Nutrients.* 2017;9(8):1–13.

65. Tong TYN, Appleby PN, Bradbury KE, et al. Risks of Ischaemic Heart Disease and Stroke in Meat Eaters, Fish Eaters, and Vegetarians Over 18 Years of Follow-Up: Results From the Prospective EPIC-Oxford Study. *BMJ.* 2019;366.

66. Enos WF, Holmes RH, Beyer J. Coronary disease among United States soldiers killed in action in Korea; preliminary report. *J Am Med Assoc.* 1953;152(12):1090–1093.

67. Strong JP, Malcom GT, Oalmann MC, Wissler RW. The PDAY Study: Natural history, risk factors, and pathobiology. *Ann N Y Acad Sci.* 1997; 811:226–237.

68. Zieske AW, Malcom GT, Strong JP. Natural history and risk factors of atherosclerosis in children and youth: the PDAY study. *Pediatr Pathol Mol Med.* 2002;21(2):213–237.

69. Desmond MA, Sobiecki J, Fewtrell M, Wells JCK. Plant-based diets for children as a means of improving adult cardiometabolic health. *Nutr Rev.* 2018;76(4):260–273.

70. Macknin M, Kong T, Weier A, et al. Plant-based, no-added-fat or American heart association diets: Impact on cardio-vascular risk in obese children with hypercholesterolemia and their parents. *J Pediatr.* 2015;166(4):953–959.e3.

71. Iacono G, Cavataio F, Montalto G, et al. Intolerance of Cow's Milk and Chronic Constipation in Children. *N Engl J Med.* 1998;339(16):1100–1104.

72. Crowley ET, Williams LT, Roberts TK, Dunstan RH, Jones PD. Does milk cause constipation? a crossover dietary trial. *Nutrients.* 2013;5(1):253–266.

73. Jakobsson I, Lindberg T. Cow's milk proteins cause infantile colic in breast-fed infants: a double-blind crossover study. *Pediatrics.* 1983;71(2):268–271.

74. Burris J, Rietkerk W, Woolf K. Acne: The Role of Medical Nutrition Therapy. *J Acad Nutr Diet.* 2013;113(3):416–430.

75. Peretti S, Mariano M, Mazzocchetti C, et al. Diet: the keystone of autism spectrum disorder? *Nutr Neurosci.* 2019;22(12):825–839.

76. Matsui MS. Update on diet and acne. *Cutis.* 2019;104(1):11–13.

77. Whiteley P. Food and the gut: Relevance to some of the autisms. *Proc Nutr Soc.* 2017;76(4):478–483.

78. North K, Golding J. A maternal vegetarian diet in pregnancy is associated with hypospadias. *BJU Int.* 2000;85(1):107–113.

79. Carmichael SL, Ma C, Feldkamp ML, et al. Nutritional factors and hypospadias risks. *Paediatr Perinat Epidemiol.* 2012;26(4):353–360.

80. De Kort CAR, Nieuwenhuijsen MJ, Mendez MA. Relationship between maternal dietary patterns and hypospadias. *Paediatr Perinat Epidemiol.* 2011;25(3):255–264. doi:10.1111/j.1365-3016.2011.01194.x

81. Martínez-González MA, Sánchez-Tainta A, Corella D, et al. A provegetarian food pattern and reduction in total mortality in the Prevención con Dieta Mediterránea (PREDIMED) study. *Am J Clin Nutr.* 2014;100 Suppl(9):320S–8S.

82. Willett, WC, Skerrett, PJ. Eat, Drink, and Be Healthy: The Harvard Medical School Guide to Healthy Eating. New York: New York: Free Press, 2017.

83. Sabaté J. The contribution of vegetarian diets to health and disease: A paradigm shift? *Am J Clin Nutr.* 2003;78(3 SUPPL.):502–507.

Chapter 2: Home

1. *Global Warming of 1.5°C. An IPCC Special Report on the impacts of global warming of 1.5°C above pre-industrial levels and related global greenhouse gas emission pathways, in the context of strengthening the global response to the threat of climate change, sustainable development, and efforts to eradicate poverty* [Masson-Delmotte, V., P. Zhai, H.-O. Pörtner, D. Roberts, J. Skea, P.R. Shukla, A. Pirani, W. Moufouma-Okia, C. Péan, R. Pidcock, S. Connors, J.B.R. Matthews, Y. Chen, X. Zhou, M.I. Gomis, E. Lonnoy, T. Maycock, M. Tignor, and T. Waterfield (eds.)]. *World Meteorological Organization, Geneva, Switzerland, 32 pp.*

2. https://www.nationalgeographic.com/environment/2018/10/ipcc-report-climate-change-impacts-forests-emissions/

3. Wallace-Wells, D. The Uninhabitable Earth: Life After Warming. New York, Tim Duggan Books, 2019.

4. https://www.nrdc.org/stories/global-climate-change-what-you-need-know

5. https://report.ipcc.ch/sr15/pdf/sr15_faq.pdf

6. https://www.wri.org/blog/2015/09/8-interactive-graphics-answer-top-climate-change-questions

7. Climate Accountability Institute. (2017). The Carbon Majors Database: CDP Carbon Majors Report 2017. Retrieved from https://6fefcbb86e61af1b2fc4-c70d8ead6ced550b4d987d7c03fcdd1d.ssl.cf3.rackcdn.com/cms/reports/documents/000/002/327/original/Carbon-Majors-Report-2017.pdf?1501833772

8. https://www.vox.com/the-goods/2018/10/12/17967738/climate-change-consumer-choices-green-renewable-energy

9. Safran Foer, Jonathan. We Are the Weather: Saving the Planet Begins at Breakfast. New York. Farrar, Straus and Giroux, 2019.

10. https://iopscience.iop.org/1748-9326/12/7/074024/downloadHRFigure/figure/erlaa7541f1

11. Poore J, Nemecek T. Reducing food's environmental impacts through producers and consumers. *Science*. 2018;360(6392):987–992.

12. Steinfeld, Henning. Livestock's Long Shadow: Environmental Issues and Options. Rome: Food and Agriculture Organization of the United Nations, 2006.

13. https://www.npr.org/sections/thesalt/2019/08/08/748416223/to-slow-global-warming-u-n-warns-agriculture-must-change

14. http://www.fao.org/3/a-a0262e.pdf

15. Gerbens-Leenes PW, Mekonnen MM, Hoekstra AY. The water footprint of poultry, pork and beef: A comparative study in different countries and production systems. *Water Resour Ind*. 2013;1–2:25–36.

16. Gerber, P.J., Steinfeld, H., Henderson, B., Mottet, A., Opio, C., Dijkman, J., Falcucci, A. & Tempio G. 2013. *Tackling Climate Change through Livestock—A Global Assessment of Emissions and Mitigation Opportunities.* Food and Agriculture Organization of the United Nations (FAO), Rome.

17. Diffenbaugh NS, Burke M. Global warming has increased global economic inequality. *Proc Natl Acad Sci U S A*. 2019; 116(20):9808–9813.

18. https://www.who.int/news-room/detail/11-09-2018-global-hunger-continues-to-rise—-new-un-report-says

19. http://www.fao.org/ag/againfo/themes/animal-welfare/news-detail/en/c/36723/

20. http://www.fao.org/3/a0701e/a0701e.pdf

21. Chai BC, van der Voort JR, Grofelnik K, Eliasdottir HG, Klöss I, Perez-Cueto FJA. Which Diet Has the Least Environmental Impact on Our Planet? A Systematic Review of Vegan, Vegetarian and Omnivorous Diets. *Sustainability*. 2019;11(15):4110.

22. Springmann M, Clark M, Mason-D'Croz D, et al. Options for keeping the food system within environmental limits. *Nature*. 2018;562(7728):519–525.

23. https://food-guide.canada.ca/en/

24. https://health.gov/sites/default/files/2019-09/Scientific-Report-of-the-2015-Dietary-Guidelines-Advisory-Committee.pdf

25. Willett W, Rockström J, Loken B, et al. Food in the Anthropocene: the EAT–Lancet Commission on healthy diets from sustainable food systems. *Lancet*. 2019;393(10170):447–492.

26. https://www.vox.com/future-perfect/2020/4/22/21228158/coronavirus-pandemic-risk-factory-farming-meat

27. https://www.nytimes.com/2020/05/21/opinion/coronavirus-meat-vegetarianism.html

Chapter 3: Heart

1. Joy, Melanie. *Beyond Beliefs: A Guide for Improving Relationships and Communication for Vegans, Vegetarians, and Meat Eaters.* Great Barrington: Steiner Books, 2018.

2. Ricard, Matthieu. *A Plea for the Animals: The Moral, Philosophical, and Evolutionary Imperative to Treat All Beings with Compassion.* Shambhala, 2016.

3. https://www.aspca.org/animal-cruelty/farm-animal-welfare

4. https://opinionator.blogs.nytimes.com/2011/04/26/who-protects-the-animals/

5. https://www.govtrack.us/congress/bills/109/s3880/text

6. https://www.theguardian.com/us-news/2015/feb/19/animal-rights-activists-challenge-federal-terrorism-charges

7. https://www.farmsanctuary.org/learn/factory-farming/the-truth-behind-humane-labels/

8. Foer, Jonathan Safran. *Eating Animals*. Back Bay Books, 2010.

9. https://www.animallaw.info/article/beyond-law-agribusiness-and-systemic-abuse-animals.

10. Leenaert, Tobias. *How to Create a Vegan World: A Pragmatic Approach.* Lantern Books, 2017.

Chapter 4: Managing Macronutrients and Fiber

1. WHO. *WHO | Diet, Nutrition and the Prevention of Chronic Diseases.* Vol No.916. Rome: World Health Organization; 2003.

2. Medicine I of. *Dietary Reference Intakes for Energy, Carbohydrate, Fiber, Fat, Fatty Acids, Cholesterol, Protein, and Amino Acids (Macronutrients).* Washington, D.C.: National Academies Press; 2005.

3. Food Guidelines–Blue Zones. https://www.bluezones.com/recipes/food-guidelines/. Accessed January 6, 2020.

4. van Dam RM, Seidell JC. Carbohydrate intake and obesity. *Eur J Clin Nutr.* 2007;61(S1):S75–S99.

5. Ferretti F, Mariani M. Simple vs. complex carbohydrate dietary patterns and the global overweight and obesity pandemic. *Int J Environ Res Public Health.* 2017;14(10).

6. Bhardwaj B, O'keefe EL, O'keefe JH. *Death by Carbs: Added Sugars and Refined Carbohydrates Cause Diabetes and Cardiovascular Disease in Asian Indians.*

7. Dinicolantonio JJ, Lucan SC, O'keefe JH. The Evidence for Saturated Fat and for Sugar Related to Coronary Heart Disease HHS Public Access. *Prog Cardiovasc Dis.* 2016;58(5):464–472.

8. Johnson RK, Appel LJ, Brands M, et al. Dietary sugars intake and cardiovascular health a scientific statement from the american heart association. *Circulation.* 2009;120(11):1011–1020.

9. Pallazola VA, Davis DM, Whelton SP, et al. A Clinician's Guide to Healthy Eating for Cardiovascular Disease Prevention. *Mayo Clin Proc Innov Qual Outcomes.* 2019;3:251–267.

10. Tappy L, Lê K-A. Metabolic Effects of Fructose and the Worldwide Increase in Obesity. *Physiol Rev.* 2010;90(1):23–46.

11. López-Alarcón M, Perichart-Perera O, Flores-Huerta S, et al. Excessive Refined Carbohydrates and Scarce Micronutrients Intakes Increase Inflammatory Mediators and Insulin Resistance in Prepubertal and Pubertal Obese Children Independently of Obesity. 2014.

12. Mehta RS, Nishihara R, Cao Y, et al. Association of dietary patterns with risk of colorectal cancer subtypes classified by Fusobacterium nucleatum in tumor tissue. *JAMA Oncol.* 2017;3(7):921–927.

13. Feng YL, Shu L, Zheng PF, et al. Dietary patterns and colorectal cancer risk: A meta-analysis. *Eur J Cancer Prev.* 2017;26(3):201–211.

14. Dixon LJ, Kabi A, Nickerson KP, McDonald C. Combinatorial effects of diet and genetics on inflammatory bowel disease pathogenesis. *Inflamm Bowel Dis.* 2015;21(4):912–922.

15. Strate LL, Keeley BR, Cao Y, Wu K, Giovannucci EL, Chan AT. Western Dietary Pattern Increases, and Prudent Dietary Pattern Decreases, Risk of Incident Diverticulitis in a Prospective Cohort Study. *Gastroenterology.* 2017;152(5):1023–1030.e2.

16. Hansen NW, Hansen AJ, Sams A. The endothelial border to health: Mechanistic evidence of the hyperglycemic culprit of inflammatory disease acceleration. *IUBMB Life.* 2017;69(3):148–161.

17. Takeuchi M, Iwaki M, Takino J, et al. Immunological detection of fructose-derived advanced glycation end-products. *Lab Invest.* 2010;90(7):1117–1127.

18. Nseir W, Nassar F, Assy N. Soft drinks consumption and nonalcoholic fatty liver disease. 2010;16(21):2579–2588.

19. Kaplan H, Thompson RC, Trumble BC, et al. Coronary atherosclerosis in indigenous South American Tsimane: a cross-sectional cohort study HHS Public Access. *Lancet.* 2017;389:1730–1739.

20. Seidelmann SB, Claggett B, Cheng S, et al. Articles Dietary carbohydrate intake and mortality: a prospective cohort study and meta-analysis. *Lancet Public Heal.* 2018;2667(18):1–10.

21. Willett W, Rockström J, Loken B, et al. Food in the Anthropocene: the EAT—Lancet Commission on healthy diets from sustainable food systems. *Lancet.* 2019;393(10170):447–492.

22. WHO/Europe | Nutrition–A healthy lifestyle. http://www.euro.who.int/en/health-topics/disease-prevention/nutrition/a-healthy-lifestyle. Accessed January 24, 2020.

23. Gonzalez Fischer C, Garnett T. *Plates, Pyramids and Planets Developments in National Healthy and Sustainable Dietary Guidelines: A State of Play Assessment.*

24. Davis B and M V. *Becoming Vegan: Comprehensive Edition.* Summertown TN: Book Publishing Company; 2014.

25. Odphp. *2015-2020 Dietary Guidelines for Americans.*; 2015.

26. Johnson RK, Appel LJ, Brands M, et al. Dietary Sugars Intake and Cardiovascular Health. *Circulation.* 2009;120(11):1011–1020.

27. Vos MB, Kaar JL, Welsh JA, et al. Added sugars and cardiovascular disease risk in children: A scientific statement from the American Heart Association. *Circulation.* 2017;135(19):e1017–e1034.

28. Powell ES, Smith-Taillie LP, Popkin BM. Added Sugars Intake Across the Distribution of US Children and Adult Consumers: 1977-2012. *J Acad Nutr Diet.* 2016;116(10):1543–1550.e1.

29. A Closer Look at Current Intakes and Recommended Shifts–2015–2020 Dietary Guidelines | health.gov. https://health .gov/dietaryguidelines/2015/guidelines/chapter-2/a-closer-look-at-current-intakes-and-recommended-shifts/. Accessed January 24, 2020.

30. Lichtenstein AH. Last Nail in the Coffin for Sugar-Sweetened Beverages: Now Let's Focus on the Hard Part. *Circulation.* 2019;139(18):2126–2128.

31. Micha R, Peñalvo JL, Cudhea F, Imamura F, Rehm CD, Mozaffarian D. Association between dietary factors and mortality from heart disease, stroke, and type 2 diabetes in the United States. *JAMA–J Am Med Assoc.* 2017;317(9).

32. Malik VS, Li Y, Pan A, et al. Long-Term Consumption of Sugar-Sweetened and Artificially Sweetened Beverages and Risk of Mortality in US Adults. *Circulation.* 2019;139(18):2113–2125.

33. Schwingshackl L, Hoffmann G, Lampousi A-M, et al. Food groups and risk of type 2 diabetes mellitus: a systematic review and meta-analysis of prospective studies. *Eur J Epidemiol.* 2017;32(5):363–375.

34. Asgari-Taee F, Zerafati-Shoae N, Dehghani M, Sadeghi M, Baradaran HR, Jazayeri S. Association of sugar sweetened beverages consumption with non-alcoholic fatty liver disease: a systematic review and meta-analysis. *Eur J Nutr.* 2019;58(5):1759–1769.

35. Cohen JFW, Rifas-Shiman SL, Young J, Oken E. Associations of Prenatal and Child Sugar Intake With Child Cognition. *Am J Prev Med.* 2018;54(6):727–735.

36. Craig WJ. Phytochemicals: Guardians of our Health. *J Am Diet Assoc.* 1997;97(10):S199–S204.

37. Slavin JL. Carbohydrates, Dietary Fiber, and Resistant Starch in White Vegetables: Links to Health Outcomes. *Adv Nutr.* 2013;4(3):351S–355S.

38. Cummings JH, Macfarlane GT EH. Prebiotic Digestion and Fermentation. *Am J Clin Nutr.* 2001;73(2 Suppl): 415S–420S.

39. Institute of Medicine. *Dietary Reference Intakes for Energy, Carbohydrate, Fiber, Fat, Fatty Acids, Cholesterol, Protein, and Amino Acids.*; 2002.

40. Quagliani D, Felt-Gunderson P. Closing America's Fiber Intake Gap: Communication Strategies From a Food and Fiber Summit. *Am J Lifestyle Med.* 11(1):80–85.

41. Ahluwalia N, Herrick KA, Rossen LM, et al. Usual nutrient intakes of US infants and toddlers generally meet or exceed Dietary Reference Intakes: findings from NHANES. 2009.

42. U.S. Department of Agriculture ARS. FoodData Central. fdc.nal.usda.gov. Published 2019.

43. Eckel RH, Jakicic JM, Miller NH, et al. 2013 AHA / ACC Guideline on Lifestyle Management to Reduce Cardiovascular Risk A Report of the American College of Cardiology / American Heart Association Task Force on Practice Guidelines. *Circulation.* 2013:1–46.

44. Brennan SF, Woodside J V., Lunny PM, Cardwell CR, Cantwell MM. Dietary fat and breast cancer mortality: A systematic review and meta-analysis. *Crit Rev Food Sci Nutr.* 2017;57(10):1999–2008.

45. Zhao J, Lyu C, Gao J, et al. Dietary fat intake and endometrial cancer risk. *Med (United States).* 2016;95(27).

46. Liss MA, Al-Bayati O, Gelfond J, et al. Higher baseline dietary fat and fatty acid intake is associated with increased risk of incident prostate cancer in the SABOR study. *Prostate Cancer Prostatic Dis.* 2019;22(2):244–251.

47. Kahleova H, Hlozkova A, Fleeman R, Fletcher K, Holubkov R, Barnard ND. Fat quantity and quality, as part of a low-fat, vegan diet, are associated with changes in body composition, insulin resistance, and insulin secretion. A 16-week randomized controlled trial. *Nutrients*. 2019;11(3).

48. von Frankenberg AD, Marina A, Song X, Callahan HS, Kratz M, Utzschneider KM. A high-fat, high-saturated fat diet decreases insulin sensitivity without changing intra-abdominal fat in weight-stable overweight and obese adults. *Eur J Nutr*. 2017;56(1):431–443.

49. Luukkonen PK, Sädevirta S, Zhou Y, et al. Saturated fat is more metabolically harmful for the human liver than unsaturated fat or simple sugars. In: *Diabetes Care*. Vol 41. American Diabetes Association Inc.; 2018:1732–1739.

50. Cândido FG, Valente FX, Grześkowiak ŁM, Moreira APB, Rocha DMUP, Alfenas R de CG. Impact of dietary fat on gut microbiota and low-grade systemic inflammation: mechanisms and clinical implications on obesity. *Int J Food Sci Nutr*. 2018;69(2):125–143.

51. Rocha DM, Caldas AP, Oliveira LL, Bressan J, Hermsdorff HH. Saturated fatty acids trigger TLR4-mediated inflammatory response. *Atherosclerosis*. 2016;244:211–215.

52. Morenga L Te, Montez JM. Health effects of saturated and trans-fatty acid intake in children and adolescents: Systematic review and meta-analysis. *PLoS One*. 2017;12(11).

53. Sacks FM, Lichtenstein AH, Wu JHY, et al. Dietary fats and cardiovascular disease: A presidential advisory from the American Heart Association. *Circulation*. 2017;136(3):e1–e23.

54. Calder PCP. Mechanisms of action of (n-3) fatty acids. *J Nutr*. 2012;142(3):592S–599S.

55. Das UN. Can essential fatty acids reduce the burden of disease(s)? *Lipids Health Dis*. 2008;7:5–9.

56. Welch A a, Shakya-shrestha S, Wareham NJ, Khaw K. Dietary intake and status of n 2 3 polyunsaturated fatty acids in a population of fish-eating and non-fish-eating meat-eaters , vegetarians , and vegans and the precursor-product ratio of a -linolenic acid to long-chain n 2 3 polyunsaturated fatty acids : *Am J Clin Nutr*. 2010;3(92):1040–1051.

57. Rosell MS, Appleby PN, Sanders T a B, Allen NE, Key TJ. Long-chain n—3 polyunsaturated fatty acids in plasma in British meat-eating , vegetarian , and vegan men 1—3. *Am J Clin Nutr*. 2005;82(2):327–334.

58. Simopoulos AP. The importance of the omega-6/omega-3 fatty acid ratio in cardiovascular disease and other chronic diseases. *Exp Biol Med*. 2008;233(6):674–688.

59. Shahidi F, Miraliakbari H. Omega-3 fatty acids in health and disease: Part 2–Health effects of omega-3 fatty acids in autoimmune diseases, mental health, and gene expression. *J Med Food*. 2005;8(2):133–148.

60. Tortosa-Caparrós E, Navas-Carrillo D, Marín F, Orenes-Piñero E. Anti-inflammatory effects of omega 3 and omega 6 polyunsaturated fatty acids in cardiovascular disease and metabolic syndrome. *Crit Rev Food Sci Nutr*. 2017;57(16):3421–3429.

61. Parziale A, Ooms G. The global fight against trans-fat: The potential role of international trade and law. *Global Health*. 2019;15(1).

62. Canada's artificial trans fats ban comes into effect—with a phase-out period | CBC News. https://www.cbc.ca/news/health/trans-fats-health-heart-disease-canada-1.4824852. Accessed February 13, 2020.

63. Artificial trans fats, widely linked to heart disease, are officially banned–The Washington Post. https://www.washingtonpost.com/news/wonk/wp/2018/06/18/artificial-trans-fats-widely-linked-to-heart-disease-are-officially-banned/. Accessed February 13, 2020.

64. Gebauer SK, Destaillats F, Dionisi F, Krauss RM, Baer DJ. Vaccenic acid and trans fatty acid isomers from partially hydrogenated oil both adversely affect LDL cholesterol: A double-blind, randomized controlled trial. *Am J Clin Nutr*. 2015;102(6):1339–1346.

65. Stender S. In equal amounts, the major ruminant trans fatty acid is as bad for LDL cholesterol as industrially produced trans fatty acids, but the latter are easier to remove from foods. *Am J Clin Nutr*. 2015;102(6):1301–1302.

66. Carson JAS, Lichtenstein AH, Anderson CAM, et al. Dietary Cholesterol and Cardiovascular Risk: A Science Advisory From the American Heart Association. *Circulation*. 2020;141(3):E39–E53.

67. Gylling H, Simonen P. Phytosterols, phytostanols, and lipoprotein metabolism. *Nutrients*. 2015;7(9):7965–7977.

68. Moumtaz S, Percival BC, Parmar D, Grootveld KL, Jansson P, Grootveld M. Toxic aldehyde generation in and food uptake from culinary oils during frying practices: peroxidative resistance of a monounsaturate-rich algae oil. *Sci Rep*. 2019;9(1):1–21.

69. Gadiraju T V, Patel Y, Gaziano JM, Djoussé L. Fried Food Consumption and Cardiovascular Health: A Review of Current Evidence.

70. Birlouez-Aragon I, Saavedra G, Tessier FJ, et al. A diet based on high-heat-treated foods promotes risk factors for diabetes mellitus and cardiovascular diseases. *Am J Clin Nutr*. 2010;91(5):1220–1226.

71. Liu G, Zong G, Wu K, et al. Meat Cooking Methods and Risk of Type 2 Diabetes: Results From Three Prospective Cohort Studies. *Diabetes Care*. 2018;41(5):1049–1060.

72. Willcox DC, Willcox BJ, Todoriki H, Suzuki M. The Okinawan Diet : Health Implications of a Low-Calorie , Nutrient-Dense, Antioxidant-Rich Dietary Pattern Low in Glycemic Load. 2009;28(4):2–6.

73. Appel LJ. Editorial: Dietary patterns and longevity expanding the blue zones. *Circulation*. 2008;118(3):214–215.

74. Barnard ND, Cohen J, Jenkins DJA, et al. A low-fat vegan diet improves glycemic control and cardiovascular risk factors in a randomized clinical trial in individuals with type 2 diabetes. *Diabetes Care*. 2006;29(8):1777–1783.

75. Esselstyn CB. Resolving the Coronary Artery Disease Epidemic Through Plant-Based Nutrition. *Prev Cardiol*. 2001;4(4):171–177.

76. Esselstyn CB, Gendy G, Doyle J, Golubic M, Roizen MF. A way to reverse CAD. *J Fam Pract*. 2014;63(7).

77. Barnard ND, Levin SM, Yokoyama Y. A Systematic Review and Meta-Analysis of Changes in Body Weight in Clinical Trials of Vegetarian Diets. *J Acad Nutr Diet*. 2015;115(6).

78. McDougall J, Thomas LE, McDougall C, et al. Effects of 7 days on an ad libitum low-fat vegan diet: The McDougall Program cohort. *Nutr J*. 2014;13(1).

79. Butte NF. Fat intake of children in relation to energy requirements. In: *American Journal of Clinical Nutrition*. Vol 72. Am J Clin Nutr; 2000.

80. Ribaya-Mercado JD, Maramag CC, Tengco LW, Dolnikowski GG, Blumberg JB, Solon FS. Carotene-rich plant foods ingested with minimal dietary fat enhance the total-body vitamin A pool size in Filipino schoolchildren as assessed by stable-isotope-dilution methodology. *Am J Clin Nutr*. 2007;85(4):1041–1049.

81. Moran NE, Johnson EJ. Closer to clarity on the effect of lipid consumption on fat-soluble vitamin and carotenoid absorption: do we need to close in further?

82. Saunders A V., Davis BC, Garg ML. Omega-3 polyunsaturated fatty acids and vegetarian diets. *Med J Aust*. 2013;199 (4):S22–S26. doi:10.5694/mjao11.11507

83. Omega-3 Fatty Acids—Health Professional Fact Sheet. https://ods.od.nih.gov/factsheets/Omega3FattyAcids -HealthProfessional/. Accessed February 12, 2020.

84. Burns-Whitmore B, Froyen E, Heskey C, Parker T, Pablo GS. Alpha-linolenic and linoleic fatty acids in the vegan diet: Do they require dietary reference intake/adequate intake special consideration? *Nutrients*. 2019;11(10).

85. Gerster H. Can adults adequately convert a-linolenic acid (18:3n-3) to eicosapentaenoic acid (20:5n-3) and doco-sahexaenoic acid (22:6n-3)? *Int J Vitam Nutr Res*. 1998;68(3):159–173.

86. Ameur A, Enroth S, Johansson A, et al. Genetic adaptation of fatty-acid metabolism: a human-specific haplotype increasing the biosynthesis of long-chain omega-3 and omega-6 fatty acids. *Am J Hum Genet*. 2012;90(5):809–820.

87. Das UN. Essential fatty acids: Biochemistry, physiology and pathology. *Biotechnol J*. 2006;1(4):420–439.

88. Simopoulos AP, Iii MF, Ph D, Worth F. Experimental Biology and Medicine. 2008.

89. Marangoni F, Colombo C, De Angelis L, et al. Cigarette smoke negatively and dose-dependently affects the bio-synthetic pathway of the n-3 polyunsaturated fatty acid series in human mammary epithelial cells. *Lipids*. 2004; 39(7):633–637.

90. Song M, Fung TT, Hu FB, et al. Association of animal and plant protein intake with all-cause and cause-specific mortality. *JAMA Intern Med*. 2016;176(10):1453–1463.

91. Budhathoki S, Sawada N, Iwasaki M, et al. Association of Animal and Plant Protein Intake with All-Cause and Cause-Specific Mortality in a Japanese Cohort. *JAMA Intern Med*. 2019;179(11):1509–1518.

92. Protein digestibility and absorption: effects of fibre, and the extent of individual variation. http://www.fao.org/3/ M2836e/M2836e00.htm. Accessed June 4, 2020.

93. Melina V, Craig W, Levin S. Position of the Academy of Nutrition and Dietetics: Vegetarian Diets. *J Acad Nutr Diet*. 2016;116(12):1970–1980.

94. Mariotti F, Gardner CD. Dietary Protein and Amino Acids in Vegetarian Diets—A Review.

95. Rizzo NS, Jaceldo-Siegl K, Sabate J, Fraser GE. Nutrient Profiles of Vegetarian and Nonvegetarian Dietary Patterns. *J Acad Nutr Diet*. 2013;113(12):1610–1619.

96. Weder S, Hoffmann M, Becker K, Alexy U, Keller M. Energy, macronutrient intake, and anthropometrics of vegetarian, vegan, and omnivorous children (1–3 years) in Germany (VeChi diet study). *Nutrients*. 2019;11(4).

97. Thane CW, Bates CJ. Dietary intakes and nutrient status of vegetarian preschool children from a British national survey. *J Hum Nutr Diet*. 2000;13(3):149–162.

98. Yen CE, Yen CH, Huang MC, Cheng CH, Huang YC. Dietary intake and nutritional status of vegetarian and omnivorous preschool children and their parents in Taiwan. *Nutr Res*. 2008;28(7):430–436.

99. Mariotti F, Gardner CD. Dietary protein and amino acids in vegetarian diets—A review. *Nutrients*. 2019;11(11).

100. Berryman CE, Lieberman HR, Fulgoni VL, Pasiakos SM. Protein intake trends and conformity with the Dietary Reference Intakes in the United States: Analysis of the National Health and Nutrition Examination Survey, 2001–2014. *Am J Clin Nutr*. 2018;108(2):405–413.

101. Campbell KJ, Abbott G, Zheng M, McNaughton SA. Early Life Protein Intake: Food Sources, Correlates, and Tracking across the First 5 Years of Life. *J Acad Nutr Diet*. 2017;117(8):1188–1197.e1.

102. Del Mar Bibiloni M, Tur JA, Morandi A, Tommasi M, Tomasselli F, Maffeis C. Protein Intake as a Risk Factor of Overweight/Obesity in 8-to 12-Year-Old Children.

103. Lind M V., Larnkjær A, MØlgaard C, Michaelsen KF. Dietary protein intake and quality in early life: Impact on growth and obesity. *Curr Opin Clin Nutr Metab Care*. 2017;20(1):71–76.

104. Patro-Gołąb B, Zalewski BM, Kołodziej M, et al. Nutritional interventions or exposures in infants and children aged up to 3 years and their effects on subsequent risk of overweight, obesity and body fat: a systematic review of systematic reviews. *Obes Rev*. 2016;17(12):1245–1257.

105. Health & Fitness—Clean Label Project. https://cleanlabelproject.org/health-fitness/. Accessed June 4, 2020.

106. Chandra-Hioe M V., Wong CHM, Arcot J. The Potential Use of Fermented Chickpea and Faba Bean Flour as Food Ingredients. *Plant Foods Hum Nutr*. 2016;71(1):90–95.

107. Drulyte D, Orlien V. The Effect of Processing on Digestion of Legume Proteins.

108. Devi CB, Kushwaha A, Kumar A. Sprouting characteristics and associated changes in nutritional composition of cowpea (Vigna unguiculata). *J Food Sci Technol*. 2015;52(10):6821–6827.

109. Rojas Allende D, Figueras Díaz F, Durán Agüero S. Ventajas y desventajas nutricionales de ser vegano o vegetariano. *Rev Chil Nutr*. 2017;44(3).

110. Nosworthy MG, Medina G, Franczyk AJ, et al. Effect of processing on the in vitro and in vivo protein quality of beans (Phaseolus vulgaris and Vicia Faba). *Nutrients*. 2018;10(6).

111. Leinonen I, Iannetta PPM, Rees RM, Russell W, Watson C, Barnes AP. Lysine Supply Is a Critical Factor in Achieving Sustainable Global Protein Economy. *Front Sustain Food Syst*. 2019;3:27.

Chapter 5: Micronutrients

1. Sobiecki JG, Appleby PN, Bradbury KE, Key TJ. High compliance with dietary recommendations in a cohort of meat eaters, fish eaters, vegetarians, and vegans: Results from the European Prospective Investigation into Cancer and Nutrition-Oxford study. *Nutr Res*. 2016;36(5):464–477.

2. Rizzo NS, Jaceldo-Siegl K, Sabate J, Fraser GE. Nutrient Profiles of Vegetarian and Nonvegetarian Dietary Patterns. *J Acad Nutr Diet*. 2013;113(12):1610–1619.

3. Kristensen NB, Madsen ML, Hansen TH, et al. Intake of macro- and micronutrients in Danish vegans. *Nutr J*. 2015;14(1).

4. Elorinne AL, Alfthan G, Erlund I, et al. Food and nutrient intake and nutritional status of Finnish vegans and non-vegetarians. *PLoS One*. 2016;11(2):1–14.

5. Schüpbach R, Wegmüller R, Berguerand C, Bui M, Herter-Aeberli I. Micronutrient status and intake in omnivores, vegetarians and vegans in Switzerland. *Eur J Nutr*. 2017;56(1).

6. Institute of Medicine (U.S.). Standing Committee on the Scientific Evaluation of Dietary Reference Intakes. Institute of Medicine (U.S.). Panel on Folate OBV, Institute of Medicine (U.S.). Subcommittee on Upper Reference Levels of Nutrients. *Dietary Reference Intakes for Thiamin, Riboflavin, Niacin, Vitamin B6, Folate, Vitamin B12, Pantothenic Acid, Biotin, and Choline.* National Academy Press; 1998.

7. Langan RC, Goodbred AJ, Luke S, Residency M. Vitamin B12 Deficiency: Recognition and Management. *Am Fam Physician.* 2017;96(6):384–389.

8. Blom HJ, Smulders Y. Overview of homocysteine and folate metabolism. With special references to cardiovascular disease and neural tube defects. *J Inherit Metab Dis.* 2011;34(1):75–81.

9. Pawlak R. Is vitamin B<inf>12</inf> deficiency a risk factor for cardiovascular disease in vegetarians? *Am J Prev Med.* 2015;48(6).

10. Chaudhry SH, Taljaard M, MacFarlane AJ, et al. The role of maternal homocysteine concentration in placenta-mediated complications: Findings from the Ottawa and Kingston birth cohort. *BMC Pregnancy Childbirth.* 2019; 19(1).

11. Watanabe F, Yabuta Y, Bito T, Teng F. Vitamin B12-containing plant food sources for vegetarians. *Nutrients.* 2014;6(5):1861–1873.

12. Rizzo G, Laganà AS, Rapisarda AMC, et al. Vitamin B12 among vegetarians: Status, assessment and supplementation. *Nutrients.* 2016;8(12).

13. Rizzo G, Laganà AS, Rapisarda AMC, et al. Vitamin B12 among Vegetarians: Status, Assessment and Supplementation. *Nutrients.* 2016;8(12):1–23.

14. Vitamin B12—Health Professional Fact Sheet. https://ods.od.nih.gov/factsheets/VitaminB12-HealthProfessional/. Accessed March 6, 2020.

15. Johnson MA. If High Folic Acid Aggravates Vitamin B12 Deficiency What Should Be Done About It? *Nutr Rev.* 2008;65(10):451–458. doi:10.1111/j.1753-4887.2007.tb00270.x

16. Briani C, Torre CD, Citton V, et al. Cobalamin deficiency: Clinical picture and radiological findings. *Nutrients.* 2013;5(11):4521–4539.

17. Bousselamti A, El Hasbaoui B, Echahdi H, Krouile Y. Psychomotor regression due to vitamin B12 deficiency. *Pan Afr Med J.* 2018;30.

18. Watanabe F, Bito T. Vitamin B12 sources and microbial interaction. *Exp Biol Med.* 2018;243(2):148–158.

19. National Institutes of Health. *Vitamin B12 Fact Sheet for Health Professionals.*; 2020.

20. U.S. Department of Agriculture ARS. FoodData Central. fdc.nal.usda.gov. Published 2019.

21. Institute of Medicine (US) Standing Committee on the Scientific Evaluation of Dietary Reference Intakes and its Panel on Folate OBV and C. *Dietary Reference Intakes for Thiamin, Riboflavin, Niacin, Vitamin B6, Folate, Vitamin B12, Pantothenic Acid, Biotin, and Choline.* National Academies Press (US); 1998.

22. Kaplan A, Zelicha H, Tsaban G, et al. Protein bioavailability of Wolffia globosa duckweed, a novel aquatic plant—A randomized controlled trial. *Clin Nutr.* 2019;38(6):2576–2582.

23. Yamada K, Yamada Y, Fukuda M, Yamada S. Bioavailability of dried asakusanori (Porphyra tenera) as a source of cobalamin (vitamin B12). *Int J Vitam Nutr Res.* 1999;69(6):412–418.

24. Institute of Medicine. National Academy of Sciences. Food and Nutrition Board. *Dietary Reference Intakes for Thiamin, Riboflavin, Niacin, Vitamin B6, Folate, Vitamin B12, Pantothenic Acid, Biotin, and Choline (1998).* Washington, D.C.: The National Academies Press; 1998.

25. Bor MV, Castel-roberts KM Von, Kauwell GPA, et al. Daily intake of 4 to 7 l g dietary vitamin B-12 is associated with steady concentrations of vitamin B-12—related biomarkers in a healthy young. *Am J Clin Nutr.* 2010;91:571–577.

26. Bolzetta F, Veronese N, De Rui M, et al. Are the Recommended Dietary Allowances for Vitamins Appropriate for Elderly People? *J Acad Nutr Diet.* 2015;115(11):1789–1797.

27. Carmel R. Efficacy and safety of fortification and supplementation with vitamin B12: Biochemical and physiological effects. In: *Food and Nutrition Bulletin.* Vol 29. Food Nutr Bull; 2008.

28. Carmel R. How I treat cobalamin (vitamin B12) deficiency. *Blood.* 2008;112(6):2214–2221.

29. Del Bo' C, Riso P, Gardana C, Brusamolino A, Battezzati A, Ciappellano S. Effect of two different sublingual dosages of vitamin B12 on cobalamin nutritional status in vegans and vegetarians with a marginal deficiency: A randomized controlled trial. *Clin Nutr*. 2019;38(2):575–583.

30. Veraldi S, Benardon S, Diani M, Barbareschi M. Acneiform eruptions caused by vitamin B12: A report of five cases and review of the literature. *J Cosmet Dermatol*. 2018;17(1):112–115.

31. Kang D, Shi B, Erfe MC, Craft N, Li H. Vitamin B 12 modulates the transcriptome of the skin microbiota in acne pathogenesis . *Sci Transl Med*. 2015;7(293):293ra103–293ra103.

32. Paul C, Brady DM. Comparative Bioavailability and Utilization of Particular Forms of B12 Supplements with Potential to Mitigate B12-related Genetic Polymorphisms. *Integr Med*. 2017;16(1):42–49.

33. Obeid R, Fedosov SN, Nexo E. Cobalamin coenzyme forms are not likely to be superior to cyano- and hydroxyl-cobalamin in prevention or treatment of cobalamin deficiency. *Mol Nutr Food Res*. 2015;59(7):1364–1372.

34. Holick MF. Resurrection of vitamin D deficiency and rickets. *J Clin Invest*. 2006;116(8):2062–2072.

35. Thacher TD, Fischer PR, Tebben PJ, et al. Increasing incidence of nutritional rickets: A population-based study in olmsted county, minnesota. *Mayo Clin Proc*. 2013;88(2):176–183.

36. Uday S, Högler W. Nutritional Rickets and Osteomalacia in the Twenty-first Century: Revised Concepts, Public Health, and Prevention Strategies. *Curr Osteoporos Rep*. 2017;15(4):293–302.

37. Medicine I of. *Dietary Reference Intakes for Calcium, Phosphorus, Magnesium, Vitamin D, and Fluoride*. Washington, D.C.: National Academies Press; 1997. doi:10.17226/5776

38. National Institutes of Health. Office of Dietary Supplements. *Vitamin D Fact Sheet for Health Professionals.*; 2019.

39. Wacker M, Holick MF. Sunlight and Vitamin D: A global perspective for health. *Derm Endocrinol*. 2013;5(1):51–108.

40. Naeem Z. Vitamin d deficiency- an ignored epidemic. *Int J Health Sci (Qassim)*. 2010;4(1):V-VI.

41. Holick MF. VITAMIN D: A D-LIGHTFUL SOLUTION FOR HEALTH. *J Investig Med*. 2011;59(6):872–880.

42. National Institutes of Health Office of Dietary Supplements. *Vitamin D - Health Professional Fact Sheet*; 2018.

43. Bolland MJ, Grey A, Gamble GD, Reid IR. The effect of vitamin D supplementation on skeletal, vascular, or cancer outcomes: A trial sequential meta-analysis. *Lancet Diabetes Endocrinol*. 2014;2(4):307–320.

44. Liu D, Fernandez BO, Hamilton A, et al. UVA irradiation of human skin vasodilates arterial vasculature and lowers blood pressure independently of nitric oxide synthase. *J Invest Dermatol*. 2014;134(7):1839–1846.

45. Weller RB. Sunlight Has Cardiovascular Benefits Independently of Vitamin D. *Blood Purif*. 2016;41(1-3):130–134.

46. Bhatnagar A. Environmental Determinants of Cardiovascular Disease. *Circ Res*. 2017;121(2):162–180.

47. Lindqvist PG. The winding path towards an inverse relationship between sun exposure and all-cause mortality. *Anticancer Res*. 2018;38(2):1173–1178.

48. Grant WB. An estimate of premature cancer mortality in the U.S. due to inadequate doses of solar ultraviolet-B radiation. *Cancer*. 2002;94(6):1867–1875.

49. Hiller TWR, O'Sullivan DE, Brenner DR, Peters CE, King WD. Solar Ultraviolet Radiation and Breast Cancer Risk: A Systematic Review and Meta-Analysis. *Environ Health Perspect*. 2020;128(1):016002.

50. Tran B, Whiteman DC, Webb PM, et al. Association between ultraviolet radiation, skin sun sensitivity and risk of pancreatic cancer. *Cancer Epidemiol*. 2013;37(6):886–892.

51. Porojnicu AC, Robsahm TE, Dahlback A, et al. Seasonal and geographical variations in lung cancer prognosis in Norway. Does Vitamin D from the sun play a role? *Lung Cancer*. 2007;55(3):263–270.

52. Wright F, Weller RB. Risks and benefits of UV radiation in older people: More of a friend than a foe? *Maturitas*. 2015;81(4):425–431.

53. Holick MF. Vitamin D deficiency. *N Engl J Med*. 2007;357(3):266–281.

54. Holick MF. Biological effects of sunlight, ultraviolet radiation, visible light, infrared radiation and Vitamin D for health. In: *Anticancer Research*. Vol 36. International Institute of Anticancer Research; 2016:1345–1356.

55. Kristensen NB, Madsen ML, Hansen TH, et al. Intake of macro- and micronutrients in Danish vegans. *Nutr J*. 2015.

56. Chan J, Jaceldo-Siegl K, Fraser GE. Serum 25-hydroxyvitamin D status of vegetarians, partial vegetarians, and nonvegetarians: The Adventist Health Study-2. In: *American Journal of Clinical Nutrition*. Vol 89. American Society for Nutrition; 2009:1686S.

57. Palacios C, Gonzalez L. Is vitamin D deficiency a major global public health problem? *J Steroid Biochem Mol Biol*. 2014;144(PART A):138-145. doi:10.1016/j.jsbmb.2013.11.003

58. Institute of Medicine of the National Academies. *Dietary Reference Intakes for Vitamin C, Vitamin E, Selenium Andd Carotenoids 2000*. Washington, DC: The National Academies Press; 2000.

59. *Dietary Reference Intakes for Vitamin A, Vitamin K, Arsenic, Boron, Chromium, Copper, Iodine, Iron, Manganese, Molybdenum, Nickel, Silicon, Vanadium, and Zinc*. National Academies Press; 2001.

60. National Institutes of Health. Dietary Supplement Fact Sheets. Office of Dietary Supplements. https://ods.od.nih.gov/factsheets/list-all/. Accessed March 6, 2020.

61. Moran N, Mohn E, Hanson N, Erdman J, Johnson E. Intrinsic and Extrinsic Factors Impacting Absorption, Metabolism, and Health Effects of Dietary Carotenoids. *Adv Nutr*. 2018;9(4):465–492.

62. Borel P, Desmarchelier C, Nowicki M, Bott R. A Combination of Single-Nucleotide Polymorphisms Is Associated with Interindividual Variability in Dietary ß-Carotene Bioavailability in Healthy Men. *J Nutr*. 2015;145(8):1740–1747.

63. Willett WC, Ludwig DS. Milk and health. *N Engl J Med*. 2020;382(7):644–654.

64. U.S. Department of Health and Human Services and U.S. Department of Agriculture. *2015 – 2020 Dietary Guidelines for Americans. 8th Edition. December 2015. Available at Https://Health.Gov/Dietaryguidelines/2015/Guidelines/*. 8th ed. USDA; 2015.

65. Konner M, Eaton SB. Paleolithic Nutrition. *Nutr Clin Pract*. 2010;25(6):594–602.

66. Ugidos-Rodríguez S, Matallana-González MC, Sánchez-Mata MC. Lactose malabsorption and intolerance: a review. *Food Funct*. 2018;9(8):4056–4068.

67. Tat D, Kenfield SA, Cowan JE, et al. Milk and other dairy foods in relation to prostate cancer recurrence: Data from the cancer of the prostate strategic urologic research endeavor (CaPSURETM). *Prostate*. 2018;78(1):32–39.

68. Vasconcelos A, Santos T, Ravasco P, Neves PM. Dairy products: Is there an impact on promotion of prostate cancer? A review of the literature. *Front Nutr*. 2019;6:62.

69. Fraser G, Miles F, Orlich M, Jaceldo-Siegl K, Mashchak A. Dairy Milk Is Associated with Increased Risk of Breast Cancer in the Adventist Health Study-2 (AHS-2) Cohort (P05-026-19). *Curr Dev Nutr*. 2019;3(Suppl 1).

70. Rizzo G, Baroni L. Soy, soy foods and their role in vegetarian diets. *Nutrients*. 2018;10(1).

71. Appleby P, Roddam A, Allen N, Key T. Comparative fracture risk in vegetarians and nonvegetarians in EPIC-Oxford. *Eur J Clin Nutr*. 2007;61(12):1400–1406.

72. Ho-Pham LT, Vu BQ, Lai TQ, Nguyen ND, Nguyen T V. Vegetarianism, bone loss, fracture and vitamin D: A longitudinal study in Asian vegans and non-vegans. *Eur J Clin Nutr*. 2012;66(1):75–82.

73. Ho-pham LT, Nguyen ND, Nguyen T V. Effect of vegetarian diets on bone mineral density : a Bayesian. 2010;(C):1–8.

74. Iguacel I, Miguel-Berges ML, Gómez-Bruton A, Moreno LA, Julián C. Veganism, vegetarianism, bone mineral density, and fracture risk: A systematic review and meta-analysis. *Nutr Rev*. 2019;77(1).

75. Karavasiloglou N, Selinger E, Gojda J, Rohrmann S, Kühn T. Differences in Bone Mineral Density between Adult Vegetarians and Nonvegetarians Become Marginal when Accounting for Differences in Anthropometric Factors. *J Nutr*. February 2020.

76. Appleby P, Roddam A, Allen N, Key T. Comparative fracture risk in vegetarians and nonvegetarians in EPIC-Oxford. *Eur J Clin Nutr*. 2007;61(12):1400–1406.

77. Chai W, Liebman M. Effect of different cooking methods on vegetable oxalate content. *J Agric Food Chem*. 2005;53(8):3027–3030.

78. Noonan, SC, Savage G. Oxalate Content of Foods and Its Effect on Humans. *Asia Pac J Clin Nutr*. 1999;8(1):64–75.

79. Calvez J, Poupin N, Chesneau C, Lassale C, Tomé D. Protein intake, calcium balance and health consequences. *Eur J Clin Nutr*. 2012;66(3):281–295.

80. Knurick JR, Johnston CS, Wherry SJ, Aguayo I. Comparison of correlates of bone mineral density in individuals adhering to lacto-ovo, vegan, or omnivore diets: A cross-sectional investigation. *Nutrients*. 2015;7(5):3416–3426.

81. Lousuebsakul-Matthews V, Thorpe DL, Knutsen R, Beeson WL, Fraser GE, Knutsen SF. Legumes and meat analogues consumption are associated with hip fracture risk independently of meat intake among Caucasian men and women: The Adventist Health Study-2. *Public Health Nutr*. 2013;17(10):2333–2343.

82. Bialo SR, Gordon CM. Underweight, overweight, and pediatric bone fragility: Impact and management. *Curr Osteoporos Rep*. 2014;12(3):319–328.

83. Fassio A, Idolazzi L, Rossini M, et al. The obesity paradox and osteoporosis. *Eat Weight Disord*. 2018;23(3):293–302.

84. Lim J, Park HS. Relationship between underweight, bone mineral density and skeletal muscle index in premenopausal Korean women. *Int J Clin Pract*. 2016;70(6):462–468.

85. Angireddy R, Kazmi HR, Srinivasan S, et al. Cytochrome c oxidase dysfunction enhances phagocytic function and osteoclast formation in macrophages. *FASEB J*. 2019;33(8):9167–9181.

86. Smoking and Bone Health | NIH Osteoporosis and Related Bone Diseases National Resource Center. https://www .bones.nih.gov/health-info/bone/osteoporosis/conditions-behaviors/bone-smoking. Accessed March 31, 2020.

87. Sampson W. Alcohol and Other Factors Affecting Osteoporosis Risk in Women. National Institue on Alcohol Abuse and Alcoholismm. https://pubs.niaaa.nih.gov/publications/arh26-4/292-298.htm. Published 2003. Accessed March 31, 2020.

88. Iodine—Health Professional Fact Sheet. https://ods.od.nih.gov/factsheets/Iodine-HealthProfessional/#en31. Accessed March 17, 2020.

89. Lewandowski TA, Peterson MK, Charnley G. Iodine supplementation and drinking-water perchlorate mitigation. *Food Chem Toxicol*. 2015;80:261–270.

90. Leung AM, LaMar A, He X, Braverman LE, Pearce EN. Iodine status and thyroid function of Boston-area vegetarians and vegans. *J Clin Endocrinol Metab*. 2011;96(8):1303–1307.

91. Lise Brantsaeter A, Katrine Knutsen H, Cathrine Johansen N, et al. Inadequate Iodine Intake in Population Groups Defined by Age, Life Stage and Vegetarian Dietary Practice in a Norwegian Convenience Sample. 2018.

92. Krajcovicova-Kudlackova M, Bučková K, Klimeš I, Šeboková E. Iodine deficiency in vegetarians and vegans. *Ann Nutr Metab*. 2003;47(5):183–185.

93. Teas J, Pino S, Critchley A, Braverman LE. Variability of iodine content in common commercially available edible seaweeds. *Thyroid*. 2004;14(10):836–841.

94. Davis B and M V. *Becoming Vegan: Comprehensive Edition*. Summertown TN: Book Publishing Company; 2014.

95. Medicine. I of. *Dietary Reference Intakes for Sodium and Potassium*. Washington, D.C.: National Academies Press; 2019.

96. JK B, P S, S S. Various Possible Toxicants Involved in Thyroid Dysfunction: A Review. *J Clin DIAGNOSTIC Res*. 2016;10(1).

97. Eastman CJ, Zimmermann MB. *The Iodine Deficiency Disorders*. MDText.com, Inc.; 2000.

98. Miller JL. Iron deficiency anemia: A common and curable disease. *Cold Spring Harb Perspect Med*. 2013;3(7).

99. McLean E, Cogswell M, Egli I, Wojdyla D, De Benoist B. Worldwide prevalence of anaemia, WHO Vitamin and Mineral Nutrition Information System, 1993–2005. *Public Health Nutr*. 2009;12(4):444–454.

100. Baker RD, Greer FR, Bhatia JJS, et al. Clinical report—Diagnosis and prevention of iron deficiency and iron-deficiency anemia in infants and young children (0–3 years of age). *Pediatrics*. 2010;126(5):1040–1050.

101. Haider LM, Schwingshackl L, Hoffmann G, Ekmekcioglu C. The effect of vegetarian diets on iron status in adults: A systematic review and meta-analysis. *Crit Rev Food Sci Nutr*. 2018;58(8).

102. Pawlak R, Berger J, Hines I. Iron Status of Vegetarian Adults: A Review of Literature. *Am J Lifestyle Med*. 2018;12(6):486–498.

103. Jin Y, He L, Chen Y, Fang Y, Yao Y. Association between serum ferritin levels and metabolic syndrome: An updated meta-analysis. *Int J Clin Exp Med*. 2015;8(8):13317–13322.

104. Orban E, Schwab S, Thorand B, Huth C. Association of iron indices and type 2 diabetes: A meta-analysis of observational studies. *Diabetes Metab Res Rev*. 2014;30(5):372–394.

105. Eftekhari MH, Mozaffari-Khosravi H, Shidfar F, Zamani A. Relation between Body Iron Status and Cardiovascular Risk Factors in Patients with Cardiovascular Disease. *Int J Prev Med*. 2013;4(8):911–916.

106. Quintana Pacheco DA, Sookthai D, Graf ME, et al. Iron status in relation to cancer risk and mortality: Findings from a population-based prospective study. *Int J Cancer*. 2018;143(3):561–569.

107. Fonseca-Nunes A, Jakszyn P, Agudo A. Iron and cancer risk—a systematic review and meta-analysis of the epidemiological evidence. *Cancer Epidemiol Biomarkers Prev*. 2014;23(1):12–31.

108. Pawlak R, Bell K. Iron Status of Vegetarian Children: A Review of Literature. *Ann Nutr Metab*. 2017;70(2).

109. Hurrell R, Egli I. Iron bioavailability and dietary reference values. *Am J Clin Nutr*. 2010;91(5):1461S–1467S.

110. Baroni L, Goggi S, Battaglino R, et al. Vegan nutrition for mothers and children: Practical tools for healthcare providers. *Nutrients*. 2019;11(1). doi:10.3390/nu11010005

111. Collings R, Harvey LJ, Hooper L, et al. The absorption of iron from whole diets : a systematic review 1–4. 2013:65–81.

112. Melina V, Craig W, Levin S. Position of the Academy of Nutrition and Dietetics: Vegetarian Diets. *J Acad Nutr Diet*. 2016;116(12):1970–1980.

113. Platel K, Srinivasan K. Bioavailability of micronutrients from plant foods: An update. *Crit Rev Food Sci Nutr*. 2016;56(10):1608–1619.

114. Zijp IM, Korver O, Tijburg LBM. Effect of tea and other dietary factors on iron absorption. *Crit Rev Food Sci Nutr*. 2000;40(5):371–398.

115. Bonsmann SSG, Walczyk T, Renggli S, Hurrell RF. Oxalic acid does not influence nonhaem iron absorption in humans: A comparison of kale and spinach meals. *Eur J Clin Nutr*. 2008;62(3):336–341.

116. Jiang T, Jeter JM, Nelson SE, Ziegler EE. Intestinal blood loss during cow milk feeding in older infants: Quantitative measurements. *Arch Pediatr Adolesc Med*. 2000;154(7):673–678.

117. Iron deficiency in children: Prevention tips for parents—Mayo Clinic. https://www.mayoclinic.org/healthy-lifestyle/childrens-health/in-depth/iron-deficiency/art-20045634. Accessed March 20, 2020.

118. Iron—Health Professional Fact Sheet. https://ods.od.nih.gov/factsheets/Iron-HealthProfessional/. Accessed March 19, 2020.

119. Manoguerra AS, Erdman AR, Booze LL, et al. Iron ingestion: an evidence-based consensus guideline for out-of-hospital management. *Clin Toxicol (Phila)*. 2005;43(6):553–570.

120. Chaudhury A, Duvoor C, Reddy Dendi VS, et al. Clinical review of antidiabetic drugs: Implications for type 2 diabetes mellitus management. *Front Endocrinol (Lausanne)*. 2017;8(JAN).

121. Prasad AS. Impact of the discovery of human zinc deficiency on health. *J Trace Elem Med Biol*. 2014;28(4):357–363.

122. Zinc—Health Professional Fact Sheet. https://ods.od.nih.gov/factsheets/Zinc-HealthProfessional/. Accessed March 22, 2020.

123. Foster M, Samman S. *Vegetarian Diets across the Lifecycle: Impact on Zinc Intake and Status*. Vol 74. 1st ed. Elsevier Inc.; 2015.

124. Foster M, Chu A, Petocz P, Samman S. Effect of vegetarian diets on zinc status: A systematic review and meta-analysis of studies in humans. *J Sci Food Agric*. 2013;93(10):2362–2371.

125. Hunt JR. Bioavailability of iron, zinc, and other trace minerals from vegetarian diets. In: *American Journal of Clinical Nutrition*. Vol 78. ; 2003.

126. Foster M, Herulah UN, Prasad A, Petocz P, Samman S. Zinc status of vegetarians during pregnancy: A systematic review of observational studies and meta-analysis of zinc intake. *Nutrients*. 2015;7(6).

127. Gibson RS, Heath ALM, Szymlek-Gay EA. Is iron and zinc nutrition a concern for vegetarian infants and young children in industrialized countries? In: *American Journal of Clinical Nutrition*. Vol 100. ; 2014.

128. Cizeikiene D, Juodeikiene G, Bartkiene E, Damasius J, Paskevicius A. Phytase activity of lactic acid bacteria and their impact on the solubility of minerals from wholemeal wheat bread. *Int J Food Sci Nutr*. 2015;66(7):736–742.

129. Lopez HW, Duclos V, Coudray C, et al. Making bread with sourdough improves mineral bioavailability from reconstituted whole wheat flour in rats. *Nutrition*. 2003;19(6):524–530.

130. Davidson TM, Smith WM. The Bradford Hill criteria and zinc-induced anosmia: A causality analysis. *Arch Otolaryngol—Head Neck Surg*. 2010;136(7):673–676.

131. Ross AC, Manson JJE, Abrams S a S, et al. *The 2011 Report on Dietary Reference Intakes for Calcium and Vitamin D from the Institute of Medicine: What Clinicians Need to Know*. Vol 96.; 2011.

132. Medicine I of. *Dietary Reference Intakes for Water, Potassium, Sodium, Chloride, and Sulfate*. Washington, D.C.: National Academies Press; 2005.

133. Palacios C. The role of nutrients in bone health, from A to Z. *Crit Rev Food Sci Nutr*. 2006;46(8):621–628.

134. Sodium (Chloride) | Linus Pauling Institute | Oregon State University. https://lpi.oregonstate.edu/mic/minerals/sodium. Accessed March 31, 2020.

Chapter 6: What Makes a Healthy Diet?

1. Hemler EC, Hu FB. Plant-Based Diets for Cardiovascular Disease Prevention: All Plant Foods Are Not Created Equal. *Curr Atheroscler Rep*. 2019;21(5).

2. Dinu M, Abbate R, Gensini GF, Casini A, Sofi F. Vegetarian, vegan diets and multiple health outcomes: A systematic review with meta-analysis of observational studies. *Crit Rev Food Sci Nutr*. 2017;57(17):3640–3649.

3. Bailey RL, West Jr. KP, Black RE. The Epidemiology of Global Micronutrient Deficiencies. *Ann Nutr Metab*. 2015;66(2):22–33.

4. *World Disasters Report Focus on Hunger and Malnutrition*.

5. Malnutrition. https://www.who.int/news-room/fact-sheets/detail/malnutrition. Accessed April 9, 2020.

6. Huang T, Yang B, Zheng J, Li G, Wahlqvist ML, Li D. Cardiovascular disease mortality and cancer incidence in vegetarians: A meta-analysis and systematic review. *Ann Nutr Metab*. 2012;60(4):233–240.

7. Kim H, Caulfield LE, Garcia-Larsen V, Steffen LM, Coresh J, Rebholz CM. Plant-Based Diets Are Associated With a Lower Risk of Incident Cardiovascular Disease, Cardiovascular Disease Mortality, and All-Cause Mortality in a General Population of Middle-Aged Adults. *J Am Heart Assoc*. 2019;8(16):e012865.

8. Appel LJ, Foti K. Sources of dietary sodium. *Circulation*. 2017;135(19):1784–1787.

9. Aune D, Giovannucci E, Boffetta P, et al. Fruit and vegetable intake and the risk of cardiovascular disease, total cancer and all-cause mortality-A systematic review and dose-response meta-analysis of prospective studies. *Int J Epidemiol*. 2017;46(3).

10. Slavin JL, Lloyd B. Health Benefits of Fruits and Vegetables. *Adv Nutr*. 2012;3(4):506–516.

11. Lee-Kwan SH, Moore L V., Blanck HM, Harris DM, Galuska D. Disparities in State-Specific Adult Fruit and Vegetable Consumption—United States, 2015. *MMWR Morb Mortal Wkly Rep*. 2017;66(45):1241–1247.

12. Moore L V., Thompson FE, Demissie Z. Percentage of Youth Meeting Federal Fruit and Vegetable Intake Recommendations, Youth Risk Behavior Surveillance System, United States and 33 States, 2013. In: *Journal of the Academy of Nutrition and Dietetics*. Vol 117. Elsevier B.V.; 2017:545–553.e3.

13. Soundararajan P, Kim JS. Anti-carcinogenic glucosinolates in cruciferous vegetables and their antagonistic effects on prevention of cancers. *Molecules*. 2018;23(11).

14. Praticò G, Gao Q, Manach C, Dragsted LO. Biomarkers of food intake for Allium vegetables Lars Dragsted. *Genes Nutr*. 2018;13(1).

15. Sytar O, Bosko P, Živčák M, Brestic M, Smetanska I. Bioactive phytochemicals and antioxidant properties of the grains and sprouts of colored wheat genotypes. *Molecules*. 2018;23(9).

16. Abellán A, Domínguez-Perles R, Moreno DA, García-Viguera C. Sorting out the value of cruciferous sprouts as sources of bioactive compounds for nutrition and health. *Nutrients*. 2019;11(2).

17. Dreher ML. Whole fruits and fruit fiber emerging health effects. *Nutrients*. 2018;10(12).

18. Yip CSC, Chan W, Fielding R. The Associations of Fruit and Vegetable Intakes with Burden of Diseases: A Systematic Review of Meta-Analyses. *J Acad Nutr Diet*. 2019;119(3):464–481.

19. Prezioso D, Strazzullo P, Lotti T, et al. Dietary treatment of urinary risk factors for renal stone formation. A review of CLU Working Group. *Arch Ital di Urol e Androl*. 2015;87(2):105–120.

20. Holzapfel NP, Holzapfel BM, Champ S, Feldthusen J, Clements J, Hutmacher DW. The potential role of lycopene for the prevention and therapy of prostate cancer: From molecular mechanisms to clinical evidence. *Int J Mol Sci*. 2013;14(7):14620–14646.

21. Jenkins DJA, Kendall CWC, Popovich DG, et al. Effect of a very-high-fiber vegetable, fruit, and nut diet on serum lipids and colonic function. *Metabolism.* 2001;50(4):494–503.

22. Du H, Bennett D, Bennett D, et al. Fresh fruit consumption in relation to incident diabetes and diabetic vascular complications: A 7-y prospective study of 0.5 million Chinese adults. *PLoS Med.* 2017;14(4).

23. Choo VL, Viguiliouk E, Blanco Mejia S, et al. Food sources of fructose-containing sugars and glycaemic control: Systematic review and meta-analysis of controlled intervention studies. *BMJ.* 2018;363.

24. Liu Q, Ayoub-Charette S, Khan TA, et al. Important Food Sources of Fructose-Containing Sugars and Incident Hypertension: A Systematic Review and Dose-Response Meta-Analysis of Prospective Cohort Studies. *J Am Heart Assoc.* 2019;8(24):e010977.

25. Wong A, Young DA, Emmanouil DE, Wong LM, Waters AR, Booth MT. Raisins and Oral Health. *J Food Sci.* 2013;78(SUPPL.1).

26. Sadler MJ. Dried fruit and dental health. *Int J Food Sci Nutr.* 2016;67(8):944–959.

27. Bolton RP, Heaton KW, Burroughs LF, Sc B. *The Role of Dietary Fiber in Satiety, Glucose, and Insulin: Studies with Fruit and Fruit Juice1' 2.* Vol 34.; 1981.

28. Faith MS, Dennison BA, Edmunds LS, Stratton HH. Fruit juice intake predicts increased adiposity gain in children from low-income families: Weight status-by-environment interaction. *Pediatrics.* 2006;118(5):2066–2075.

29. Aune D, Keum N, Giovannucci E, et al. Whole grain consumption and risk of cardiovascular disease, cancer, and all cause and cause specific mortality: Systematic review and dose-response meta-analysis of prospective studies. *BMJ.* 2016;353.

30. Myers JP, Antoniou MN, Blumberg B, et al. Concerns over use of glyphosate-based herbicides and risks associated with exposures: A consensus statement. *Environ Heal A Glob Access Sci Source.* 2016;15(1):1–13.

31. Temkin A. Breakfast With a Dose of Roundup? | Children's Health Initiative | EWG. https://www.ewg.org/childrens health/glyphosateincereal/. Published 2018. Accessed January 10, 2020.

32. Song M, Fung TT, Hu FB, et al. Association of animal and plant protein intake with all-cause and cause-specific mortality. *JAMA Intern Med.* 2016;176(10):1453–1463.

33. Budhathoki S, Sawada N, Iwasaki M, et al. Association of Animal and Plant Protein Intake with All-Cause and Cause-Specific Mortality in a Japanese Cohort. *JAMA Intern Med.* 2019;179(11):1509–1518.

34. Yau T, Dan X, Ng CCW, Ng TB. Lectins with potential for anti-cancer therapy. *Molecules.* 2015;20(3):3791–3810.

35. Sugizaki CSA, Naves MM V. Potential prebiotic properties of nuts and edible seeds and their relationship to obesity. *Nutrients.* 2018;10(11).

36. De Souza RGM, Schincaglia RM, Pimente GD, Mota JF. Nuts and human health outcomes: A systematic review. *Nutrients.* 2017;9(12).

Chapter 7: Pregnancy and Lactation

1. Koletzko B, Cremer M, Flothkötter M, et al. Diet and Lifestyle before and during Pregnancy–Practical Recommendations of the Germany-wide Healthy Start–Young Family Network. *Geburtshilfe Frauenheilkd.* 2018;78(12): 1262–1282.

2. Planning for Pregnancy | Preconception Care | CDC. https://www.cdc.gov/preconception/planning.html. Accessed April 18, 2020.

3. Procter RD SB, Campbell RD CG. FROM THE ACADEMY Position Paper Position of the Academy of Nutrition and Dietetics: Nutrition and Lifestyle for a Healthy Pregnancy Outcome POSITION STATEMENT. 2014.

4. Stephenson J, Heslehurst N, Hall J, et al. Before the beginning: nutrition and lifestyle in the preconception period and its importance for future health. *Lancet.* 2018;391(10132):1830–1841.

5. Dörsam AF, Preißl H, Micali N, Lörcher SB, Zipfel S, Giel KE. The impact of maternal eating disorders on dietary intake and eating patterns during pregnancy: A systematic review. *Nutrients.* 2019;11(4).

6. Bibbins-Domingo K, Grossman DC, Curry SJ, et al. Folic acid supplementation for the prevention of neural tube defects US preventive services task force recommendation statement. *JAMA–J Am Med Assoc.* 2017;317(2):183–189.

7. Landrigan PJ. Pesticides and Human Reproduction. *JAMA Intern Med*. 2018;178(1):26–27.

8. Morris A. Reproductive endocrinology: Exposure to pesticide residues linked to adverse pregnancy outcomes. *Nat Rev Endocrinol*. 2018;14(1):4.

9. Bommarito PA, Martin E, Fry RC. Effects of prenatal exposure to endocrine disruptors and toxic metals on the fetal epigenome. *Epigenomics*. 2017;9(3):333–350.

10. Wahlang B. Exposure to persistent organic pollutants: Impact on women's health. *Rev Environ Health*. 2018;33(4):331–348.

11. Smarr MM, Grantz KL, Zhang C, et al. Persistent organic pollutants and pregnancy complications. *Sci Total Environ*. 2016;551-552:285-291.

12. Sferruzzi-Perri AN, Camm EJ. The programming power of the placenta. *Front Physiol*. 2016;7(MAR).

13. Melina V, Craig W, Levin S. Position of the Academy of Nutrition and Dietetics: Vegetarian Diets. *J Acad Nutr Diet*. 2016;116(12):1970-1980.

14. Baroni L, Goggi S, Battaglino R, et al. Vegan nutrition for mothers and children: Practical tools for healthcare providers. *Nutrients*. 2019;11(1).

15. Pistollato F, Sumalla Cano S, Elio I, Masias Vergara M, Giampieri F, Battino M. Plant-Based and Plant-Rich Diet Patterns during Gestation: Beneficial Effects and Possible Shortcomings. *Adv Nutr An Int Rev J*. 2015;6(5).

16. Carter JP, Furman T, Robert Hutcheson H. Preeclampsia and reproductive performance in a community of vegans. *South Med J*. 1987;80(6):692–697.

17. Kominiarek MA, Rajan P. Nutrition Recommendations in Pregnancy and Lactation. *Med Clin North Am*. 2016;100(6):1199–1215.

18. Wen T, Lv Y. Inadequate gestational weight gain and adverse pregnancy outcomes among normal weight women in China. *Int J Clin Exp Med*. 2015;8(2):2881–2886.

19. Viecceli C, Remonti LR, Hirakata VN, et al. Weight gain adequacy and pregnancy outcomes in gestational diabetes: a meta-analysis. *Obes Rev*. 2017;18(5):567–580.

20. Middleton P, Gomersall JC, Gould JF, Shepherd E, Olsen SF, Makrides M. Omega-3 fatty acid addition during pregnancy. *Cochrane Database Syst Rev*. 2018;2018(11).

21. Burns-Whitmore B, Froyen E, Heskey C, Parker T, Pablo GS. Alpha-linolenic and linoleic fatty acids in the vegan diet: Do they require dietary reference intake/adequate intake special consideration? *Nutrients*. 2019;11(10).

22. Davis BC, Kris-Etherton PM. Achieving optimal essential fatty acid status in vegetarians : current knowledge and practical implications 1—3. *Am J Clin Nutr*. 2003;78:640–646.

23. Koletzko B, Lien E, Agostoni C, et al. The roles of long-chain polyunsaturated fatty acids in pregnancy, lactation and infancy: Review of current knowledge and consensus recommendations. *J Perinat Med*. 2008;36(1):5–14.

24. Food and Agriculture Organization of the United Nations. Fats and fatty acids in human nutrition: Report of an expert consultation. In: *FAO Food and Nutrition Paper 91*. ; 2010.

25. Saunders A V., Davis BC, Garg ML. Omega-3 polyunsaturated fatty acids and vegetarian diets. *Med J Aust*. 2013;199(4):S22–S26.

26. Nordgren TM, Lyden E, Anderson-Berry A, Hanson C. Omega-3 fatty acid intake of pregnant women and women of childbearing age in the united states: Potential for deficiency? *Nutrients*. 2017;9(3).

27. Advice about Eating Fish | FDA. https://www.fda.gov/food/consumers/advice-about-eating-fish. Accessed April 20, 2020.

28. Valera-Gran D, Navarrete-Muñoz EM, De La Hera MG, et al. Effect of maternal high dosages of folic acid supplements on neurocognitive development in children at 4–5 y of age: The prospective birth cohort Infancia y Medio Ambiente (INMA) study. *Am J Clin Nutr*. 2017;106(3):878–887.

29. Sebastiani G, Barbero AH, Borrás-Novel C, et al. The effects of vegetarian and vegan diet during pregnancy on the health of mothers and offspring. *Nutrients*. 2019;11(3).

30. Langan RC, Goodbred AJ, Luke S, Residency M. Vitamin B12 Deficiency: Recognition and Management. *Am Fam Physician*. 2017;96(6):384–389.

31. Olson SR, Deloughery TG, Taylor JA. Time to Abandon the Serum Cobalamin Level for Diagnosing Vitamin B12 Deficiency. *Blood*. 2016;128(22):2447–2447.

32. Stabler SP. Vitamin B 12 Deficiency.

33. Agnoli C, Baroni L, Bertini I, et al. Position paper on vegetarian diets from the working group of the Italian Society of Human Nutrition. *Nutr Metab Cardiovasc Dis*. 2017;27(12).

34. Korsmo HW, Jiang X, Caudill MA. Choline: Exploring the growing science on its benefits for moms and babies. *Nutrients*. 2019;11(8).

35. Agarwal S, Kovilam O, Agrawal DK. Vitamin D and its impact on maternal-fetal outcomes in pregnancy: A critical review. *Crit Rev Food Sci Nutr*. 2018;58(5):755–769.

36. Palacios C, Kostiuk LK, Peña-Rosas JP. Vitamin D supplementation for women during pregnancy. *Cochrane Database Syst Rev*. 2019;2019(7).

37. Baroni L, Goggi S, Battaglino R, et al. nutrients Vegan Nutrition for Mothers and Children: Practical Tools for Healthcare Providers. 2018.

38. Hofmeyr GJ, Lawrie TA, Atallah ÁN, Torloni MR. Calcium supplementation during pregnancy for preventing hypertensive disorders and related problems. *Cochrane Database Syst Rev*. 2018;2018(10).

39. Iron—Health Professional Fact Sheet. https://ods.od.nih.gov/factsheets/Iron-HealthProfessional/. Accessed March 19, 2020.

40. Introduction–Routine Iron Supplementation and Screening for Iron Deficiency Anemia in Pregnant Women–NCBI Bookshelf. https://www.ncbi.nlm.nih.gov/books/NBK285987/. Accessed April 22, 2020.

41. *Dietary Reference Intakes for Vitamin A, Vitamin K, Arsenic, Boron, Chromium, Copper, Iodine, Iron, Manganese, Molybdenum, Nickel, Silicon, Vanadium, and Zinc*. National Academies Press; 2001.

42. Lee SY, Pearce EN. Reproductive endocrinology: Iodine intake in pregnancy—even a little excess is too much. *Nat Rev Endocrinol*. 2015;11(5):260–261.

43. Edwards SM, Cunningham SA, Dunlop AL, Corwin EJ. The Maternal Gut Microbiome during Pregnancy. *MCN Am J Matern Nurs*. 2017;42(6):310–316.

44. Guide to healthy pregnancy–Canada.ca. https://www.canada.ca/en/public-health/services/pregnancy/guide -healthy-pregnancy.html. Accessed April 24, 2020.

45. Eating for Two–Nutrition During Pregnancy–MedBroadcast.com. https://www.medbroadcast.com/healthfeature /gethealthfeature/eating-for-two—-nutrition-during-pregnancy?_ga=2.29929791.1039075782.1587746231 -312428333.1587409629. Accessed April 24, 2020.

46. Dermott A. Safe herbal teas during pregnancy. Healthline Parenthood. https://www.healthline.com/health /pregnancy/safe-herbal-teas. Published 2016.

47. Pope E, Koren G, Bozzo P. Sugar substitutes during pregnancy. *Can Fam Physician*. 2014;60(11):1003–1005.

48. Sharma A, Amarnath S, Thulasimani M, Ramaswamy S. Artificial sweeteners as a sugar substitute: Are they really safe? *Indian J Pharmacol*. 2016;48(3):237–240.

49. Caffeine and pregnancy–Canada.ca. https://www.canada.ca/en/public-health/services/pregnancy/caffeine.html. Accessed April 24, 2020.

50. Rhee J, Kim R, Kim Y, et al. Maternal caffeine consumption during pregnancy and risk of low birth weight: A dose-response meta-analysis of observational studies. *PLoS One*. 2015;10(7).

51. Vitamin A—Health Professional Fact Sheet. https://ods.od.nih.gov/factsheets/VitaminA-HealthProfessional/. Accessed February 29, 2020.

52. Rumbold A, Ota E, Hori H, Miyazaki C, Crowther CA. Vitamin E supplementation in pregnancy. *Cochrane Database Syst Rev*. 2015;2016(3).

53. O'Donnell A, McParlin C, Robson SC, et al. Treatments for hyperemesis gravidarum and nausea and vomiting in pregnancy: A systematic review and economic assessment. *Health Technol Assess (Rockv)*. 2016;20(74):vii–268.

54. Dean E. Morning sickness. *Nurs Stand*. 2016;30(50):15.

55. Fujimura T, Lum SZC, Nagata Y, Kawamoto S, Oyoshi MK. Influences of maternal factors over offspring allergies and the application for food allergy. *Front Immunol*. 2019;10(AUG).

56. Hörnell A, Lagström H, Lande B, Thorsdottir I. Breastfeeding, introduction of other foods and effects on health: a systematic literature review for the 5th Nordic Nutrition Recommendations. *Food Nutr Res*. 2013;57(1):20823.

57. Sattari M, Serwint JR, Levine DM. Maternal Implications of Breastfeeding: A Review for the Internist. *Am J Med*. 2019;132(8):912–920.

58. Binns C, Lee M, Low WY. The Long-Term Public Health Benefits of Breastfeeding. *Asia-Pacific J Public Heal*. 2016;28(1):7–14.

59. Mosca F, Giannì ML. Human milk: composition and health benefits. *Pediatr Med Chir*. 2017;39(2):155.

60. Calcium I of M (US) C to RDRI for VD and, Ross AC, Taylor CL, Yaktine AL, Valle HB Del. *Dietary Reference Intakes for Calcium and Vitamin D*. National Academies Press; 2011.

61. Institute of Medicine. National Academy of Sciences. Food and Nutrition Board. *Dietary Reference Intakes for Thiamin, Riboflavin, Niacin, Vitamin B6, Folate, Vitamin B12, Pantothenic Acid, Biotin, and Choline (1998)*. Washington, D.C.: The National Academies Press; 1998.

62. Institute of Medicine of the National Academies. *Dietary Reference Intakes for Vitamin C, Vitamin E, Selenium Andd Carotenoids 2000*. Washington, DC: The National Academies Press; 2000.

63. *Consensus Study Report HIGHLIGHTS Dietary Reference Intakes for Sodium and Potassium*.; 2019.

64. Norén K. Levels Of Organochlorine Contaminants In Human Milk In Relation To The Dietary Habits Of The Mothers. *Acta Pædiatrica*. 1983;72(6):811–816.

65. van Kaam AH, Koopman-Esseboom C, Sulkers EJ, Sauer PJ, van der Paauw CG, Tuinstra LG. [Polychlorobiphenyls in human milk, adipose tissue, plasma and umbilical cord blood; levels and correlates]. *Ned Tijdschr Geneeskd*. 1991;135(31):1399–1403.

66. Hergenrather J, Hlady G, Wallace, B SE. Pollutants in Breast Milk of Vegetarians. *N Engl J Med*. 1981;304(13):792.

Chapter 8: Childhood and Adolescence

1. Melina V, Craig W, Levin S. Position of the Academy of Nutrition and Dietetics: Vegetarian Diets. *J Acad Nutr Diet*. 2016;116(12):1970–1980.

2. Sabate J, Lindsted KD, Harris RD, Sanchez A. Attained height of lacto-ovo vegetarian children and adolescents. *Eur J Clin Nutr*. 1991;45(1):51–58.

3. O'Connell JM, Dibley MJ, Sierra J, Wallace B, Marks JS, Yip R. Growth of vegetarian children: The Farm Study. *Pediatrics*. 1989;84(3):475–481.

4. Sanders TA. Growth and development of British vegan children | The American Journal of Clinical Nutrition | Oxford Academic. *Am J Clin Nutr*. 1988:822–825.

5. Mikkilä V, Räsänen L, Raitakari OT, Pietinen P, Viikari J. Consistent dietary patterns identified from childhood to adulthood: The Cardiovascular Risk in Young Finns Study. *Br J Nutr*. 2005;93(6):923–931.

6. Li J, Wang Y. Tracking of Dietary Intake Patterns Is Associated with Baseline Characteristics of Urban Low-Income African-American Adolescents. *J Nutr*. 2008;138(1):94–100.

7. Ambrosini GL, Emmett PM, Northstone K, Jebb SA. Tracking a dietary pattern associated with increased adiposity in childhood and adolescence. *Obesity*. 2014;22(2):458–465.

8. Maynard M, Gunnell D, Ness AR, Abraham L, Bates CJ, Blane D. Health-Related Behaviours What influences diet in early old age? Prospective and cross-sectional analyses of the Boyd Orr cohort. *Eur J Public Health*. 2005;16(3):315–323.

9. Center for Chronic Disease Prevention N, Promotion H, of Nutrition D, Activity P. *Breastfeeding Report Card, Progressing Toward National Breastfeeding Goals: United States / 2013*.

10. Brown CRL, Dodds L, Legge A, Bryanton J, Semenic S. Factors influencing the reasons why mothers stop breastfeeding. *Can J Public Heal*. 2014;105(3).

11. Eidelman AI, Schanler RJ. Breastfeeding and the use of human milk. *Pediatrics*. 2012;129(3):e827–e841.

12. van den Elsen LWJ, Garssen J, Burcelin R, Verhasselt V. Shaping the gut microbiota by breastfeeding: The gateway to allergy prevention? *Front Pediatr.* 2019;7(FEB):47.

13. Weaning from the breast. *Paediatr Child Health.* 2004;9(4):249.

14. Abrams SA, Landers S, Noble LM, Poindexter BB. Donor human milk for the high- risk infant: Preparation, safety, and usage options in the United States. *Pediatrics.* 2017;139(1).

15. Wagner CL, Greer FR. Prevention of rickets and vitamin D deficiency in infants, children, and adolescents. *Pediatrics.* 2008;122(5):1142–1152.

16. Questions & Answers for Consumers Concerning Infant Formula | FDA. https://www.fda.gov/food/people-risk -foodborne-illness/questions-answers-consumers-concerning-infant-formula#2. Accessed May 3, 2020.

17. Choosing an Infant Formula–HealthyChildren.org. https://www.healthychildren.org/English/ages-stages/baby /formula-feeding/Pages/Choosing-an-Infant-Formula.aspx. Accessed May 3, 2020.

18. Leung AK, Sauve RS. Whole cow's milk in infancy. *Paediatr Child Health.* 2003;8(7):419.

19. Where We Stand: Soy Formulas–HealthyChildren.org. https://www.healthychildren.org/English/ages-stages/baby/ formula-feeding/Pages/Where-We-Stand-Soy-Formulas.aspx. Accessed May 3, 2020.

20. Fang X, Wang L, Wu C, et al. Sex Hormones, Gonadotropins, and Sex Hormone-binding Globulin in Infants Fed Breast Milk, Cow Milk Formula, or Soy Formula. *Sci Rep.* 2017;7(1).

21. Sinai T, Ben-Avraham S, Guelmann-Mizrahi I, et al. Consumption of soy-based infant formula is not associated with early onset of puberty. *Eur J Nutr.* 2019;58(2):681–687.

22. Testa I, Salvatori C, Di Cara G, et al. Soy-Based Infant Formula: Are Phyto-Oestrogens Still in Doubt? *Front Nutr.* 2018;5.

23. Bhatia J, Greer F. Use of soy protein-based formulas in infant feeding. *Pediatrics.* 2008;121(5):1062–1068.

24. Fanni D, Ambu R, Gerosa C, et al. Aluminum exposure and toxicity in neonates: A practical guide to halt aluminum overload in the prenatal and perinatal periods. *World J Pediatr.* 2014;10(2):101–107.

25. Shinwell ED, Gorodischer R. Totally vegetarian diets and infant nutrition. *Pediatrics.* 1982;70(4):582–586.

26. Zmora E, Gorodischer R, Bar-Ziv J. Multiple Nutritional Deficiencies in Infants From a Strict Vegetarian Community. *Am J Dis Child.* 1979;133(2):141–144.

27. Davis SA, Knol LL, Crowe-White KM, Turner LW, McKinley E. Homemade infant formula recipes may contain harmful ingredients: A quantitative content analysis of blogs. *Public Health Nutr.* 2020;23(8).

28. DIMaggio DiM, Cox A, Porto AF. Updates in infant nutrition. *Pediatr Rev.* 2017;38(10):449–460.

29. U.S. Department of Agriculture ARS. FoodData Central. fdc.nal.usda.gov. Published 2019.

30. D'Auria E, Bergamini M, Staiano A, et al. Baby-led weaning: What a systematic review of the literature adds on. *Ital J Pediatr.* 2018;44(1).

31. Atiaga O, Nunes LM, Otero XL. Effect of cooking on arsenic concentration in rice. *Environ Sci Pollut Res.* 2020;27 (10):10757–10765.

32. Greer FR, Sicherer SH, Wesley Burks A, et al. The effects of early nutritional interventions on the development of atopic disease in infants and children: The role of maternal dietary restriction, breastfeeding, hydrolyzed formulas, and timing of introduction of allergenic complementary foods. *Pediatrics.* 2019;143(4).

33. Abrams EM, Hildebrand K, Blair B, Chan ES. Timing of introduction of allergenic solids for infants at high risk. *Paediatr Child Health.* 2019;24(1):56.

34. Choi YY, Ludwig A, Harris JL. US toddler milk sales and associations with marketing practices. *Public Health Nutr.* 2020;23(6):1127–1135. doi:10.1017/S1368980019003756

35. Silk® Plant-Based Products: Almondmilk, Soymilk, Coconutmilk, Oatmilk. https://silk.com/plant-based-products/. Accessed May 25, 2020.

36. Dairy-Free Plant-Based Milk Alternatives | Ripple Foods. https://www.ripplefoods.com/plant-milk/. Accessed May 25, 2020.

37. Willett WC, Ludwig DS. Milk and health. *N Engl J Med.* 2020;382(7):644–654.

38. Mennella JA, Trabulsi JC. Complementary foods and flavor experiences: Setting the foundation. *Ann Nutr Metab.* 2012;60(SUPPL. 2):40–50.

39. John KA, Cogswell ME, Zhao L, Maalouf J, Gunn JP, Merritt RK. US consumer attitudes toward sodium in baby and toddler foods. *Appetite.* 2016;103:171–175.

40. Your Toddler May Be Getting Too Much Salt—Health Essentials from Cleveland Clinic. https://health.cleveland clinic.org/your-toddler-may-be-getting-too-much-salt/. Accessed May 8, 2020.

41. Medicine. I of. *Dietary Reference Intakes for Sodium and Potassium.* Washington, D.C.: National Academies Press; 2019.

42. Vos MB, Kaar JL, Welsh JA, et al. Added sugars and cardiovascular disease risk in children: A scientific statement from the American Heart Association. *Circulation.* 2017;135(19):e1017–e1034.

43. Institute of Medicine. *Dietary Reference Intakes for Energy, Carbohydrate, Fiber, Fat, Fatty Acids, Cholesterol, Protein, and Amino Acids.*; 2002.

44. Costa CS, Del-Ponte B, Assunção MCF, Santos IS. Consumption of ultra-processed foods and body fat during childhood and adolescence: A systematic review. *Public Health Nutr.* 2018;21(1):148–159.

45. Park S, Cho SC, Hong YC, et al. Association between dietary behaviors and attention-deficit/hyperactivity disorder and learning disabilities in school-aged children. *Psychiatry Res.* 2012;198(3):468–476.

46. Sadeghirad B, Duhaney T, Motaghipisheh S, Campbell NRC, Johnston BC. Influence of unhealthy food and beverage marketing on children's dietary intake and preference: a systematic review and meta-analysis of randomized trials. *Obes Rev.* 2016;17(10):945–959.

47. Heart and Stroke Foundation of Canada. *The Kids Are Not Alright. 2017 Report on the Health of Canadians.*; 2017.

48. Das JK, Salam RA, Thornburg KL, et al. Nutrition in adolescents: physiology, metabolism, and nutritional needs. *Ann N Y Acad Sci.* 2017;1393(1):21–33.

49. Hagan J, Shaw JS, Duncan PM. *BF Nutrition 4th Edition Supervision AAP.*; 2017.

50. U.S. Department of Health and Human Services and U.S. Department of Agriculture. *2015—2020 Dietary Guidelines for Americans. 8th Edition. December 2015. Available at Https://Health.Gov/Dietaryguidelines/2015/Guidelines/.* 8th ed. USDA; 2015.

51. Kimmons J, Gillespie C, Seymour J, Serdula M, Blanck HM. Fruit and vegetable intake among adolescents and adults in the United States: Percentage meeting individualized recommendations. *MedGenMed Medscape Gen Med.* 2009;11(1):26.

52. Kranz S, Brauchla M, Slavin JL, Miller KB. What Do We Know about Dietary Fiber Intake in Children and Health? The Effects of Fiber Intake on Constipation, Obesity, and Diabetes in Children. *Adv Nutr.* 2012;3(1):47–53.

53. Larson N, Neumark-Sztainer D, Adam HM. Adolescent nutrition. *Pediatr Rev.* 2009;30(12):494–496.

54. How Much Junk Food Do Teenagers Eat?–The New York Times. https://www.nytimes.com/2015/09/22/health /how-much-junk-food-do-teenagers-eat.html. Accessed May 18, 2020.

55. Pereira MA, Kartashov AI, Ebbeling CB, et al. Fast-food habits, weight gain, and insulin resistance (the CARDIA study): 15-year prospective analysis. *Lancet.* 2005;365(9453):36–42.

56. Segovia-Siapco G, Burkholder-Cooley N, Haddad Tabrizi S, Sabaté J. Beyond meat: A comparison of the dietary intakes of vegetarian and non-vegetarian adolescents. *Front Nutr.* 2019;6.

57. Mountjoy M, Sundgot-Borgen J, Burke L, et al. The IOC consensus statement: Beyond the Female Athlete Triad-Relative Energy Deficiency in Sport (RED-S). *Br J Sports Med.* 2014;48(7):491–497.

58. Desbrow B, McCormack J, Burke LM, et al. Sports dietitians australia position statement: Sports nutrition for the adolescent athlete. *Int J Sport Nutr Exerc Metab.* 2014;24(5):570–584.

59. Clénin GE, Cordes M, Huber A, et al. Iron deficiency in sports–definition, influence on performance and therapy. *Schweizerische Zeitschrift fur Sport und Sport.* 2016;64(1):6–18.

60. Lynn D, Umari T, Dellavalle R, Dunnick C. The epidemiology of acne vulgaris in late adolescence. *Adolesc Health Med Ther.* 2016;7:13.

61. Juhl CR, Bergholdt HKM, Miller IM, Jemec GBE, Kanters JK, Ellervik C. Dairy intake and acne vulgaris: A systematic review and meta-analysis of 78,529 children, adolescents, and young adults. *Nutrients.* 2018;10(8).

62. Zouboulis CC, Jourdan E, Picardo M. Acne is an inflammatory disease and alterations of sebum composition initiate acne lesions. *J Eur Acad Dermatology Venereol.* 2014;28(5):527–532.

63. Kucharska A, Szmurło A, Sinska B. Significance of diet in treated and untreated acne vulgaris. *Postep Dermatologii i Alergol.* 2016;33(2):81–86.

64. Isgin-Atici K, Buyuktuncer Z, Akgül S, Kanbur N. Adolescents with premenstrual syndrome: Not only what you eat but also how you eat matters! *J Pediatr Endocrinol Metab.* 2018;31(11):1231–1239.

65. Hashim MS, Obaideen AA, Jahrami HA, et al. Premenstrual syndrome is associated with dietary and lifestyle behaviors among university students: A cross-sectional study from sharjah, UAE. *Nutrients.* 2019;11(8).

66. Barnard ND, Scialli AR, Hurlock D, Bertron P. Diet and sex-hormone binding globulin, dysmenorrhea, and pre-menstrual symptoms. *Obstet Gynecol.* 2000;95(2):245–250.

67. Najafi N, Khalkhali H, Moghaddam Tabrizi F, Zarrin R. Major dietary patterns in relation to menstrual pain: A nested case control study. *BMC Womens Health.* 2018;18(1).

68. Bielecka GJ, Mizgier M, Kedzia W. Metrorrhagia iuvenilis and Premenstrual Syndrome as frequent problems of adolescent gynecology with aspects of diet therapy. *Ginekol Pol.* 2019;90(7):423–429.

69. Isgin-Atici K, Kanbur N, Akgül S, Buyuktuncer Z. Diet quality in adolescents with premenstrual syndrome: A cross-sectional study. *Nutr Diet.* 2019.

70. Hansen SO, Knudsen UB. Endometriosis, dysmenorrhoea and diet. *Eur J Obstet Gynecol Reprod Biol.* 2013;169 (2):162–171.

71. Sohrabi N, Kashanian M, Ghafoori SS, Malakouti SK. Evaluation of the effect of omega-3 fatty acids in the treatment of premenstrual syndrome: " A pilot trial." *Complement Ther Med.* 2013;21(3):141–146.

72. Messina M. Soy and health update: Evaluation of the clinical and epidemiologic literature. *Nutrients.* 2016;8(12).

73. Rudloff S, Bührer C, Jochum F, et al. Vegetarian diets in childhood and adolescence. *Mol Cell Pediatr.* 2019;6(1).

74. Slavin J. Fiber and Prebiotics: Mechanisms and Health Benefits. 2013:1417–1435.

75. Bell V, Ferrão J, Fernandes T. *Fermented Food Guidelines for Children.* Vol 2.; 2018.

76. Roberts JR, Karr CJ, Paulson JA, et al. Pesticide exposure in children. *Pediatrics.* 2012;130(6):e1757–e1763.

77. Bradman A, Quirós-Alcalá L, Castorina R, et al. Effect of Organic Diet Intervention on Pesticide Exposures in Young Children Living in Low-Income Urban and Agricultural Communities. *Environ Health Perspect.* 2015;123(10):1086–1093.

78. Barański M, Średnicka-Tober D, Volakakis N, et al. Higher antioxidant and lower cadmium concentrations and lower incidence of pesticide residues in organically grown crops: A systematic literature review and meta-analyses. *Br J Nutr.* 2014;112(5):794–811.

79. Babies Bright Futures H. *A National Investigation Finds 95 Percent of Baby Foods Tested Contain Toxic Chemicals That Lower Babies' IQ, Including Arsenic and Lead Report Includes Safer Choices for Parents, Manufacturers and Retailers Seeking Healthy Foods for Infants.*; 2019.

80. Ashraf MA. Persistent organic pollutants (POPs): a global issue, a global challenge. *Environ Sci Pollut Res.* 2017;24 (5):4223–4227.

81. Guo W, Pan B, Sakkiah S, et al. Persistent organic pollutants in food: Contamination sources, health effects and detection methods. *Int J Environ Res Public Health.* 2019;16(22).

82. Gill V, Kumar V, Singh K, Kumar A, Kim JJ. Advanced glycation end products (AGEs) may be a striking link between modern diet and health. *Biomolecules.* 2019;9(12).

83. Barzegar F, Kamankesh M, Mohammadi A. Heterocyclic aromatic amines in cooked food: A review on formation, health risk-toxicology and their analytical techniques. *Food Chem.* 2019;280:240–254.

84. Bansal V, Kumar P, Kwon EE, Kim KH. Review of the quantification techniques for polycyclic aromatic hydrocarbons (PAHs) in food products. *Crit Rev Food Sci Nutr.* 2017;57(15):3297–3312.

85. Semla M, Goc Z, Martiniaková M, Omelka R, Formicki G. Acrylamide: a common food toxin related to physiological functions and health. *Physiol Res.* 2017;66(2):205–217.

86. Sansano M, Juan-Borrás M, Escriche I, Andrés A, Heredia A. Effect of Pretreatments and Air-Frying, a Novel Technology, on Acrylamide Generation in Fried Potatoes. *J Food Sci.* 2015;80(5):T1120–T1128.

87. Grohs MN, Reynolds JE, Liu J, et al. Prenatal maternal and childhood bisphenol a exposure and brain structure and behavior of young children. *Environ Heal A Glob Access Sci Source.* 2019;18(1).

88. Braun JM, Hauser R. Bisphenol A and children's health. *Curr Opin Pediatr.* 2011;23(2):233–239.

89. Baker RD, Greer FR, Bhatia JJS, et al. Clinical report–Diagnosis and prevention of iron deficiency and iron-deficiency anemia in infants and young children (0–3 years of age). *Pediatrics.* 2010;126(5):1040–1050.

90. AAP: Screen for lipids with nonfasting total cholesterol and HDL | MDedge Pediatrics. https://www.mdedge.com /pediatrics/article/103949/endocrinology/aap-screen-lipids-nonfasting-total-cholesterol-and-hdl. Accessed June 9, 2020.

91. Detection of Lead Poisoning. https://www.aap.org/en-us/advocacy-and-policy/aap-health-initiatives/lead-exposure /Pages/Detection-of-Lead-Poisoning.aspx. Accessed June 9, 2020.

Chapter 9: Principles of Feeding: Setting The Table

1. Satter E. Hierarchy of Food Needs. *J Nutr Educ Behav.* 2007;39(5 SUPPL.).

2. Kerzner B, Milano K, MacLean WC, Berall G, Stuart S, Chatoor I. A practical approach to classifying and managing feeding difficulties. *Pediatrics.* 2015;135(2):344–353.

3. Black MM, Aboud FE. The Journal of Nutrition Symposium: Responsive Feeding-Promoting Healthy Growth and Development for Infants and Toddlers Responsive Feeding Is Embedded in a Theoretical Framework of Responsive Parenting 1–3. *J Nutr.* 2011;141:490–494.

4. Vollmer RL. Parental feeding style changes the relationships between children's food preferences and food parenting practices: The case for comprehensive food parenting interventions by pediatric healthcare professionals. *J Spec Pediatr Nurs.* 2019;24(1).

5. Satter E. Feeding dynamics: Helping children to eat well. *J Pediatr Heal Care.* 1995;9(4):178–184.

6. Mennella JA, Jagnow CP, Beauchamp GK. Prenatal and postnatal flavor learning by human infants. *Pediatrics.* 2001;107(6):E88.

7. Birch LL, Doub AE. Learning to eat: Birth to age 2 y. *Am J Clin Nutr.* 2014;99(3):723–728.

8. Harris G, Mason S. Are There Sensitive Periods for Food Acceptance in Infancy? *Curr Nutr Rep.* 2017;6(2):190–196.

9. Van der Horst K. Overcoming picky eating. Eating enjoyment as a central aspect of children's eating behaviors. *Appetite.* 2012;58(2):567–574.

10. Mitchell GL, Farrow C, Haycraft E, Meyer C. Parental influences on children's eating behaviour and characteristics of successful parent focussed interventions. *Appetite.* 2013;60(1):85–94.

11. Satter, E. *Secrets of Feeding a Healthy Family: How to Eat, How to Raise Good Eaters, How to Cook.* Madison, WI: Kelcy Press, 2008.

12. Rowell K, McGlothlin J. *Helping Your Child with Extreme Picky Eating: A Step-by-Step Guide for Overcoming Selective Eating, Food Aversion, and Feeding Disorders.* Oakland, CA: New Harbinger Publications, Inc., 2015.

Chapter 10: Family Meals

1. McCullough MB, Robson SM, Stark LJ. A Review of the Structural Characteristics of Family Meals with Children in the United States. *Adv Nutr An Int Rev J.* 2016;7(4):627–640.

2. https://thefamilydinnerproject.org/

3. Fishel, AK. *Home for Dinner: Mixing Food, Fun, and Conversation for a Happier Family and Healthier Kids.* New York, NY: American Management Association, 2015.

4. Satter, E. *Secrets of Feeding a Healthy Family: How to Eat, How to Raise Good Eaters, How to Cook.* Madison, WI: Kelcy Press, 2008.

5. Snow CE, Beals DE. Mealtime talk that supports literacy development. *New Dir Child Adolesc Dev.* 2006;2006 (111):51–66.

6. The National Center on Addiction and Substance Abuse at Columbia University (CASA), *The Importance of Family Dinners IV*, 2007

7. Neumark-Sztainer D, Larson NI, Fulkerson JA, Eisenberg ME, Story M. Family meals and adolescents: What have we learned from Project EAT (Eating Among Teens)? *Public Health Nutr.* 2010;13(7):1113–1121

8. Neumark-Sztainer D, Eisenberg ME, Fulkerson JA, Story M, Larson NI. Family Meals and Disordered Eating in Adolescents. *Arch Pediatr Adolesc Med.* 2008;162(1):17.

9. Hammons AJ, Fiese BH. Is frequency of shared family meals related to the nutritional health of children and adolescents? *Pediatrics.* 2011;127(6):1565–1574.

10. Fulkerson JA, Story M, Mellin A, Leffert N, Neumark-Sztainer D, French SA. Family Dinner Meal Frequency and Adolescent Development: Relationships with Developmental Assets and High-Risk Behaviors. *J Adolesc Heal.* 2006;39(3):337–345.

11. Utter J, Denny S, Robinson E, Fleming T, Ameratunga S, Grant S. Family meals and the well-being of adolescents. *J Paediatr Child Health.* 2013;49(11):906–911.

12. The National Center on Addiction and Substance Abuse at Columbia University (CASA) *The Importance of Family Dinners VII*, 2012.

13. Utter J, Larson N, Berge JM, Eisenberg ME, Fulkerson JA, Neumark-Sztainer D. Family meals among parents: Associations with nutritional, social and emotional wellbeing. *Prev Med (Baltim).* 2018;113:7–12.

14. Eisenberg ME, Olson RE, Neumark-Sztainer D, Story M, Bearinger LH. Correlations between family meals and psychosocial well-being among adolescents. *Arch Pediatr Adolesc Med.* 2004;158(8):792–796.

15. https://www.acpeds.org/the-college-speaks/position-statements/parenting-issues/the-benefits-of-the-family-table

16. Duke MP, Fivush R, Lazarus A, Bohanek J. Of Ketchup and Kin : Dinnertime Conversations as a Major Source of Family Knowledge , Family Adjustment , and Family Resilience. 2003;(26).

17. Skeer MR, Ballard EL. Are Family Meals as Good for Youth as We Think They Are? A Review of the Literature on Family Meals as They Pertain to Adolescent Risk Prevention. *J Youth Adolesc.* 2013;42(7):943-963.

18. https://www.theatlantic.com/health/archive/2019/10/work-its-whats-for-dinner/599770/

19. Hennessy E, Dwyer L, Oh A, Patrick H. Promoting family meals: a review of existing interventions and opportunities for future research. *Adolesc Health Med Ther.* 2015;115.

20. https://www.nytimes.com/guides/well/make-most-of-family-table

21. Fiese BH, Schwartz M. Reclaiming the Family Table: Mealtimes and Child Health and Wellbeing. *Soc Policy Rep.* 2008;22(4):1–20.

22. Dwyer RJ, Kushlev K, Dunn EW. Smartphone Use Undermines Enjoyment of Face-to-Face Social Interactions. *Journal of Experimental Social Psychology.* 2018; 78:233–239.

23. Fulkerson JA, Larson N, Horning M, Neumark-Sztainer D. A review of associations between family or shared meal frequency and dietary and weight status outcomes across the lifespan. *J Nutr Educ Behav.* 2014;46(1):2–19.

Chapter 11: Weighty Matters

1. Rowell K, McGlothlin J. *Helping Your Child with Extreme Picky Eating: A Step-by-Step Guide for Overcoming Selective Eating, Food Aversion, and Feeding Disorders.* Oakland, CA: New Harbinger Publications, Inc., 2015

2. https://www.cdc.gov/growthcharts/data/set1clinical/cj41l021.pdf

3. Rothman KJ. BMI-related errors in the measurement of obesity. *Int J Obes.* 2008;32:S56–S59.

4. https://www.nytimes.com/interactive/projects/cp/summer-of-science-2015/latest/how-often-is-bmi-misleading?smid=tw-nytimes&smtyp=cur

5. Reilly JJ. Diagnostic Accuracy of the BMI for Age in Paediatrics. *Int J Obes.* 2006;30(4):595–597.

6. Thompson HR, Madsen KA. The Report Card on BMI Report Cards. *Curr Obes Rep.* 2017;6(2):163–167.

7. Golden NH, Schneider M, Wood C. Preventing Obesity and Eating Disorders in Adolescents. *Pediatrics.* 2016;138(3).

8. Hales CM, Carroll MD, Fryar CD, Ogden CL. Prevalence of Obesity Among Adults and Youth: United States, 2015–2016. NCHS data brief, no 288. Hyattsville, MD: National Center for Health Statistics.

9. https://www.who.int/en/news-room/fact-sheets/detail/obesity-and-overweight

10. Geserick M, Vogel M, Gausche R, et al. Acceleration of BMI in early childhood and risk of sustained obesity. *N Engl J Med.* 2018;379(14):1303–1312

11. Freedman DS, Khan LK, Serdula MK, Dietz WH, Srinivasan SR, Berenson GS. The relation of childhood BMI to adult adiposity: The Bogalusa heart study. Pediatrics. 2005;115(1): 22–27.

12. Steinberger J, Moran A, Hong CP, Jacobs DR, Sinaiko AR. Adiposity in childhood predicts obesity and insulin resistance in young adulthood. *J Pediatr.* 2001;138(4):469–473.

13. Reilly JJ. Health consequences of obesity. *Arch Dis Child.* 2003;88(9):748–752.

14. Afshin A, Forouzanfar MH, Reitsma MB, et al. Health Effects of Overweight and Obesity in 195 Countries Over 25 years. *N Engl J Med.* 2017;377(1):13–27.

15. U.S. Department of Health and Human Services. Managing Overweight and Obesity in Adults: Systematic Evidence Review from the Obesity Expert Panel. *Natl Hear Lung, Blood Inst.* 2013:501.

16. Cook S, Kavey REW. Dyslipidemia and Pediatric Obesity. *Pediatr Clin North Am.* 2011;58(6):1363–1373.

17. Koskinen J, Juonala M, Dwyer T, et al. Impact of Lipid Measurements in Youth in Addition to Conventional Clinic-Based Risk Factors on Predicting Preclinical Atherosclerosis in Adulthood. *Circulation.* 2018;137(12):1246–1255.

18. Turer CB, Brady TM, De Ferranti SD. Obesity, hypertension, and dyslipidemia in childhood are key modifiable antecedents of adult cardiovascular disease: A call to action. *Circulation.* 2018;137(12):1256–1259.

19. Hannon TS. Childhood Obesity and Type 2 Diabetes Mellitus. *Pediatrics.* 2005;116(2):473–480.

20. Must A, Anderson SE. Effects of obesity on morbidity in children and adolescents. *Nutr Clin Care.* 2003;6(1): 4–12.

21. Harriger JA, Thompson JK. Psychological consequences of obesity: Weight bias and body image in overweight and obese youth. *Int Rev Psychiatry.* 2012;24(3):247–253.

22. The Academy of Eating Disorders (AED) BEDA, (BEDA), The Eating Disorders Coalition for Research, Policy & Action (EDC) F, Empowered And Supporting Treatment of Eating Disorders (F.E.A.S.T.) ST, Initiative for the Prevention of Eating Disorders (S.T.R.I.P.E.D.) and Kendrin Sonneville S, RD U of MS of PH. Facts and Concerns About School-Based BMI Screening, Surveillance and Reporting. *http://eatingdisorderscoalition.org.s208556.gridserver.com /couch/uploads/file/School%20Based%20BMI.pdf.* 2012:1–4. http://link.springer.com/10.1007/s13679-017-0259-6.

23. Satter, E. *Your Child's Weight: Helping Without Harming.* Madison, WI: Kelcy Press, 2005.

24. Neumark-Sztainer D. *I'm Like So Fat: Helping Your Teen Make Healthy Choices about Eating and Exercise in a Weight-Obsessed World.* New York, NY: The Guildford Press, 2005.

25. Neumark-Sztainer D. Preventing Obesity and Eating Disorders in Adolescents: What Can Health Care Providers Do? *J Adolesc Heal.* 2009;44(3):206–213.

26. Hingle M, Kunkel D. Childhood Obesity and the Media. *Pediatr Clin North Am.* 2012;59(3):677–692.

27. Sabaté J, Wien M. Vegetarian diets and childhood obesity prevention. *Am J Clin Nutr.* 2010;91:1525S-1529S.

28. Tiwari A, Aggarwal A, Tang W, Drewnowski A. Cooking at Home: A Strategy to Comply With U.S. Dietary Guidelines at No Extra Cost. *Am J Prev Med.* 2017;52(5):616–624.

29. Tumin R, Anderson SE. Television, Home-Cooked Meals, and Family Meal Frequency: Associations with Adult Obesity. *J Acad Nutr Diet.* 2017;117(6):937–945.

30. American Psychiatric Association. *Diagnostic and Statistical Manual of Mental Disorders.* 5th ed. Arlington, VA: American Psychiatric Publishing; 2013.

31. Rosen DS, Blythe MJ, Braverman PK, et al. Clinical report–Identification and management of eating disorders in children and adolescents. *Pediatrics.* 2010;126(6):1240–1253.

32. https://www.nationaleatingdisorders.org/statistics-research-eating-disorders

33. Get the facts on eating disorders. National Eating Disorders Association website. http://www.nationaleating disorders.org/get-facts-eating-disorders

34. Bardone-Cone AM, Fitzsimmons-Craft EE, Harney MB, et al. The inter-relationships between vegetarianism and eating disorders among females. *J Acad Nutr Diet.* 2012;112(8):1247–1252.

35. Amit M. Vegetarian diets in children and adolescents. *Paediatr Child Health*. 2010;15(5):303–314.

36. Connor MAO, Touyz SW, Dunn SM, Beumont PJ V. Vegetarianism in anorexia nervosa? A review of 116 consecutive cases. 1987; 147:540–542.

37. Lindeman M, Stark K, Latvala K. Vegetarianism and eating-disordered thinking. *Eat Disord*. 2000;8(2):157–165.

38. Bas M, Karabudak, E, Kiziltan G. Vegetarianism and eating disorders: association between eating attitudes and other psychological factors among Turkish adolescents. *Appetite*. 2005;44(3):309–315.

39. Klopp SA, Heiss CJ, Smith HS. Self-reported vegetarianism may be a marker for college women at risk for disordered eating. *J Am Diet Assoc*. 2003;103(6):745–747.

40. Neumark-Sztainer D, Story M, Resnick MD, Blum RW. Adolescent vegetarians. A behavioral profile of a school-based population in Minnesota. *Arch Pediatr Adolesc Med*. 1997;151(8):833–838.

41. Robinson-O'Brien R, Perry CL, Wall MM, Story M, Neumark-Sztainer D. Adolescent and young adult vegetarianism: better dietary intake and weight outcomes but increased risk of disordered eating behaviors. *J Am Diet Assoc*. 2009;109(4):648–655.

42. Forestell CA, Spaeth AM, Kane SA. To eat or not to eat red meat. A closer look at the relationship between restrained eating and vegetarianism in college females. *Appetite*. 2012;58(1):319–325.

43. Timko CA, Hormes JM, Chubski J. Will the real vegetarian please stand up? An investigation of dietary restraint and eating disorder symptoms in vegetarians versus non-vegetarians. *Appetite*. 2012;58(3):982–990.

Index

Note: an *f* indicates a figure; a *t* indicates a table.

A

Acceptable Macronutrient Distribution Range (ADMR), 76, 76*t*
Acne, 28, 226
ADMR. *See* Acceptable Macronutrient Distribution Range (ADMR)
Adolescent growth and plant–based diet, 218–226
  addiction and substance abuse, 257–258
  athlete nutrition, 223–226
  sample menus, 321*t*, 322*t*
Adventist Health Study, 15–16, 24, 25, 84–85, 94
ALA. *See* Alpha-linoleic acid (ALA)
Alpha-linoleic acid (ALA), 69*f*, 71
  content in common foods, 80*t*
  sufficient intake in plant-based diet, 77–80, 80*t*
American Heart Association, 28, 60, 70, 72, 221
American Society for the Prevention of Cruelty to Animals (ASPCA), 46
Amino acids, 81, 88–90
Animal agriculture, 37–42
Animal compassion, 43–52
Animal consumption, 37–42
  ethics, 43–52
ASPCA. *See* American Society for the Prevention of Cruelty to Animals (ASPCA)
Atherosclerosis, 28

B

B12 vitamin (cobalamin), 96–103, 110*t*
  deficiency, 98–99
  forms, 102–103
  importance, 96–97
  pregnancy needs, 178–179
  reliable sources, 99–100
  sufficient intake, 97–98, 100–102, 102*t*
  supplements for children, 232–233
Banana Walnut Pancakes, 339
Better Broth Base, 349
Bisphenol A (BPA), 88, 231
Black Bean, Corn, and Salsa Soup, 354
"Blue Zones," 23–24, 45, 56, 58–59, 116
BMI. *See* Body Mass Index (BMI)
Body Mass Index (BMI), 24, 268–269, 278
Bone health, 120–121
BPA. *See* Bisphenol A (BPA)
Breakfast
  Banana Walnut Pancakes, 339
  Cranberry Orange Almond Muffins, 338
  Creamy Steel Cut Oats, 332
  Essential Overnight Oats, 333
  Golden Scrambled Tofu and Vegetables, 336
  Pumpkin Muffins, 337
  Smart Start Smoothie Bowl, 334
  Smoothies, 335
Breastfeeding, 187–190
  milk for infants, 194–196, 198–199*t*
  milk for toddlers, 208
  recommended dietary allowances, 189–190*t*
Buetner, Dan, 23
Build Your Own Full-Meal Salad, 344–345
Burger Night, 366–367
Burkitt, Dr. Denis, 63

C

CAFOs. *See* Concentrated animal feeding operations (CAFOs)
"Cage-free" farming, 48–49
Calciferol, 103–107
  deficiency, 106–107

importance, 103–104
sunshine as source, 106
sufficient intake, 104–105
Calcium, 114–121, 136*t*
    adolescent consumption, 222, 225
    dairy as source, 115–116, 118*t*
    importance, 115
    nondairy sources, 117–118, 118–119*t*
    pregnancy needs, 180
    sufficient intake, 116–121
Cancer, 26–27
Carbohydrates, 55, 57–63
    adjusting intake, 59
    health issues, 58–59
    importance, 57–58
    refined, 58–59
    starches, 58–59, 62–63
    sugars, 58–61
Cardiovascular health, 25–26
Carrot Raisin Salad, 342
CDC. *See* Centers for Disease Control and
        Prevention (CDC)
Centers for Disease Control and Prevention (CDC),
        41
Children, 191–234
    adolescents and plant-based diet, 218–226
    allergies, 187, 203–204
    calcium intake, 119–120
    children and plant-based diet, 214–218
    eating disorders, 278–283
    fat intake, 74–75, 76*t*, 80*t*
    fiber intake, 65–67
    food safety, 229–231
    growth and development, 15–19, 266–267
    health issues, 28–30
    infants and plant-based diet, 193–206
    iron intake, 130–131
    lab tests, 233–234
    obesity and health consequences, 270–273
    protein intake, 82, 83*t*, 85
    safety of plant-based diet, 13–14
    sample menus, 320*t*
    school lunches, 217–218
    solid food introduction, 199–206, 205–206*t*
    soy intake, 227
    supplements, 232–233, 233*t*
    toddlers and plant-based diet, 206–214
    transition to plant-based diet, 285–301
    weight and healthy management, 273–283
Cholesterol, 72–73
Choline, 179
Climate change, 33–42
    global inequality, 37–38
Cobalamin, 96–103

deficiency, 98–99
forms, 102–103
importance, 96–97
reliable sources, 99–100
sufficient intake, 97–98, 100–102, 102*t*
Coconut, 167
Colon health, 28
Complete diet, 9, 9*t*
Concentrated animal feeding operations (CAFOs),
        46–48
COVID-19, 41
Cranberry Orange Almond Muffins, 338
Creamy Broccoli Soup, 353
Creamy Steel Cut Oats, 332
Crispy Tofu Fingers, 362
Curried Chickpea Salad Spread, 341
Curried Red Lentil Soup, 351

D

DGA. *See* Dietary Guidelines for America (DGA)
DHA. *See* Docosahexaenoic acid (DHA)
Dips, Dressings, and Spreads, 356–361
    Dilly Dip, 358
    Ginger Miso Sauce, 357
    Lemon Tahini Dressing, 356
    Spinach Artichoke Dip, 359
    Velvety Cheeze Sauce, 361
    White Bean, Garlic, and Lemon Spread, 360
Diabetes, 26
Dietary Guidelines for Americans (DGA), 19–20, 40,
        53, 69, 220
Dilly Dip, 358
Docosahexaenoic acid (DHA), 69*f*, 78–81, 80*t*
D vitamin (calciferol), 103–107, 111*t*
    adolescent consumption, 225
    deficiency, 106–107
    importance, 103–104
    pregnancy needs, 179–180
    sunshine as source, 106
    sufficient intake, 104–105
    supplements for children, 232–233

E

Eating disorders, 278–283
Edamame with Lime and Sea Salt, 379
Eicosapentaenoic acid (EPA), 69*f*, 78–81, 80*t*
Enriched grains, 159
EPA. *See* Eicosapentaenoic acid (EPA)
Essential Overnight Oats, 333
European Prospective Investigation into Cancer and
        Nutrition (EPIC–Oxford), 23, 94, 117

F

Factory farming, 41–42, 46–48

Family meals, 253–264, 313–322
    adjusting to plant-based diet, 285–301
    budget meals, 316
    communication, 258
    importance, 255–259
    obstacles, 259–260
    strategies, 260–264, 313–315
Farm Sanctuary, 48–49
Farm Study, 15
Fat, 55, 67–81
    acceptable quantity in diet, 75–77
    adolescent consumption, 225
    ADMR at various ages, 76t
    highest quality, 73–74
    importance, 67–68
    intake for toddlers, 213
    nut and seed content, 167
    sources in children's diet, 74–75
    triglycerides, 58
    types, 68–73, 69f
Fat–soluble vitamins, 95
Feeding principles, 237–351
    adolescent participation, 242–243
    child participation, 242
    feeding difficulties, 245–248
    infant participation, 240–242
    maladaptive practices, 243–244
    strategies, 249–251
    styles and practices, 239–245
    toddler participation, 242
Fermented foods, 228
Fiber, 55, 63–67
    content in common foods, 66t
    dietary reference intakes for, 64–65t
Fischel, Anne, 254
5 Quick Smoothies, 335
Berry Bliss Smoothie, 335
Chocolate Peanut Butter Smoothie, 335
Citrus Kale Smoothie, 335
Pumpkin Pie Smoothie, 335
Tropical Glow Smoothie, 335
Flexitarian diet, 9, 9t
Folate, 171
    pregnancy needs, 177–178
Food
    consumption and environmental impact, 33–42
    macronutrients and fiber in, 55–92
Food and Agriculture Organization, 39, 53
Food labels, 152
Food marketing, 152, 216–217, 275
Fortified foods, 20–21, 99, 102t
"Free-range" farming, 48–50
Fructose, 158
Fruitarian diet, 86

Fruit Compotes
    Blueberry and Green Apple Compote, 340
    Italian Prune Plum Compote, 340
    Mixed Berry Compote, 340
    Raspberry Vanilla Compote, 340
Fruit juice, 158–159
Full-Meal Salad, 344–345

G

Gas production, 163
Ginger Miso Sauce, 357
Gluten, 161
Glyphosate, 161
Goitrogens, 125
Golden Scrambled Tofu and Vegetables, 336
Goodall, Jane, 46
Grains, 159–161
    use in cooking, 328–329, 329t
"Grass-fed" farming, 48–49
Greenhouse gas emissions, 34–36, 38–40
Growth charts, 266–267
Gut health, 27

H

Healthy Eating Index (HEI), 19–20
Heavy metals, 230
Heede, Richard, 35
HEI. See Healthy Eating Index (HEI)
Heme iron, 127
Hemoglobin, 126
Holidays, 297–298
Hypospadias, 29–30

I

Infant growth and plant-based diet, 193–206
    sample menus, 318–319t
Iodine, 121–125, 138t
    content in common foods, 123–124t
    deficiency, 122–123
    importance, 122
    pregnancy needs, 181–182
    sources, 123–124
    sufficient intake, 124–125
Iron, 125–131, 139t
    adolescent consumption, 222, 225
    content in common foods, 129–130t
    deficiency, 127
    importance, 126–127
    pregnancy needs, 181
    sufficient intake, 130–131
    types in food, 127–128

J

Joy, Melanie, 45

K

Keto diet, 55–56
Kind Shepherd's Pie, 376–377
Kitchen utensils and tools, 311–313, 312–313*f*
Kwashiorkor, 85

L

LA. *See* Linoleic acid (LA)
Lacto-ovo-vegetarian diet, 9, 9*t*
Lacto-vegetarian diet, 9*t*
Lectins, 164–165
Legumes, 90–91, 91*t*, 162–165
    use in cooking, 326–327, 327–328*t*
Lemon Tahini Dressing, 356
Lemony Chickpea Pasta with Mushrooms and
        Broccoli, 372–373
Lentil, Wheat Berry, and Roasted Veggie Salad, 348
Linoleic acid (LA), 69*f*, 71
    reduction in diet, 79
Long-chain polyunsaturated fatty acids, 71–72
Low-fat diets, 76–77
Lysine, 86–87*t*, 89–90

M

Macronutrients, 55–63
    carbohydrates, 57–63
    definition, 55–56
Mains, 362–379
    Burger Night, 366–367
    Crispy Tofu Fingers, 362
    Kind Shepherd's Pie, 376–377
    Lemony Chickpea Pasta with Mushrooms and
        Broccoli, 372–373
    Peanut Dragon Bowl, 370–371
    Taco Night, 368–369
    Tofu Tikka Masala, 363
    Tofu Stir-Fry, 364–365
    Ultimate Veggie Lasagna, The, 374–375
Malnutrition, 146
Mango Avocado Black Bean Salad, 343
Marasmus, 85
Meat reducers, 51
Menus, 317–322
    adolescent athletes, 322*t*
    adolescents, 321*t*
    children, 320*t*
    infants, 318–319*t*
    planning and shopping, 306–308
    toddlers, 319*t*
Microbiome health, 27, 29
Micronutrient-related malnutrition, 146
Micronutrients, 93–143
    definition, 93

intake in dietary patterns, 94–95
    minerals, 113–143
    vitamins, 95–113
Milk, 28
    breast milk alternatives, 196–198
    calcium content, 115–116
    infant consumption, 194–199, 198–199*t*
    toddler consumption, 208–211, 209–210*t*
Minerals, 113–143
    calcium, 114–121
    definition, 113
    iodine, 121–125
    iron, 125–131
    kinds, 136–143*t*
    zinc, 132–136
Monounsaturated fat, 69*f*, 70–71
Morning sickness, 186–187
Mortality, 23–28
Myoglobin, 126

N

NAFLD. *See* Non-alcoholic Fatty Liver Disease
        (NAFLD)
Neurodevelopmental disorders, 29
Non-alcoholic Fatty Liver Disease (NAFLD), 28
Non-heme iron, 128
Not Your Everyday Kale Salad, 346
Nuts, 165–167

O

Oil, 324–326
Omega-3 fatty acids, 69*t*, 71, 165, 166
    content in common foods, 66*t*
    pregnancy needs, 176–177
    sufficient intake in plant diet, 77–80, 80*t*
Omega-6 fatty acids, 69*f*, 71
    reduction in diet, 79
Organic foods, 229
Overconsumption, 146–147
Ovo-vegetarian diet, 9*t*
Oxalates, 118

P

Paleo diet, 55–56
Peanut Dragon Bowl, 370–371
Pediatrician, 298–300
Persistent Organic Pollutants (POPs), 230
Pescatarian, 9, 9*t*
Pescovegetarian diet, 77
Pesticides, 229
Photosynthesis, 57
Phytosterols, 73
Plant-based diet, 8–9, 55–56
    adjusting family meals, 285–301

balance, 145–167
budget meals, 316
calcium, 116–117
childhood and adolescence, 191–234
definitions, 9t
easy meals, 315–316t
effects on children's health, 28–30
environmental impact, 33–42
feeding principles, 237–251
growth and development in children, 15–19
health benefits, 7–32
nutritional needs for children, 13–14, 17
optimization, 30–31
pediatrician and discouragement, 298–300
pregnancy and lactation concerns, 169–190
protective qualities, 23–28
protein, 84–90
recipes, 323–391
safety for children, 13–14, 18
shopping and preparation, 305–315
variations, 8–13
whole plant foods, 11
Plant-based dietary index, 10–11
Plant-Based Plate, 147–167, 149f, 150t, 171, 211
fruits, 156–159
grains and starches, 159–161
legumes, 162–165
nuts and seeds, 165–167
pregnancy and breastfeeding option, 183t
vegetables, 153–156
Plant-exclusive diet, 9, 9t
Plastics, 231
Polyunsaturated fat, 69t, 71–72
types, 71
Prasad, Dr. Ananda, 132
Prebiotics, 227–229
Pregnancy, 169–190
B12 vitamin, 178–179
calcium, 180
choline, 179
D vitamin, 179–180
folate, 177–178
iodine, 181–182
iron, 181
morning sickness, 186–187
omega-3 fatty acids, 176–177
nutrients, 174–175
preconception and plant-based diet, 170–172
pregnancy and plant-based diet, 172–187
protein, 175–176
recommended dietary allowances, 189–190t
supplement intake, 184t, 186
unsafe foods, 184–185t
weight gain, 174t

zinc, 182–183
Probiotics, 227–229
Processed foods, 11–13, 151
categories, 12t
family discussion of, 12–13
Protein, 55, 81–92
adolescent consumption, 222
amino acids and plants, 88–90
animal versus plant, 90–91, 91t
content in common foods, 86–87t
importance, 81–82
pregnancy needs, 175–176
sufficient intake in plant diet, 82–87, 83t, 90
Protein powders, 88
Pseudograins, 159
Pseudovegetarianism, 279, 282
Pumpkin Muffins, 337
Pure vegetarian diet, 9, 9t

R

Rainbow Spiral Noodle Salad, 347
Raw vegan diet, 9, 9t, 227
Recipes, 323–391
breakfast, 332–340
dips, dressing, and spreads, 356–361
mains, 362–377
salads, 341–348
snacks and sweets, 378–391
soups, 349–355
Refined carbohydrates, 58–59
Restaurants, 295–297
Restrained eating, 280
Ricard, Matthieu, 45–46, 48
Roasted Chickpeas, 378
Roasted Pepper and Tomato Soup, 355
Rustic Lentil Soup, 350

S

Sabaté, Joan, 30–31
Salads
Carrot Raisin Salad, 342
Curried Chickpea Salad Spread, 341
Full-Meal Salad, 344–345
Lentil, Wheat Berry, and Roasted Veggie Salad, 348
Mango, Avocado, Black Bean Salad, 343
Not Your Everyday Kale Salad, 346
Rainbow Spiral Noodle Salad, 347
Satter, Ellyn, 240, 248
Saturated fat, 69–70, 69f
School lunches, 217–218
Seeds, 165–167
Semi-vegetarian diet, 9, 9t
Skin cancer, 106

Smart Start Smoothie Bowl, 334
Smoothies
Berry Bliss Smoothie, 335
Chocolate Peanut Butter Smoothie, 335
Citrus Kale Smoothie, 335
Pumpkin Pie Smoothie, 335
Snacks and Sweets
    Edamame with Lime and Sea Salt, 379
    Roasted Chickpeas, 378
SnackWell's brand, 272
Sodium, 124, 142t, 151
    intake for toddlers, 213
    use in cooking, 324–326
Soups
    Better Broth Base, 349
    Black Bean, Corn, and Salsa Soup, 354
    Creamy Broccoli Soup, 353
    Curried Red Lentil Soup, 351
    Roasted Pepper and Tomato Soup, 355
    Rustic Lentil Soup, 350
    Split Pea Soup, 352
Spinach Artichoke Dip, 359
Split Pea Soup, 352
Starches, 58–59, 62–63, 159–161
Sterols, 72–73
Stocking plant-based food, 309–311, 310–311f
Stroke, 25
Sugar, 58–59
    intake for toddlers, 213
    use in cooking, 324–326
Supplements, 102t, 184t, 186
    child consumption, 232–233, 233t
    adolescent consumption, 225, 233t
Sustainable diet, 39–40

T

Taco Night, 368–369
Toddler growth and plant-based diet, 206–214
    sample menus, 319t
Trans fatty acids, 72
Transition to plant-based diet, 285–301
Tofu Stir-Fry, 364–365
Tofu Tikka Masala, 363
Triglycerides, 68

U

Ultimate Veggie Lasagna, The, 374–375
Undernutrition, 146
United States Department of Agriculture (USDA),
    148
Urinary tract infection, 28
USDA. See United States Department of Agriculture
    (USDA)

V

Vegan diet, 9, 9t, 50–51
Vegetables, 153–156
Vegetarian and Vegan Children Study, 16–17, 85
Velvety Cheeze Sauce, 361
Vitamins, 95–113
    B12, 96–103
    D, 103–107
    kinds, 107–112t

W

Water, 151
Water-soluble vitamins, 95
Watson, Donald, 50
Watson, Dorothy, 50
Weight, 265–283
    body mass index, 268–269
    growth charts, 266–268, 267f
    healthy management, 273–283
    obesity in children, 270–272
    pregnancy goals, 174t
    underweight, 269–270
Western diet, 19–21, 145
Wet markets, 41
White Bean, Garlic, and Lemon Spread, 360
WHO. See World Health Organization (WHO)
Whole food, plant-based diet, 10
Wiesel, Elie, 46
World Health Organization (WHO), 38, 41, 53, 56,
    60, 122, 182

Z

Zinc, 132–136, 143t
    content in common foods, 134t
    deficiency, 133
    importance, 132
    pregnancy needs, 182–183
    sources, 133–134
    sufficient intake in plant-based diets, 135–136

About the Authors

R eshma Shah, MD, MPH, is a board-certified pediatrician and an affiliate clinical instructor at Stanford University School of Medicine. She received her undergraduate and graduate degrees from Johns Hopkins University and her medical degree from Drexel University College of Medicine. She has additional training and certification in plant-based nutrition and cooking. She lives in the Bay Area with her husband and two children. Most Sundays, you can find her at the local farmers market where she finds inspiration for weekly family meals.

B renda Davis, RD, is widely regarded as a rock star of plant-based nutrition. She has been a featured speaker at medical and nutrition conferences around the world and is the prolific author of 11 vegetarian and vegan nutrition classics, including *Becoming Vegan: Comprehensive Edition* and *Becoming Vegan: Express Edition*. In 2007, she was inducted into the Vegetarian Hall of Fame. She lives in Calgary with her husband, Paul. She has two grown children and two beautiful grandchildren.